Clinical Aspects in Nephrology and Kidney Transplantation

Clinical Aspects in Nephrology and Kidney Transplantation

Editor: Reagen Hu

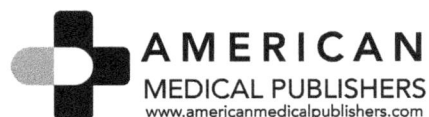

AMERICAN
MEDICAL PUBLISHERS
www.americanmedicalpublishers.com

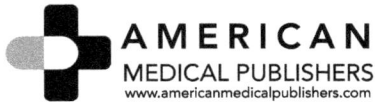

AMERICAN
MEDICAL PUBLISHERS
www.americanmedicalpublishers.com

Cataloging-in-Publication Data

Clinical aspects in nephrology and kidney transplantation / edited by Reagen Hu.
p. cm.
Includes bibliographical references and index.
ISBN 978-1-63927-631-8
1. Nephrology. 2. Kidneys--Transplantation. 3. Kidneys--Disease--Diagnosis.
4. Kidneys--Diseases--Treatment. 5. Clinical medicine. I. Hu, Reagen.
RC902 .C473 2023
616.61--dc23

© American Medical Publishers, 2023

American Medical Publishers,
41 Flatbush Avenue,
1st Floor, New York,
NY 11217, USA

ISBN 978-1-63927-631-8 (Hardback)

Contents

Preface

Nephrology is the study of kidneys which includes studying their normal function, diseases associated with them, maintaining their health, and treatment of related diseases through medication, kidney transplant, diet and dialysis procedure. Kidney transplant is the process of transplanting a healthy kidney into a patient having last stage kidney disease. It is broadly categorized as living donor or deceased donor transplantation based on the donor's source. Prior to kidney transplant, an individual with last stage kidney disease should undergo a complete medical examination for ensuring that they are healthy and can undergo organ transplant surgery. Patients who undergo kidney transplant usually live longer and have better quality of life, as compared to people who receive dialysis treatment. This book unravels the recent studies in the field of nephrology. It is a valuable compilation of topics, ranging from the basic to the most complex advancements in kidney transplantation. The readers would gain knowledge that would broaden their perspective in this area of medicine.

This book is the end result of constructive efforts and intensive research done by experts in this field. The aim of this book is to enlighten the readers with recent information in this area of research. The information provided in this profound book would serve as a valuable reference to students and researchers in this field.

At the end, I would like to thank all the authors for devoting their precious time and providing their valuable contribution to this book. I would also like to express my gratitude to my fellow colleagues who encouraged me throughout the process.

Editor

Dietary Assessment and Self-Management Using Information Technology in Order to Improve Outcomes in Kidney Transplant Recipients

Fernanda G. Rodrigues [1,2,*](ID), Martin H. de Borst [2](ID) and Ita P. Heilberg [1,3](ID)

1   Nutrition Post Graduation Program, Universidade Federal de São Paulo, São Paulo 04023-900, Brazil; ita.heilberg@gmail.com
2   Department of Nephrology, University of Groningen, University Medical Center Groningen, 9713 Groningen, The Netherlands; m.h.de.borst@umcg.nl
3   Nephrology Division, Universidade Federal de São Paulo, São Paulo 04023-900, Brazil
*   Correspondence: fernanda.gr91@gmail.com

Abstract: Big data and artificial intelligence (AI) will transform the way research in nephrology is carried out and consequently improve the performance of clinical practice in nephrology and transplantation. Managing long-term health outcomes in kidney transplant recipients (KTR) includes the improvement of modifiable factors, such as diet. Self-management using information technology (IT) aims to facilitate lifestyle changes, manage symptoms and treatment in the course of chronic kidney disease (CKD) or any chronic condition. The advantages of health mobile applications further include the capacity of data compilation and yielding responses to numerous research questions in nephrology and transplantation. However, studies investigating the employment of such applications in KTR and its impact in kidney transplant outcomes are still lacking. The specific advantages of dietary assessment and self-management using IT in order to improve outcomes in KTR are presently discussed. This Special Issue features a great set of articles regarding IT approaches to improve kidney allograft survival and posttransplant outcomes in all areas.

Keywords: kidney transplantation; nutrition; self-management; information technology

Kidney transplantation is considered the preferred treatment for most patients with end-stage renal disease (ESRD) [1] in view of the improved quality of life, survival rates and cost-effectiveness in comparison to chronic dialysis treatment [2]. Notwithstanding the advance in overall one-year kidney allograft survival brought by innovative surgical techniques and immunosuppressive protocols [3], the survival of kidney transplant recipients (KTRs) continues to be significantly lower than individuals of a similar age in the general population [4].

Managing long-term health outcomes in KTR includes the improvement of modifiable factors such as diet. Although specific dietary recommendations for KTR are still lacking [5], recent large cohort studies have disclosed novel and interesting findings that assist the comprehension and attainment of new knowledge regarding nutrition and post-transplant outcomes [6–9]. The adherence to dietary patterns, such as DASH (dietary approach to stop hypertension) and Mediterranean diet, has been positively associated with better kidney graft outcomes and lower risk of all-cause mortality [7,8]. Large KTR cohort studies investigating specific food groups have demonstrated that the intake of fish, known to be rich in omega-3 fatty acids, was inversely associated with risks of long-term cardiovascular and all-cause mortality [6,10]. Moreover, vegetable intake was associated with a lower risk of post-transplantation diabetes mellitus and cardiovascular mortality [9]. Weight gain and other metabolic comorbidities are frequent in KTR [11] and have been associated with graft loss [12]. These findings shed light on the importance of adequate nutrition after transplantation.

Recently, a qualitative study in KTR by Boslooper-Meulenbelt et al. [13] has reported the lack of food literacy as a barrier to a good-quality dietary pattern, emphasizing the importance of accessible and understandable nutritional interventions following kidney transplant. Furthermore, the authors emphasize that specific attention for dietary transition barriers is required for KTR, especially considering their previous dietary restrictions imposed by chronic kidney disease (CKD). Self-management using information technology (IT) aims to facilitate lifestyle changes, manage symptoms and treatment in the course of CKD or any chronic condition [14]. Several health-related mobile applications contain functionalities that are effective and highly promising for nutrition-related health outcomes [14,15]. A study performed in CKD patients used a web application to help individuals in pre-dialysis, in dialysis and posttransplant to make decisions according to diet restrictions and phosphate binder dosage [16]. The results of this research have shown that this application increased the patients' insight and understanding related to an appropriate CKD-specific diet, besides improving the ability to provide decision support regarding diet and binder intake [16]. A study evaluating twenty-one renal diet-related mobile applications disclosed that the technical quality and health literacy demand of the apps were acceptable, although more than half of the apps did not contain accurate, evidence-based renal diet information [17]. The most important characteristics of a renal diet tailored to KTR should consist of an adequate energy to prevent either protein–energy wasting or overweight/obesity; adequate protein intake to improve quality of life and survival rates, to better control serum phosphorus and ameliorate lipid profile; phosphorus intake to avoid hyperphosphatemia in the late period post-transplantation, which in turn leads to or worsens pre-existent CKD–MBD (mineral bone disorder); adequate potassium intake to reduce the risk of hyperkalemia, associated with cardiac arrhythmia and sudden death; control of sodium intake to avoid increases in blood pressure and cardiovascular risk [18]. The suggested modifiable dietary elements in post-kidney transplantation are summarized in Table 1. Kosa et al. [19] have demonstrated in a systematic review that a mobile application with focus on engaging patients and encouraging healthy self-management of CKD was beneficial to ameliorate the adherence to dietary restrictions pertaining to sodium, potassium, phosphorus, protein, calories, and fluid.

Recently, the employment of mobile health technology application aimed at managing and monitoring medication for KTR has proved useful for these patients [20]. However, it seems that the quality of online information for transplant health care still needs improvements [21]. A recent clinical trial has shown that a web-based intervention with individual telemedicine couching for three months was able to cause reduction in dietary sodium in CKD patients, including KTR, when compared to regular routine care [22]. Despite the foreseen advantages of a better control of food intake by KTR, there are only a few studies investigating the use of a dietary self-management application in KTR to date.

Besides intervention, the advantages of health mobile applications should include the capacity of data compilation. A recent review has disclosed that the methods for dietary assessment using technology has several advantages, encompassing the use of minimal resources and cost-savings, the enhanced veracity of dietary intake reports, besides more engagement and feedback from patients [23]. Given that more than half of the global population is currently connected to the internet, the usage of electronic health records can empower the patients in their dietary decision-making process, and in exchange, contribute to the development of large datasets that can be used by researchers to answer numerous pertinent research questions in nephrology and transplantation, as exemplified above. In recent years, the artificial intelligence (AI) field has substantially changed the way digital data are analyzed and used [24], and it will similarly transform the way research in nephrology is carried out, improving clinical practice in nephrology and transplantation [25]. For this to happen, future AI models must be integrative, gathering diversified data to provide superior accuracy and tenacity [24].

This Special Issue presents a great set of articles regarding IT approaches to improve kidney allograft survival and posttransplant outcomes. Further prospective and multi-center validation studies are needed to fully elucidate how KTR can benefit from IT use, particularly in relation to functionalities targeted to facilitate dietary self-management tasks. Future research is also required to enlighten how IT applications in KTR can be translated into improvements in clinical outcomes in post-transplantation.

Table 1. Suggested modifiable dietary elements for a post-kidney transplant in metabolically stable patients with preserved graft function.

Energy	Energy consumption must be maintained between 25 and 35 kcal/kg body weight per day based on age, sex, level of physical activity, body composition, weight status goals and eGFR level.
Protein	Protein intake must be adjusted according to graft function and eGFR level. The amount of dietary protein intake may vary between 0.55 and 1.0 g/kg body weight per day.
Phosphorus	Dietary phosphorus intake must be adjusted to maintain serum phosphate levels within the normal range.
Potassium	Dietary potassium intake is aimed to maintain serum potassium within the normal range and has to be adjusted according to eGFR level.
Sodium	Sodium intake must be adjusted to less than 100 mmol/d (or <2.3 g/d).

eGFR—estimate glomerular filtration rate.

References

1. Abecassis, M.; Bartlett, S.T.; Collins, A.J.; Davis, C.L.; Delmonico, F.L.; Friedewald, J.J.; Hays, R.; Howard, A.; Jones, E.; Leichtman, A.B.; et al. Kidney Transplantation as Primary Therapy for End-Stage Renal Disease: A National Kidney Foundation/Kidney Disease Outcomes Quality Initiative (NKF/KDOQI™) Conference. *Clin. J. Am. Soc. Nephrol.* **2008**, *3*, 471–480. [CrossRef] [PubMed]

2. Tonelli, M.; Wiebe, N.; Knoll, G.; Bello, A.; Browne, S.; Jadhav, D.; Klarenbach, S.; Gill, J. Systematic Review: Kidney Transplantation Compared With Dialysis in Clinically Relevant Outcomes. *Arab. Archaeol. Epigr.* **2011**, *11*, 2093–2109. [CrossRef]

3. Laupacis, A.; Keown, P.; Pus, N.; Krueger, H.; Ferguson, B.; Wong, C.; Muirhead, N. A study of the quality of life and cost-utility of renal transplantation. *Kidney Int.* **1996**, *50*, 235–242. [CrossRef]

4. Oterdoom, L.H.; De Vries, A.P.J.; Van Ree, R.M.; Gansevoort, R.T.; Van Son, W.J.; Van Der Heide, J.J.H.; Navis, G.; De Jong, P.E.; Gans, R.O.B.; Bakker, S.J.L. N-Terminal Pro-B-Type Natriuretic Peptide and Mortality in Renal Transplant Recipients Versus the General Population. *Transplantation* **2009**, *87*, 1562–1570. [CrossRef] [PubMed]

5. Kasiske, B.L.; Zeier, M.G.; Chapman, J.R.; Craig, J.C.; Ekberg, H.; Garvey, C.A.; Green, M.D.; Jha, V.; Josephson, M.A.; Kiberd, B.A.; et al. KDIGO clinical practice guideline for the care of kidney transplant recipients: A summary. *Kidney Int.* **2010**, *77*, 299–311. [CrossRef]

6. Gomes-Neto, A.W.; Sotomayor, C.G.; Pranger, I.G.; Berg, E.V.D.; Gans, R.O.B.; Soedamah-Muthu, S.S.; Navis, G.; Bakker, S.J.L. Intake of Marine-Derived Omega-3 Polyunsaturated Fatty Acids and Mortality in Renal Transplant Recipients. *Nutrient* **2017**, *9*, 363. [CrossRef]

7. Osté, M.C.J.; Gomes-Neto, A.W.; Corpeleijn, E.; Gans, R.O.B.; De Borst, M.H.; Berg, E.V.D.; Soedamah-Muthu, S.S.; Kromhout, D.; Navis, G.J.; Bakker, S.J.L. Dietary Approach to Stop Hypertension (DASH) diet and risk of renal function decline and all-cause mortality in renal transplant recipients. *Arab. Archaeol. Epigr.* **2018**, *18*, 2523–2533. [CrossRef] [PubMed]

8. Gomes-Neto, A.W.; Osté, M.C.; Sotomayor, C.G.; Berg, E.V.D.; Geleijnse, J.M.; Berger, S.P.; Gans, R.O.; Bakker, S.J.L.; Navis, G.J. Mediterranean Style Diet and Kidney Function Loss in Kidney Transplant Recipients. *Clin. J. Am. Soc. Nephrol.* **2020**, *15*, 238–246. [CrossRef]

9. Gomes-Neto, A.W.; Osté, M.C.; Sotomayor, C.G.; vd Berg, E.; Geleijnse, J.M.; Gans, R.O.; Navis, G.J. Fruit and vegetable intake and risk of post trans plantation diabetes in renal transplant recipients. *Diabetes Care* **2019**, *42*, 1645–1652. [CrossRef]

10. Baia, L.; Berg, E.V.D.; Vervloet, M.; Heilberg, I.; Navis, G.; Bakker, S.; Geleijnse, J.; Kromhout, D.; Soedamah-Muthu, S.; De Borst, M.H. Fish and omega-3 fatty acid intake in relation to circulating fibroblast growth factor 23 levels in renal transplant recipients. *Nutr. Metab. Cardiovasc. Dis.* **2014**, *24*, 1310–1316. [CrossRef]

11. Baxmann, A.C.; Menon, V.B.; Pestana, J.L.; Carvalho, A.B.; Heilberg, I.P. Overweight and body fat are predictors of hypovitaminosis D in renal transplant patients. *Clin. Kidney J.* **2014**, *8*, 49–53. [CrossRef] [PubMed]

12. González, A.L.; Pérez, R.G.; Soto, J.B.; Castillo, R.F. Study of weight and body mass index on graft loss after transplant over 5 years of evolution. *Int. J. Med Sci.* **2020**, *17*, 2306–2311. [CrossRef] [PubMed]

13. Boslooper-Meulenbelt, K.; Patijn, O.; Battjes-Fries, M.C.E.; Haisma, H.; Pot, G.K.; Navis, G.J.; Meulenbelt, B.; Fries, B. Pot Barriers and Facilitators of Fruit and Vegetable Consumption in Renal Transplant Recipients, Family Members and Healthcare Professionals—A Focus Group Study. *Nutrient* **2019**, *11*, 2427. [CrossRef]

14. Donald, M.; Kahlon, B.K.; Beanlands, H.; Straus, S.; Ronksley, P.; Herrington, G.; Tong, A.; Grill, A.; Waldvogel, B.; Large, A.C.; et al. Self-management interventions for adults with chronic kidney disease: A scoping review. *BMJ Open* **2018**, *8*, e019814. [CrossRef] [PubMed]

15. Villinger, K.; Wahl, D.R.; Boeing, H.; Schupp, H.T.; Renner, B. The effectiveness of app-based mobile interventions on nutrition behaviours and nutrition-related health outcomes: A systematic review and meta-analysis. *Obes. Rev.* **2019**, *20*, 1465–1484. [CrossRef] [PubMed]

16. Heiden, S.; Buus, A.A.; Jensen, M.H.; Hejlesen, O.K. A diet management information and communication system to help chronic kidney patients cope with diet restrictions. *Stud. Heal. Technol. informatics* **2013**, *192*, 543–547.

17. Lambert, K.; Mullan, J.; Mansfield, K.; Owen, P. Should We Recommend Renal Diet–Related Apps to Our Patients? An Evaluation of the Quality and Health Literacy Demand of Renal Diet–Related Mobile Applications. *J. Ren. Nutr.* **2017**, *27*, 430–438. [CrossRef] [PubMed]

18. Ikizler, T.A.; Burrowes, J.D.; Byham-Gray, L.D.; Campbell, K.L.; Carrero, J.-J.; Chan, W.; Fouque, D.; Friedman, A.N.; Ghaddar, S.; Goldstein-Fuchs, D.J.; et al. KDOQI Clinical Practice Guideline for Nutrition in CKD: 2020 Update. *Am. J. Kidney Dis.* **2020**, *76*, S1–S107. [CrossRef]

19. Kosa, S.D.; Monize, J.; D'Souza, M.; Joshi, A.; Philip, K.; Reza, S.; Samra, S.; Serrago, B.; Thabane, L.; Gafni, A.; et al. Nutritional Mobile Applications for CKD Patients: Systematic Review. *Kidney Int. Rep.* **2019**, *4*, 399–407. [CrossRef]

20. Browning, R.B.; McGillicuddy, J.W.; Treiber, F.A.; Taber, D.J. Kidney transplant recipients' attitudes about using mobile health technology for managing and monitoring medication therapy. *J. Am. Pharm. Assoc.* **2016**, *56*, 450–454. [CrossRef]

21. Van Klaveren, C.W.; De Jong, P.G.M.; Hendriks, A.R.; Luk, F.; De Vries, A.P.J.; Van Der Boog, P.J.M.; Reinders, M.E.J. Content, Delivery Modes, and Social-Epistemological Dimensions of Online Information for Renal Transplant Patients and Living Donors during the COVID-19 Pandemic: Lessons Learned (Preprint). *J. Med. Internet Res.* **2020**. [CrossRef]

22. Humalda, J.K.; Klaassen, G.; De Vries, H.; Meuleman, Y.; Verschuur, L.C.; Straathof, E.J.; Laverman, G.D.; Bos, W.J.W.; Van Der Boog, P.J.; Vermeulen, K.M.; et al. A Self-management Approach for Dietary Sodium Restriction in Patients With CKD: A Randomized Controlled Trial. *Am. J. Kidney Dis.* **2020**, *75*, 847–856. [CrossRef]

23. Eldridge, A.L.; Piernas, C.; Illner, A.-K.; Gibney, M.J.; Gurinović, M.A.; De Vries, J.H.; Cade, J.E. Evaluation of New Technology-Based Tools for Dietary Intake Assessment—An ILSI Europe Dietary Intake and Exposure Task Force Evaluation. *Nutrient* **2018**, *11*, 55. [CrossRef] [PubMed]

24. Rashidi, P.; Bihorac, A. Artificial intelligence approaches to improve kidney care. *Nat. Rev. Nephrol.* **2020**, *16*, 71–72. [CrossRef] [PubMed]

25. Thongprayoon, C.; Kaewput, W.; Kovvuru, K.; Hansrivijit, P.; Kanduri, S.R.; Bathini, T.; Chewcharat, A.; Leeaphorn, N.; Gonzalez-Suarez, M.L.; Cheungpasitporn, W. Promises of Big Data and Artificial Intelligence in Nephrology and Transplantation. *J. Clin. Med.* **2020**, *9*, 1107. [CrossRef] [PubMed]

Is there Decreasing Public Interest in Renal Transplantation? A Google Trends™ Analysis

Andreas Kronbichler [1,*], Maria Effenberger [2,*], Jae Il Shin [3,4,5], Christian Koppelstätter [1], Sara Denicolò [1], Michael Rudnicki [1], Hannes Neuwirt [1], Maria José Soler [6], Kate Stevens [7], Annette Bruchfeld [8], Herbert Tilg [2], Gert Mayer [1] and Paul Perco [1]

[1]   Department of Internal Medicine IV (Nephrology and Hypertension), Medical University Innsbruck, Anichstrasse 35, 6020 Innsbruck, Austria; christian.koppelstaetter@tirol-kliniken.at (C.K.); sara.denicolo@i-med.ac.at (S.D.); michael.rudnicki@i-med.ac.at (M.R.); hannes.neuwirt@i-med.ac.at (H.N.); gert.mayer@i-med.ac.at (G.M.); paul.perco@i-med.ac.at (P.P.)
[2]   Department of Internal Medicine I (Gastroenterology, Hepatology, Endocrinology and Metabolism), Medical University Innsbruck, Anichstrasse 35, 6020 Innsbruck, Austria; herbert.tilg@i-med.ac.at
[3]   Department of Pediatrics, Yonsei University College of Medicine, 03722 Seoul, Korea; shinji@yuhs.ac
[4]   Department of Pediatric Nephrology, Severance Children's Hospital, Seoul 03722, Korea
[5]   Institute of Kidney Disease Research, Yonsei University College of Medicine, Seoul 03722, Korea
[6]   Department of Nephrology, Hospital Universitari Vall d'Hebron, Nephrology Research Group, Vall d'Hebron Research Institute (VHIR), 08035 Barcelona, Spain; mjsoler01@gmail.com
[7]   Glasgow Renal and Transplant Unit, Queen Elizabeth University Hospital, Glasgow G51 4TF, UK; kate.stevens@glasgow.ac.uk
[8]   Department of Clinical Sciences Interventions and Technology (CLINTEC), Division of Renal Medicine, Karolinska Institutet, Karolinska University Hospital, 171 77 Stockholm, Sweden; annette.bruchfeld@ki.se
*   Correspondence: andreas.kronbichler@i-med.ac.at (A.K.); Maria.effenberger@tirol-kliniken.at (M.E.)

Abstract: Background and objectives: Renal transplantation is the preferred form of renal replacement therapy for the majority of patients with end stage renal disease (ESRD). The Internet is a key tool for people seeking healthcare-related information. This current work explored the interest in kidney transplantation based on Internet search queries using Google Trends™. Design, setting, participants, and measurements: We performed a Google Trends™ search with the search term "kidney transplantation" between 2004 (year of inception) and 2018. We retrieved and analyzed data on the worldwide trend as well as data from the United Network for Organ Sharing (UNOS), the Organización Nacional de Trasplantes (ONT), the Eurotransplant area, and the National Health Service (NHS) Transplant Register. Google Trends™ indices were investigated and compared to the numbers of performed kidney transplants, which were extracted from the respective official websites of UNOS, ONT, Eurotransplant, and the NHS. Results: During an investigational period of 15 years, there was a significant decrease of the worldwide Google Trends™ index from 76.3 to 25.4, corresponding to an absolute reduction of −50.9% and a relative reduction by −66.7%. The trend was even more pronounced for the UNOS area (−75.2%), while in the same time period the number of transplanted kidneys in the UNOS area increased by 21.9%. Events of public interest had an impact on the search queries in the year of occurrence, as shown by an increase in the Google Trends™ index by 39.2% in the year 2005 in Austria when a person of public interest received his second live donor kidney transplant. Conclusions: This study indicates a decreased public interest in kidney transplantation. There is a clear need to raise public awareness, since transplantation represents the best form of renal replacement therapy for patients with ESRD. Information should be provided on social media, with a special focus on readability and equitable access, as well as on web pages.

Keywords: kidney transplantation; transplant numbers; live donors; public awareness; Google Trends^{TM}

1. Introduction

Kidney transplantation is considered to be the optimal form of renal replacement therapy and has a positive impact on quality of life, survival rates of the recipients, and overall is considered cost-effective [1]. Due to organ shortage and longer waiting time, death on the waiting list is a serious concern and criteria for suitable organs have been extended. There are several advantages of live donor transplantation compared with deceased donor transplantation including lower risk of rejection, reduced waiting time for transplantation, and improved allograft and overall survival [2]. The frequency of live kidney donation is stable in the United States (US), while increasing in the Eurotransplant area and in the United Kingdom (UK) over the last 15 years. Despite these efforts there are currently 94,621 patients on the kidney waiting list in the US according to the United Network for Organ Sharing (UNOS), 10,791 (at the end of 2018) potential recipients in the Eurotransplant area and as of March 2019, approximately 5000 patients were waiting for a kidney transplant in the UK. Analysis of different surveys among the public revealed barriers towards live kidney transplantation [3], and strategies to overcome these barriers are necessary to increase the number of transplants.

Google Trends^{TM} generates data on spatial and temporal patterns according to specified keywords. A study comparing the reliability of Google Trends^{TM} in two settings, more common diseases with low media coverage and less common diseases with higher media coverage, found that Google Trends^{TM} seems to be influenced by media presence rather than by true epidemiological burden of one disease [4]. Several studies using Google Trends^{TM} data have been conducted recently. One of these investigated the influence of meteorological variables on relative search volumes for pain and found that selected local weather conditions were associated with online search volumes for specific musculoskeletal pain symptoms [5]. Analysis of Google Trends^{TM} search volume queries not only holds great promise in medicine, but also in other areas of research. Analysis of northern Europeans' (Finland, Germany, Norway, Ireland, and the UK) web searching behavior on Mediterranean tourist destinations revealed a relationship between thermal conditions and the searching behavior, and the authors observed no time lag between the prevalence of thermal conditions and searching of the keywords [6].

In transplant medicine, public awareness is key to promote discussion around organ donation, both live and deceased. In the current study, we investigate the public interest in kidney transplantation using data on Internet search queries extracted from the Google Trends^{TM} tool.

2. Materials and Methods

2.1. Retrieving Transplantation Numbers for UNOS, ONT, and Eurotransplant

Data were retrieved by accessing the respective websites of the transplant organizations ((https://unos.org) for the UNOS, (http://www.ont.es) for the Organización Nacional de Trasplantes (ONT), (https://www.eurotransplant.org) for the Eurotransplant countries, and (https://www.nhsbt.nhs.uk) for the UK.

Information about live and deceased donor kidney transplantation over a period of 15 years (2004–2018) for the following countries was extracted from the web pages as stated above: United States of America (UNOS), Spain (ONT), Austria, Belgium, Croatia, Germany, Hungary, Slovenia, and the Netherlands (belonging to the Eurotransplant countries), and the UK (NHS Transplant Register).

2.2. Retrieving Google Trends^{TM} Data on Kidney Transplantation

The Google Trends^{TM} tool (https://trends.google.com/trends/) was used to retrieve data on Internet user search activities in the context of kidney transplantation. Google Trends^{TM} is a freely accessible tool that enables researchers to study trends and patterns of Google search queries [7]. It was implemented in 2004 and data on Internet search queries are available since then on a monthly basis. Google Trends™ expresses the absolute number of searches relative to the total number of searches over the defined period of interest. The retrieved Google Trends™ index ranges from 0 to 100, with 100 being the highest relative search term activity for the specified search query in any given month [7]. Thus, a search index of 50 indicates that the search activity for kidney transplantation was 50% of that seen at the time when search activity was most intense [7].

Worldwide Google Trends™ indices were retrieved between January 2004 and December 2018 using the search term "kidney transplantation". We retrieved Google Trends™ indices for the US, Spain, the following European countries being part of the Eurotransplant network, namely Austria, Belgium, Croatia, Germany, Hungary, Slovenia, and the Netherlands, and the UK. No Google Trends™ indices could be retrieved for Luxembourg. Whereas the worldwide search was performed in English, the individual searches in the respective countries were performed in the official languages (see Table S1).

2.3. Data Analysis

Annual average Google Trends™ indices were calculated based on the monthly data downloaded from the Google Trends™ webpage. Time-lag correlations between transplant numbers and Google Trends™ indices were calculated using the ccf function of the tseries R package using a time lag between −3 and +3. The ggplot2 R package was used to generate all graphics. R version 3.4.1 was used for all analyses.

None of the queries in the Google database for this study can be associated to a particular individual. The database retains no information about the identity, Internet protocol address or specific physical location of any user. Furthermore, any original web search logs older than nine months are anonymized in accordance with Google's privacy policy (www.google.com/privacypolicy.html).

3. Results

The worldwide search query using Google Trends™ highlighted a decrease from an index of 76.3 in 2004 to 25.4 in 2018 (absolute reduction −50.9, or a relative reduction of −66.7%, see Figure 1). This trend was particularly confirmed in the US, with a decrease of the Google Trends™ index from an index of 68.4 to 17.0 (absolute reduction −51.4, relative reduction of −75.2%) over time. While an initial sharp decrease in search results was observed from an index of 68.4 to 37.6 (absolute reduction −30.8, relative reduction of −45.0%) within two years, there was a further decrease by 54.8% over the following thirteen years. In the same period of time, UNOS reported an increase of deceased donor kidney transplants from 16,007 in 2004 to 21,167 in 2018 (+32.2%); within the same period the live donor kidney transplantation rate remained stable (6648 in 2004 and 6442 in 2018, −3.1%). A similar search tendency of a decreased Google Trends™ index was found for the Eurotransplant area and the UK. There was a modest increase in Google Trends™ search queries in Spain, with a very low number in 2004 (index of 8.3) and 10.1 in 2018 (absolute increase +1.8, or a relative increase of +21.7%). In the same time-period the number of transplanted kidneys increased from 2125 to 3313 (+55.9%). In smaller countries, it is likely that events of interest to the public lead to an increase in search queries in that particular year. This for example might explain the increase in search queries in Austria in 2005 when a person of public interest received a second live-related kidney transplant in the same year. We observed an increase of Google Trends™ search queries from an index of 26.3 in 2004 to 36.6 in 2005 (absolute increase +10.3 or relative increase of +39.2%). In the following years, a decrease was found with an index of 12.9 in 2018 (absolute reduction −13.4 or a relative decrease of −51.0%). Similar curves were observed in all Eurotransplant countries, even in countries with a higher number of live-related kidney transplants, for example, the Netherlands (48.1% in 2004 and 40.0% in 2018), where more web-based information retrieval might be expected. Online searches assessed by Google Trends™ decreased from 49.3 to 37.8 (−11.5, or −23.3%) over 15 years. In Germany a decrease from 52.4 to 30.7 (−21.7, or −41.4%) was found in the same period, with even more pronounced reductions observed in Belgium (from 21.5 to 8.1, corresponding to a decrease of 13.4, or −62.3%) and Hungary (from 8.3 to 2.6, absolute reduction of −5.7 or relative reduction by −68.7%). In the UK, Google Trends™ indices decreased from 33.25 to 7.58 with an absolute reduction of 25.67 and a relative reduction of −77.2%, mirroring the decrease observed in the US. An overview of Google Trends™ changes over time and number of transplants (deceased donor and live donor transplantation) in the respective countries is highlighted in Table 1, Table S2, and Figure 2.

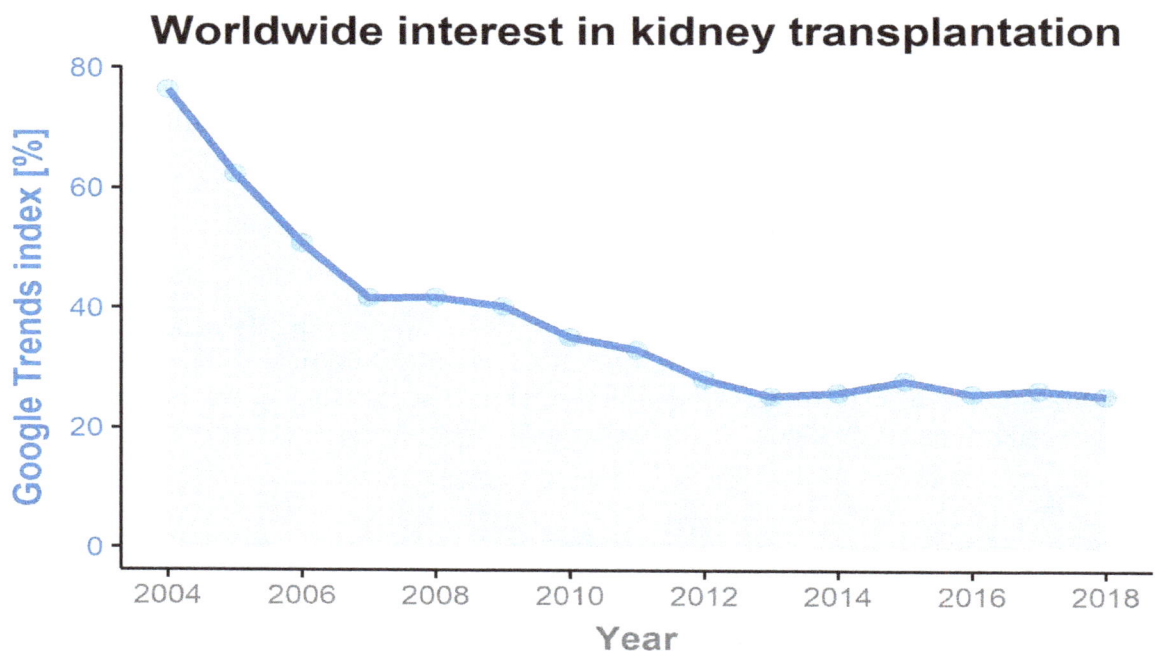

Figure 1. A worldwide decrease in the Google Trends™ indices from inception to 2018 was found. During a period of 15 years, the index decreased from 76.3 to 25.4, corresponding to a change of −66.7%.

We used correlation analysis to compare the Google Trends™ indices to the number of transplants over time and found negative correlations in particular for the UK, Belgium, and Austria, but also for Hungary, Slovenia, Germany, and the US. Spain is the only country where both transplant numbers as well as Google Trends™ indices show positive correlations above 0.5 (Figure 3).

Is there Decreasing Public Interest in Renal Transplantation? A Google TrendsTM Analysis

9

Table 1. The respective year, number of search queries using Google Trends[TM], and the total number of kidney transplantations performed (deceased donor and living donor).

Year.	World GT.	US GT.	US Tx.	UK GT.	UK Tx.	ESP GT.	ESP Tx.	B GT.	B Tx.	NL GT.	NL Tx.	GER GT.	GER Tx.	AUT GT.	AUT Tx.	SLO GT.	SLO Tx.	H GT.	H Tx.	CRO GT.	CRO Tx.
2004	76.3.	68.4	22,655	33.25	1836.	8.3	2125	21.5	235	49.3	520	52.4	1991	26.3	253	17.4	35	8.3	0	0.0	0
2005	62.3	49.1	23,057	36.75	1783.	0.0	2200	28.4	260	53.5	762	40.0	2165	36.6	255	14.8	20	5.8	0	0.0	0
2006	50.8	37.6	23,530	30.67	1915.	4.0	2157	18.6	324	32.8	752	31.5	2206	30.3	303	19.5	30	8.2	0	18.8	0
2007	41.6	33.8	22,677	20.58	2130.	0.0	2211	16.9	338	32.4	968	36.7	2336	26.6	299	8.5	22	8.3	0	21.0	26
2008	41.8	29.8	22,489	15.00	2282	9.3	2229	11.6	325	31.3	1012	30.8	2257	26.9	273	9.2	34	3.3	0	4.7	46
2009	40.3	32.6	23,216	16.08	2495.	5.7	2328	13.3	335	31.8	1036	28.4	2317	22.8	331	9.0	31	7.4	0	10.2	57
2010	35.1	24.1	23,178	14.00	2694.	5.3	2225	12.4	313	31.8	1151	28.7	2512	17.8	300	8.2	38	2.8	0	11.2	70
2011	33.1	25.7	22,589	11.83	2686.	10.3	2498	10.1	338	33.3	1091	32.6	2660	13.2	293	9.0	29	3.7	0	8.3	47
2012	28.2	21.9	22,106	10.50	2799.	9.8	2551	10.6	373	37.5	1215	30.0	2471	17.2	307	8.8	39	3.8	13	9.6	57
2013	25.4	19.6	22,629	8.67	3001.	8.0	2552	8.9	361	33.9	1273	30.8	2241	17.7	321	8.5	40	3.8	120	7.5	46
2014	25.9	16.2	22,646	9.58	3259.	8.9	2678	8.0	353	35.1	1321	33.5	2021	15.0	336	8.3	37	3.9	276	8.7	57
2015	27.9	20.2	23,506	7.50	3121.	9.3	2905	10.5	374	28.2	1280.	30.0	2089	12.3	305	10.7	43	3.1	242	8.3	53
2016	25.8	17.6	24,689	8.50	3268.	8.9	2997	6.1	380	28.8	1348	29.5	1957	14.3	324	11.5	35	3.9	238	6.8	52
2017	26.3	15.1	25,660	9.75	3351.	11.0	3269	8.7	386	30.5	1329	34.2	1814	12.7	330	10.8	32	2.8	218	8.0	50
2018	25.4	17.0	27,609	7.58	3608.	10.1	3313	8.1	373	37.8	1274	30.7	2130	12.9	320	11.2	37	2.6	244	8.8	43
Change (%).	-66.7	-75.1	+21.9.	-77.2	+196.5	+21.7	+55.9	-62.3	+58.7	-23.3	+245.0	-41.4	+7.0	-51.0	+26.5	-35.6	+5.7	-68.7	-	-	-

Abbreviations: GT (Google Trends[TM]), US (United States of America), UK (United Kingdom), ESP (Spain), B (Belgium), NL (the Netherlands), GER (Germany), AUT (Austria), SLO (Slovenia), H (Hungary), CRO (Croatia), Tx. (transplants).

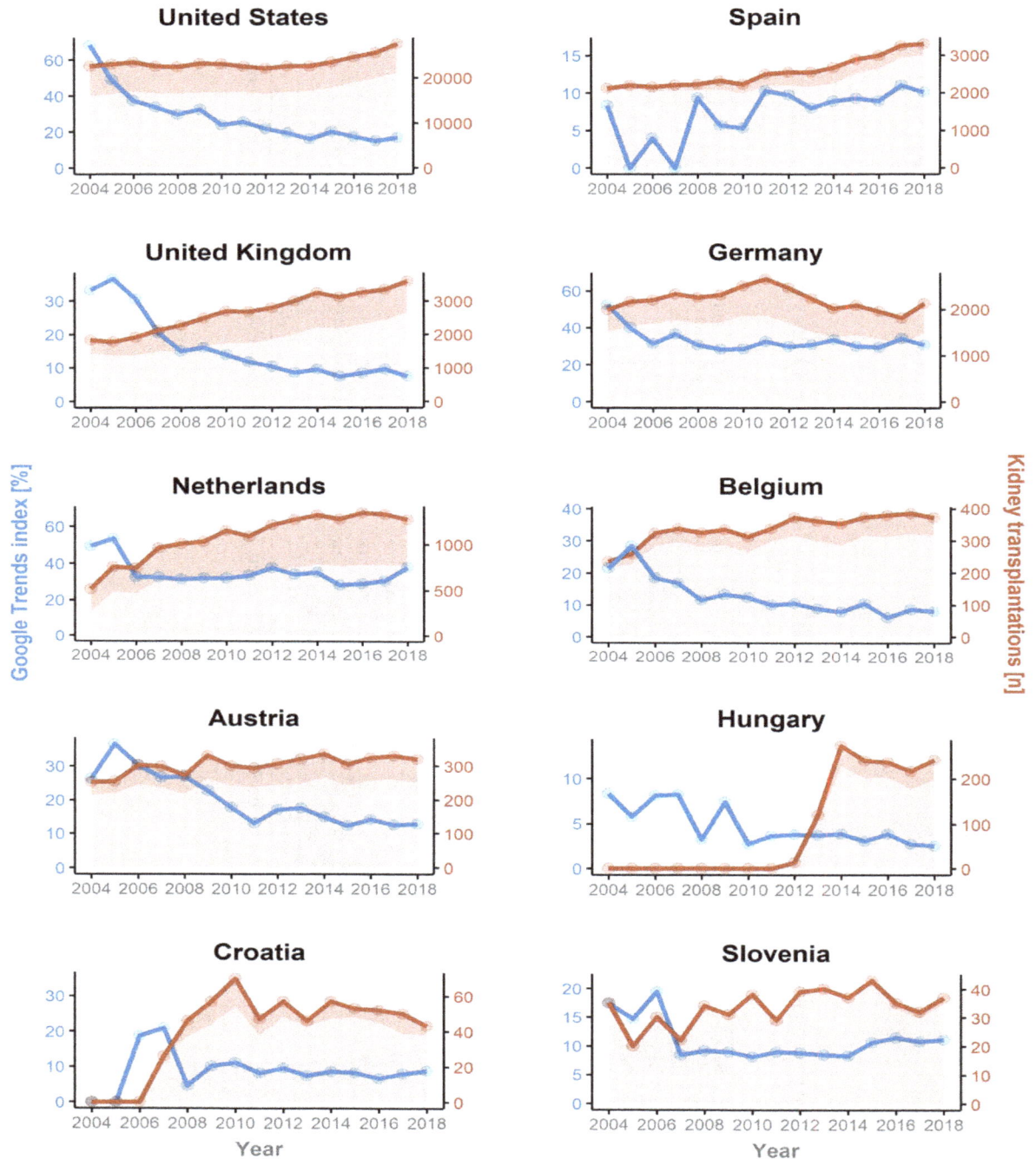

Figure 2. The respective numbers of renal transplants (red line) and the Google Trends™ indices (blue line) are given for the United Nations of Organ Sharing (UNOS), the Organización Nacional de Trasplantes (ONT), the Eurotransplant areas, and the UK National Register. Numbers of deceased and living donor transplants are indicated by light and dark red areas. While there was a marginal increase in the Google Trends™ index observed in Spain, the curves obtained from the UNOS, Eurotransplant areas, and the UK National Register mirror the worldwide trend.

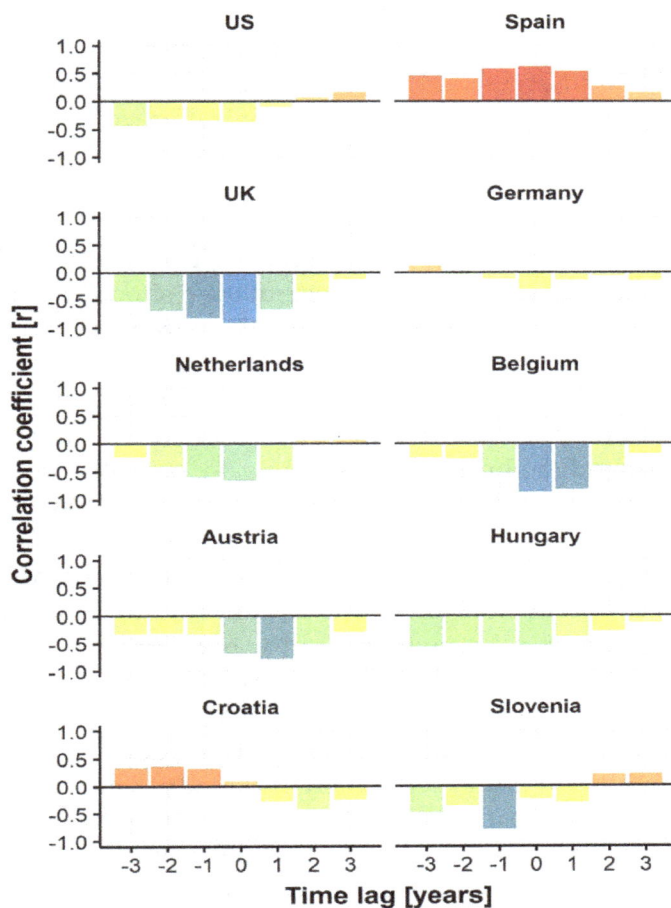

Figure 3. Time-lag correlations of Google Trends^{TM} indices and number of performed transplants for the countries under study. Negative correlations between Google Trends^{TM} indices and number of transplants are highlighted in green to blue whereas positive correlations are given in orange to red.

4. Discussion

To our knowledge, this is the first study investigating the trend of search queries for kidney transplantation. We observed a global decrease in public interest regarding kidney transplant, in particular in the UNOS, the Eurotransplant areas, and the UK. There is a global increase in transplanted kidneys, however, an increase in waiting time and a shortage of kidney donors highlight the demand [8]. Kidney transplant is the optimal form of renal replacement therapy for patients with end stage renal disease, improving both quality and quantity of life. Whilst this is true for both live and deceased organ donation, recipients of a live donor kidney transplant demonstrate better outcomes at both, one and five-years post transplantation [9]. Thus, raising and maintaining awareness about kidney transplants is imperative. How can we achieve this essential goal? Along with strategies discussed below, supra-national alliances such as the European Kidney Health Alliance (EKHA) are essential.

Efforts should be made to increase the number of live kidney donor transplants which are performed [9]. To help overcome hurdles like lack of awareness, particularly in populations with lower rates of live donor kidney transplants, namely ethnic minority populations and in groups who suffer from socioeconomic deprivation [10,11], successful campaigns have been orchestrated using both traditional media as well as online media, and community-based venues. By using Google Analytics^{TM}, the authors found an eight-fold increase in traffic to the Infórmate website, a website developed by the Northwestern University faculty in partnership with the National Kidney Foundation, compared to the pre-campaign period [12]. Website exposure was associated with a significant knowledge score increase between pretest and posttest assessments, which was maintained at a follow-up assessment at three weeks [13]. Readability and accessibility of online living donor and deceased donor recipient material is essential. An analysis of the top ten websites for both revealed that the reading level for the living donor materials was 12.54, while it was 12.87 for the deceased donor materials, corresponding to a university level. Overall, the readability of online material remains too high for the corresponding health literacy rates among potential kidney transplant recipients [14]. Whilst the readability must be increased, Information Score (IS) assessment also revealed a poor quality of many websites and that more input from transplant physicians is needed. Information should be freely available in multiple languages, as well as in Braille format and as audio text. Generally, websites belonging to academic institutions have higher IS than professional, or commercial websites [15]. Among 46 Italian YouTube® videos analyzed for usefulness to inform about live donor kidney transplantation, only a minority (15.2%) were categorized to contain useful information for the general population [16].

Kidney transplant knowledge should be improved in potential recipients. The Knowledge Assessment of Renal Transplantation (KART) contains 15 items including basic information about the procedure, prognosis, and insurance issues, and has an acceptable evidenced reliability. The KART distinguished patients who spent more or less than one hour receiving different types of education, including communication between doctors and medical staff, reading brochures, browsing the Internet, and watching videos [17]. Limited knowledge is not only present among patients but is also evident amongst medical students. In total, 96% were aware of the possibility of live donor kidney transplantation, but only 8% of the surveyed students were registered as potential donors in this South African study [18]. Similarly, a study from Leeds found that students had a basic understanding of organ donation and transplantation but lack detailed knowledge, such as understanding the criteria which are commonly used for brain death testing [19]. A study from India reporting on 200 interviews found that awareness will promote organ donation and there is a need for effective campaigns that educate people with relevant information, since a majority (59%) believed that donated organs might be misused, abused, or misappropriated [20].

Potential kidney transplant donors and recipients and those who have donated or received a transplant should be invited to share their experience online, in person, and on social media platforms. A survey involving 199 patients revealed that half use social media (52.3%, not further specified which channels were used) and most reported to be willing to post information about live kidney donation on their social networks (51%) [21]. Renal patients' organizations must also be supported and encouraged to provide information via social media.

Transplant physicians, surgeons, and nursing staff may also use social media to increase awareness of kidney transplantation. A survey among members of the American Society of Transplant Surgeons indicated that among 299 physicians who completed the survey, 59% use social media to communicate with surgeons, 57% with transplant professionals, 21% with transplant recipients, 16% with living donors, and 15% with waitlisted candidates. Younger age and fewer years of experience in transplantation were significantly associated with a stronger belief that social media may be influential in living organ donation [22].

Religious differences in mixed communities may play a role. In a Dutch study, the impact of religion on live donor kidney transplantation was assessed. The authors reported that religion is not perceived as an obstacle to live donation in the Netherlands. However, there is a necessity for increased clarity and awareness for different religions with respect to live donation [23]. While most of the patients seemed to favor live donor kidney transplantation, a variety of potentially modifiable barriers were identified, including inadequate patient education, emotional factors, restrictive social influences, and suboptimal communication [24].

Altruistic live donation will play an increasing role in the future. Social media is used to facilitate transplantation (i.e., through websites such as MatchingDonors.com), which was implemented as early as 1994. An organ registration fee is one of the ethical concerns of such strategies. Facebook and

Twitter are freely available platforms to communicate with others within groups and via hashtags and offer the opportunity to connect with potential live donors [25]. Moorlock et al. critically assessed the so-called "identifiable victim effect" and proposed that institutionally organized personal case-based campaigns aimed at promoting specific recipients for directed donation, despite its ethical concerns, should be preferred to facilitate altruistic live donation [26]. Building a framework for social media and organ donation is necessary and recommendations for transplant hospitals have been issued [27]. Programs such as the Kidney Coach Program (KCP) need to be implemented in the clinical practice to equip individuals (candidates and advocates for candidates) with tools to identify potential donors, which enables individuals to discuss donation with people in their social network [28].

Amongst countries participating in the Eurotransplant program, different legal strategies are employed; for instance, in Germany a potential donor needs to declare willingness to be registered as a deceased donor or 'opt in' [29]. This can increase the time it takes to ascertain suitability and thus delay transplant surgery. It also means that there are likely to be many willing donors, who simply do not register but if the system were 'opt out' would be very willing to be organ donors. Furthermore, 'opt in' systems for deceased donor donation lead to ongoing political debate which one might anticipate would help to raise awareness. When this was assessed via a Google Trends™ search, the decrease in the Google Trends™ index mirrored the changes observed in other Eurotransplant countries and thus this ongoing debate did not influence the public interest as assessed by Google Trends™. By the end of 2020, the organ donation laws in the UK will have moved from an 'opt in' system for deceased donor organ donation to an 'opt out' system (i.e., a deemed authorization system, applicable to the vast majority of the population with some notable exceptions). Northern Ireland is excepted from this change and the donation system there remains 'opt in' [30]. A significant factor in this change in legislation is the result of campaigning and lobbying from a nine-year old boy, Max Johnson, and his family. Max was awaiting a heart transplant which he ultimately received from Keira Ball, a nine-year old girl whose parents selflessly agreed to donate her organs. The legislation is to be commonly referred to as Max and Keira's Law [31].

Whilst this study shows a decreasing interest in web-based information over time in most areas, the number of live kidney donations increased in the ONT, the Eurotransplant areas, and the UK, while it was almost stable over time in the UNOS area (−3.1% from 2004 to 2018). This highlights that in most countries information from the treating physicians is more important than from the World Wide Web. A scoping review addressed strategies to increase live kidney donation and found that recipient-based education that reaches friends and family has the best evidence of being effective [32]. In contrast to the global trend, the Google Trends™ search highlighted an increase in search queries in Spain. In the same time period, the number of live and deceased kidney transplantation increased by 480.3% and 46.3%. It is tempting to speculate that either a sharp increase in transplant numbers or the implementation of non-heart-beating donation increased public interest [33].

This study has a few limitations. While Google Trends™ captures Google search queries and might act as a surrogate for public interest, Google is not the only available search engine next to other social media networks being used to search for information on the Internet. Previous work by others however indicates that Google Trends™ is a very valid measure of public interest. Additionally, the results obtained from Google Trends™ represent only relative numbers with no information on the absolute interest being available. We restricted our analysis to countries with an excellent documentation of transplant numbers and excluded countries from Asia and Africa, although they were included in the worldwide Google Trends™ analysis.

In conclusion, our Google Trends™ analysis found a decreasing public interest in renal transplantation. Strategies to inform the general population about unmet needs in the transplant setting (i.e., reduction of the waiting list time and live kidney donation) need to be utilized by all involved in the care of patients with kidney disease, by the patients themselves, and by national societies and academic institutions. Easily accessible information must be provided which is coherent and available in multiple languages including Braille and audio text. The message conveyed should be consistent and the information should be made available on multiple platforms including webpages, social media, and paper format. This may help reduce barriers in accessing information for different groups and improve outcomes according to the principles of patient-centered care.

Author Contributions: Conceptualization, A.K., M.E., and P.P. Data curation, A.K., M.E., and P.P. Formal analysis, P.P. Investigation, P.P. Supervision, A.K., M.E., and P.P., Validation, A.K., M.E., J.I.S., C.K., S.D., M.R., H.N., M.J.S., K.S., A.B., H.T., G.M., and P.P. Visualization, P.P. Writing—original draft A.K., M.E., J.I.S., C.K., S.D., M.R., H.N., M.J.S., K.S., A.B., H.T., G.M., and P.P. Writing—review & editing, A.K., M.E., J.I.S., C.K., S.D., M.R., H.N., M.J.S., K.S., A.B., H.T., G.M., and P.P. All authors have read and agreed to the published version of the manuscript.

References

1. Shrestha:, B.; Haylor, J.; Raftery, A. Historical perspectives in kidney transplantation: An updated review. *Prog. Transplant.* **2015**, *25*, 64–76. [CrossRef]
2. Reese, P.P.; Boudville, N.; Garg, A.X. Living kidney donation: Outcomes, ethics, and uncertainty. *Lancet* **2015**, *385*, 2003–2013. [CrossRef]
3. Tong, A.; Chapman, J.R.; Wong, G.; Josephson, M.A.; Craig, J.C. Public awareness and attitudes to living organ donation: Systematic review and integrative synthesis. *Transplantation* **2013**, *96*, 429–437. [CrossRef] [PubMed]
4. Cervellin, G.; Comelli, I.; Lippi, G. Is Google Trends a reliable tool for digital epidemiology? Insights from different clinical settings. *J. Epidemiol. Glob. Health* **2017**, *7*, 185–189. [CrossRef]
5. Telfer, S.; Obradovich, N. Local weather is associated with rates of online searches for musculoskeletal pain symptoms. *PLoS ONE* **2017**, *12*, e0181266. [CrossRef] [PubMed]
6. Charalampopoulos, I.; Nastos, P.T.; Didaskalou, E. Human Thermal Conditions and North Europeans' Web Searching Behavior (Google Trends) on Mediterranean Touristic Destinations. *Urban Sci.* **2017**, *1*, 8. [CrossRef]
7. Arora, V.S.; McKee, M.; Stuckler, D. Google Trends: Opportunities and limitations in health and health policy research. *Health Policy* **2019**, *123*, 338–341. [CrossRef]
8. Andre, M.; Huang, E.; Everly, M.; Bunnapradist, S. The UNOS Renal Transplant Registry: Review of the Last Decade. *Clin. Transpl.* **2014**, 1–12.
9. Terasaki, P.I.; Cecka, J.M.; Gjertson, D.W.; Takemoto, S. High survival rates of kidney transplants from spousal and living unrelated donors. *N. Engl. J. Med.* **1995**, *333*, 333–336. [CrossRef] [PubMed]
10. Bratton, C.; Chavin, K.; Baliga, P. Racial disparities in organ donation and why. *Curr. Opin. Organ. Transpl.* **2011**, *16*, 243–249. [CrossRef]
11. Reed, R.D.; Sawinski, D.; Shelton, B.A.; MacLennan, P.A.; Hanaway, M.; Kumar, V.; Long, D.; Gaston, R.S.; Kilgore, M.L.; Julian, B.A.; et al. Population Health, Ethnicity, and Rate of Living Donor Kidney Transplantation. *Transplantation* **2018**, *102*, 2080–2087. [CrossRef] [PubMed]
12. Gordon, E.J.; Shand, J.; Black, A. Google analytics of a pilot mass and social media campaign targeting Hispanics about living kidney donation. *Internet Interv.* **2016**, *6*, 40–49. [CrossRef]
13. Gordon, E.J.; Feinglass, J.; Carney, P.; Vera, K.; Olivero, M.; Black, A.; O'Connor, K.; MacLean, J.; Nichols, S.; Sageshima, J.; et al. A Culturally Targeted Website for Hispanics/Latinos About Living Kidney Donation and Transplantation: A Randomized Controlled Trial of Increased Knowledge. *Transplantation* **2016**, *100*, 1149–1160. [CrossRef]
14. Zhou, E.P.; Kiwanuka, E.; Morrissey, P.E. Online patient resources for deceased donor and live donor kidney recipients: A comparative analysis of readability. *Clin. Kidney J.* **2018**, *11*, 559–563. [CrossRef] [PubMed]
15. Hanif, F.; Abayasekara, K.; Willcocks, L.; Jolly, E.C.; Jamieson, N.V.; Praseedom, R.K.; Goodacre, J.A.; Read, J.C.; Chaudhry, A.; Gibbs, P. The quality of information about kidney transplantation on the World Wide Web. *Clin. Transpl.* **2007**, *21*, 371–376. [CrossRef]
16. Bert, F.; Gualano, M.R.; Scozzari, G.; Alesina, M.; Amoroso, A.; Siliquini, R. YouTube((R)): An ally or an enemy in the promotion of living donor kidney transplantation? *Health Inform. J.* **2018**, *24*, 103–110. [CrossRef] [PubMed]

17. Peipert, J.D.; Hays, R.D.; Kawakita, S.; Beaumont, J.L.; Waterman, A.D. Measurement Characteristics of the Knowledge Assessment of Renal Transplantation. *Transplantation* **2019**, *103*, 565–572. [CrossRef]

18. Sobnach, S.; Borkum, M.; Hoffman, R.; Muller, E.; McCurdie, F.; Millar, A.; Numanoglu, A.; Kahn, D. Medical students' knowledge about organ transplantation: A South African perspective. *Transpl. Proc.* **2010**, *42*, 3368–3371. [CrossRef] [PubMed]

19. Bedi, K.K.; Hakeem, A.R.; Dave, R.; Lewington, A.; Sanfey, H.; Ahmad, N. Survey of the knowledge, perception, and attitude of medical students at the University of Leeds toward organ donation and transplantation. *Transpl. Proc.* **2015**, *47*, 247–260. [CrossRef]

20. Balwani, M.R.; Gumber, M.R.; Shah, P.R.; Kute, V.B.; Patel, H.V.; Engineer, D.P.; Gera, D.N.; Godhani, U.; Shah, M.; Trivedi, H.L. Attitude and awareness towards organ donation in western India. *Ren. Fail.* **2015**, *37*, 582–588. [CrossRef]

21. Kazley, A.S.; Hamidi, B.; Balliet, W.; Baliga, P. Social Media Use Among Living Kidney Donors and Recipients: Survey on Current Practice and Potential. *J. Med. Internet Res.* **2016**, *18*, e328. [CrossRef]

22. Henderson, M.L.; Adler, J.T.; Van Pilsum Rasmussen, S.E.; Thomas, A.G.; Herron, P.D.; Waldram, M.M.; Ruck, J.M.; Purnell, T.S.; DiBrito, S.R.; Holscher, C.M.; et al. How Should Social Media Be Used in Transplantation? A Survey of the American Society of Transplant Surgeons. *Transplantation* **2019**, *103*, 573–580. [CrossRef]

23. Ismail, S.Y.; Massey, E.K.; Luchtenburg, A.E.; Claassens, L.; Zuidema, W.C.; Busschbach, J.J.; Weimar, W. Religious attitudes towards living kidney donation among Dutch renal patients. *Med. Health Care Philos.* **2012**, *15*, 221–227. [CrossRef]

24. Ismail, S.Y.; Claassens, L.; Luchtenburg, A.E.; Roodnat, J.I.; Zuidema, W.C.; Weimar, W.; Busschbach, J.J.; Massey, E.K. Living donor kidney transplantation among ethnic minorities in the Netherlands: A model for breaking the hurdles. *Patient Educ. Couns.* **2013**, *90*, 118–124. [CrossRef] [PubMed]

25. Henderson, M.L. Social Media in the Identification of Living Kidney Donors: Platforms, Tools, and Strategies. *Curr. Transpl. Rep.* **2018**, *5*, 19–26. [CrossRef] [PubMed]

26. Moorlock, G.; Draper, H. Empathy, social media, and directed altruistic living organ donation. *Bioethics* **2018**, *32*, 289–297. [CrossRef] [PubMed]

27. Henderson, M.L.; Clayville, K.A.; Fisher, J.S.; Kuntz, K.K.; Mysel, H.; Purnell, T.S.; Schaffer, R.L.; Sherman, L.A.; Willock, E.P.; Gordon, E.J. Social media and organ donation: Ethically navigating the next frontier. *Am. J. Transpl.* **2017**, *17*, 2803–2809. [CrossRef] [PubMed]

28. LaPointe Rudow, D.; Geatrakas, S.; Armenti, J.; Tomback, A.; Khaim, R.; Porcello, L.; Pan, S.; Arvelakis, A.; Shapiro, R. Increasing living donation by implementing the Kidney Coach Program. *Clin. Transpl.* **2019**, *33*, e13471. [CrossRef] [PubMed]

29. Metz, C.; Hoppe, N. Organ transplantation in Germany: Regulating scandals and scandalous regulation. *Eur. J. Health Law* **2013**, *20*, 113–116. [CrossRef]

30. Organ Donation Laws. Available online: https://www.organdonation.nhs.uk/uk-laws/ (accessed on 7 April 2020).

31. Max, Heart Transplant Recipient and Campaigner. Available online: https://www.organdonation.nhs.uk/helping-you-to-decide/real-life-stories/people-who-have-benefitted-from-receiving-a-transplant/max-heart-transplant-recipient-and-campaigner/ (accessed on 7 April 2020).

32. Barnieh, L.; Collister, D.; Manns, B.; Lam, N.N.; Shojai, S.; Lorenzetti, D.; Gill, J.S.; Klarenbach, S. A Scoping Review for Strategies to Increase Living Kidney Donation. *Clin. J. Am. Soc. Nephrol.* **2017**, *12*, 1518–1527. [CrossRef]

33. Gentil, M.A.; Castro de la Nuez, P.; Gonzalez-Corvillo, C.; de Gracia, M.C.; Cabello, M.; Mazuecos, M.A.; Rodriguez-Benot, A.; Ballesteros, L.; Osuna, A.; Alonso, M. Non-Heart-Beating Donor Kidney Transplantation Survival Is Similar to Donation After Brain Death: Comparative Study With Controls in a Regional Program. *Transpl. Proc.* **2016**, *48*, 2867–2870. [CrossRef] [PubMed]

3

A Low Tacrolimus Concentration/Dose Ratio Increases the Risk for the Development of Acute Calcineurin Inhibitor-Induced Nephrotoxicity

Gerold Thölking [1,2,*,†], Katharina Schütte-Nütgen [1,†], Julia Schmitz [1], Alexandros Rovas [1], Maximilian Dahmen [1], Joachim Bautz [1], Ulrich Jehn [1], Hermann Pavenstädt [1], Barbara Heitplatz [3], Veerle Van Marck [3], Barbara Suwelack [1] and Stefan Reuter [1,*]

[1] Department of Medicine D, Division of General Internal Medicine, Nephrology and Rheumatology, University Hospital of Münster, 48149 Münster, Germany; Katharina.schuette-nuetgen@ukmuenster.de (K.S.-N.); schmitzjulia.js@googlemail.com (J.S.); Alexandros.rovas@ukmuenster.de (A.R.); Maximilian.dahmen@ukmuenster.de (M.D.); joachim.bautz@ukmuenster.de (J.B.); ulrich.jehn@ukmuenster.de (U.J.); herman.pavenstaedt@ukmuenster.de (H.P.); Barbara.Suwelack@ukmuenster.de (B.S.)

[2] Department of Internal Medicine and Nephrology, University Hospital of Münster, Marienhospital Steinfurt, 48565 Steinfurt, Germany

[3] Gerhard-Domagk-Institute of Pathology, University Hospital of Münster, 48149 Münster, Germany; barbara.heitplatz@ukmuenster.de (B.H.); veerle.vanmarck@ukmuenster.de (V.V.M.)

* Correspondence: Gerold.Thoelking@ukmuenster.de (G.T.); Stefan.Reuter@ukmuenster.de (S.R.);

† These authors contributed equally to this work.

Abstract: Fast tacrolimus metabolism is linked to inferior outcomes such as rejection and lower renal function after kidney transplantation. Renal calcineurin-inhibitor toxicity is a common adverse effect of tacrolimus therapy. The present contribution hypothesized that tacrolimus-induced nephrotoxicity is related to a low concentration/dose (C/D) ratio. We analyzed renal tubular epithelial cell cultures and 55 consecutive kidney transplant biopsy samples with tacrolimus-induced toxicity, the C/D ratio, C0, C2, and C4 Tac levels, pulse wave velocity analyses, and sublingual endothelial glycocalyx dimensions in the selected kidney transplant patients. A low C/D ratio (C/D ratio < 1.05 ng/mL×1/mg) was linked with higher C2 tacrolimus blood concentrations (19.2 ± 8.7 µg/L vs. 12.2 ± 5.2 µg/L respectively; $p = 0.001$) and higher degrees of nephrotoxicity despite comparable trough levels (6.3 ± 2.4 µg/L vs. 6.6 ± 2.2 µg/L respectively; $p = 0.669$). However, the tacrolimus metabolism rate did not affect the pulse wave velocity or glycocalyx in patients. In renal tubular epithelial cells exposed to tacrolimus according to a fast metabolism pharmacokinetic profile it led to reduced viability and increased Fn14 expression. We conclude from our data that the C/D ratio may be an appropriate tool for identifying patients at risk of developing calcineurin-inhibitor toxicity.

Keywords: calcineurin inhibitor nephrotoxcity; tacrolimus; C/D ratio; tacrolimus metabolism; kidney transplantation

1. Introduction

Although the calcineurin inhibitor (CNI) tacrolimus (Tac) is effective in preventing graft rejection after transplantation, its therapeutic window is narrow. Furthermore, Tac exhibits a high intra- and inter-individual variability in pharmacokinetics (PK) and pharmacodynamics [1]. Tac-related adverse effects are common even in patients with Tac trough levels within the intended therapeutic range, despite meticulous therapeutic drug monitoring. CNI-induced nephrotoxicity (CNIT) especially remains a severe issue during CNI treatment [2]. While acute CNIT comprises isometric tubular vacuolization, acute arteriolopathy, and thrombotic microangiopathy, the features of chronic CNIT include interstitial fibrosis and tubular atrophy, arteriolar hyalinosis, tubular microcalcifications, and global glomerulosclerosis [2]. Unfortunately, there are no specific molecular markers of CNIT, but it was recently experimentally shown that, e.g., the TWEAK/Fn14 pathway, is critically involved in the pathogenesis of CNIT [3]. Although it is known that overexposure to Tac causes CNIT trough level-dependently, even patients presenting with Tac trough levels within the therapeutic range (5–15 µg/L) are vulnerable to developing both acute or chronic CNIT [4–9]. This indicates the possibility of additional causative factors.

Using the concentration/dose (C/D) ratio, a strong association between a fast Tac metabolism rate/fast oral Tac clearance (C/D ratio < 1.05 µg/L×1/mg) and reduced renal function within the first month following renal transplantation (RTx) can be demonstrated [9]. Other studies found comparable outcomes; even after liver transplantation [7,10–14]. However, this effect cannot be observed, if considerably higher C/D-ratio cut-offs are chosen [15]. The Tac metabolism effect on renal function was detectable even five years after RTx and was also associated with increased mortality in patients with a low C/D ratio [16].

What are the reasons for these findings? Apart from an increased susceptibility of fast metabolizers to BK virus infections, these patients more frequently required indication biopsies that revealed higher rates of rejections and acute CNIT [9,16,17]. Therefore, we hypothesized that the C/D ratio as a simple estimate of the Tac metabolism correlates with the severity of CNIT.

2. Experimental Section

2.1. Patients and Histology

At first, the study was conducted to answer the question if there is an association between histological findings of acute CNIT and the corresponding Tac C/D ratio at the time of biopsy. We hypothesized that a C/D ratio <1.05 ng/mL×1/mg is associated with acute CNIT. To prove the hypothesis, we performed a histological reevaluation of all for-cause RTx-biopsy samples that showed acute CNIT in our center between 2007 and 2016. Only samples with definite histological signs of acute CNIT (isometric vacuolization of tubular epithelial cells) were included in the study. Biopsy samples with isometric vacuolization that could be attributed to other causes were excluded from the evaluation.

Two pathologists, independently and blinded, categorized the graft biopsies in the following groups: <10%, 10–25%, 25–50%, and ≥50% of tubules showing isometric vacuolization of the cytoplasm (Figure 1A–D). In case of different assessment of the pathologists, mean values were taken. Due to limited sample numbers, for final analysis two categories were considered: samples with <25% and with ≥25% affected tubular cells ($n = 35$ and $n = 20$, respectively).

The C/D ratio was calculated by the Tac blood trough concentrations and the corresponding Tac doses on the day of the renal biopsy. C/D ratio values < 1.05 ng/mL×1/mg defined patients as fast Tac metabolizers (patients with fast oral clearance), values ≥ 1.05 ng/mL×1/mg characterized slow metabolizers (patients with slow oral clearance) as published before [8,13]. Only 12 h Tac trough levels were used for this analysis.

After confirmation of our first hypothesis, we secondly designed a prospective part of the study to address the question, if CNIT could be related to Tac peak levels. We hypothesized, that patients with a fast oral Tac clearance develop higher Tac peak levels than patients with a slow oral Tac clearance. Therefore, C0 and C2 Tac levels were determined in an additional cohort of 56 RTx patients. Additionally, we assessed C4 levels and the area under the curve (AUC) in 25 of these 56 individuals. For C0, 12 h trough levels were assessed. C2 was assessed 2 h and C4 4 h after intake of the morning dose, respectively. Whole blood was analyzed for Tac (automated tacrolimus (TACR) assay; Dimension Clinical Chemistry System; Siemens Healthcare Diagnostic GmbH; Eschborn; Germany). In addition, a cell culture model using supra-therapeutic Tac concentrations was used to mimic the different Tac profiles of patients with fast and slow oral Tac clearance (see below).

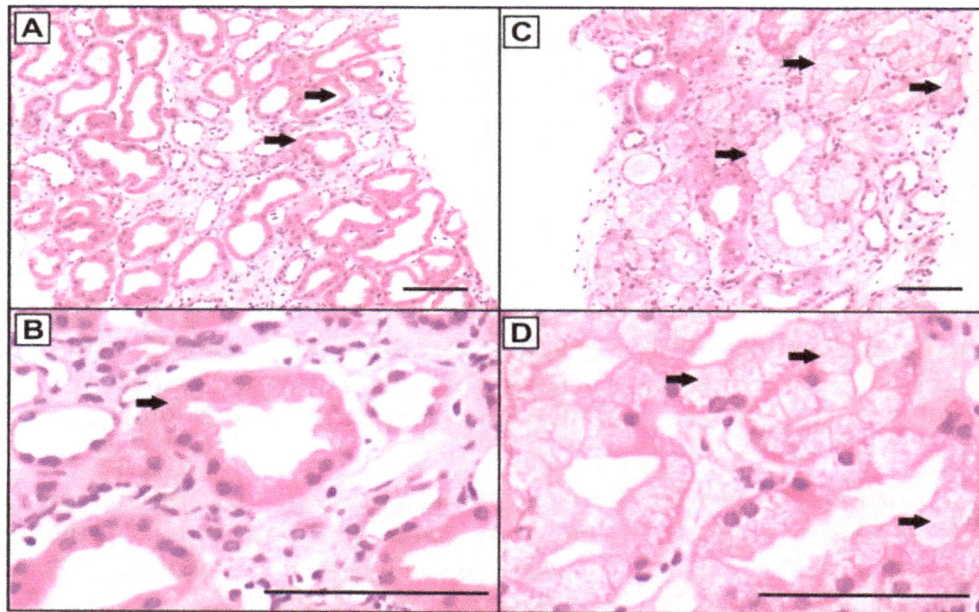

Figure 1. Examples of Hematoxylin and Eosin (HE)-stained sections of kidney transplant biopsies with different overall scores of isometric vacuolization (arrows) as a marker of calcineurin inhibitor-induced nephrotoxicity. (**A**): < 25% of the tubular epithelial cells, (**B**): magnification of A, (**C**) ≥ 25% of the tubular epithelial cells, and (**D**): magnification of C (bars: 100 μm).

All patients received an induction therapy with basiliximab or anti T-lymphocyte antibody and an immunosuppressive regimen containing immediate release tacrolimus (Prograf©), mycophenolate (CellCept©/Myfortic©), and prednisolone (Soludecortin H© /Decortin H©).

Patients' demographics were taken from the clinical hospital database and are presented in Table 1, and Tables S1 and S2.

Table 1. Patient characteristic: Histological analysis.

CNI Nephrotoxicity	x < 25% (n = 35)	x ≥ 25% (n = 20)	p-Value
Age (years, mean ± SD)	57.8 ± 12.4	50.2 ± 20.2	0.014 [a]
Male sex, n (%)	24 (68.6)	12 (60)	0.566 [b]
BMI (kg/m^2, mean ± SD)	25.5 ± 5.2	25.6 ± 5.3	0.981 [a]
Prednisolone dose (mg, mean ± SD)	10.0 ± 6.3	14.9 ± 17.5	0.239 [a]
Living donor transplantation, n (%)	26 (74.3)	14 (70)	0.761 [b]
ESP, n (%)	9 (25.7)	1 (5)	0.075 [b]
Combined RTx + liver Tx, n (%)	3 (8.6)	1 (5)	1 [b]
Previous Tx, n (%)	3 (8.6)	0	0.293 [b]
ABOi, n (%)	4 (11.4)	2 (10)	1 [b]
CIT (hours, mean ± SD)	9.2 ± 5.0	8.5 ± 5.0	0.669 [a]
WIT (min, mean ± SD)	32.5 ± 8.1	32.5 ± 5.4	0.418 [a]
DGF	11 (31.4)	2 (10)	0.107 [b]
Donor data			
Male donor sex, n (%)	13 (47,1)	14 (70)	0.026 [b]
Donor age (years, mean ± SD)	61.1 ± 15.7	52.2±14.7	0.073 [a]
Time from RTx to biopsy (days)	63 (3–2877)	223 (10–5057)	0.059 [c]

Patients with a CNI nephrotoxicity < 25% were observed to be older and received more female allografts; CNI, calcineurin inhibitor; BMI, body mass index; ESP, European senior program; RTx, renal transplantation, Tx, transplantation; ABOi, ABO incompatible transplantation; CIT, cold ischemia time, WIT, warm ischemia time, DGF, delayed graft function; [a] Student's t-test; [b] Fisher's exact test; [c] Mann–Whitney U test.

The study was performed in accordance with the Declaration of Helsinki and approved by the local ethics committee (Ethik Kommission der Ärztekammer Westfalen-Lippe und der Medizinischen Fakultät der Westfälischen Wilhelms-Universität, 2017-407-f-S). Prior to analysis, all patient data were anonymized. Written informed consent with regard to recording their clinical data was given by all participants at the time of transplantation or inclusion into the study. Recipients aged <18 years, pregnant women, or patients with uncontrolled infection, tumor, or hypertension were excluded from the study.

2.2. Assessment of Pulse Wave Velocity and Glycocalyx

Besides tubular changes tacrolimus toxicity comprises vascular effects (vasoconstriction, arteriolopathy) as well. After having linked tubular changes with the Tac oral clearance in patients and a cell culture model, respectively, we conducted a second prospective study to assess potential Tac metabolism-related vascular changes. Therefore, we measured pulse wave velocity (PVW) and the glycocalyx as surrogate parameters of endothelial dysfunction/arterial stiffness in 120 stable RTx outpatients (30 patients with a C/D ratio < 1.05 ng/mL×1/mg and 90 patients with a C/D ratio ≥ 1.05 ng/mL×1/mg). Arterial stiffness was assessed as pulse wave velocity (PWV) using cuff-based oscillometry (Mobil-O-Graph, IEM, Stolberg, Germany) [18,19]. Subjects rested for 10 min at 23 °C before the baseline hemodynamic measurements were performed. Initially, brachial systolic blood pressure (mmHg) was measured. Two sequential measurements separated by a 5-min interval were obtained. The mean PWV was used for the analysis only if the PWV difference between the assessments was <0.5 m/sec. Otherwise, a third measure was conducted and the median of all values was calculated as published before [20]. An experienced single operator performed the measurements.

Furthermore, we prospectively assessed the dynamic lateral red blood cell movement into the glycocalyx that is expressed as the perfused boundary region (PBR) (in μm) in a subset of 28 (14 fast metabolizer) stable and matched RTx patients using bedside real-time intravital microscopy [21]. The sublingual microvasculature was visualized and examined with the use of GlycoCheckTM Software, coupled to a sidestream dark field (SDF) camera (CapiScope HVCS, KK Technology, Honiton, UK) by an experienced single operator, as thoroughly described before [21]. Briefly, the SDF camera uses stroboscopic diodes (540 nm) to detect the hemoglobin of the red blood cells (RBC). The GlycoCheck software allows automatic video recording when predefined image quality criteria (motion, intensity, focus) are met. The software automatically identifies all available micro-vessels with a diameter between 5 to 25 μm and marks vascular segments every 10 μm along the assessed microvasculature. Before further analysis of the videos, it performs an automatic quality check (Figure 2C). Invalid vascular segments are marked with yellow and automatically discarded, while all valid vascular segments (green lines) are subjected to further analysis. The software measures the PBR (in μm); an inverse parameter of glycocalyx dimensions. Specifically, the dynamic lateral RBC movement towards the endothelial wall is assessed in an average of about 3000 different vascular segments with a diameter from 5 to 25 μm (Figure 2B,C). An impaired endothelial glycocalyx allows RBCs to penetrate more deeply towards the endothelium, which translates into higher PBR values.

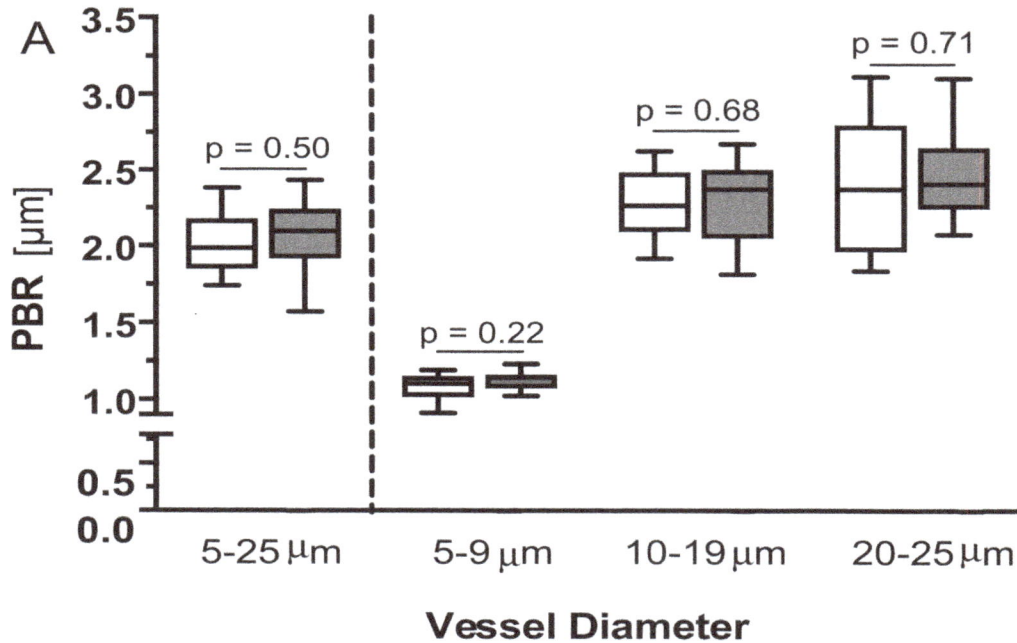

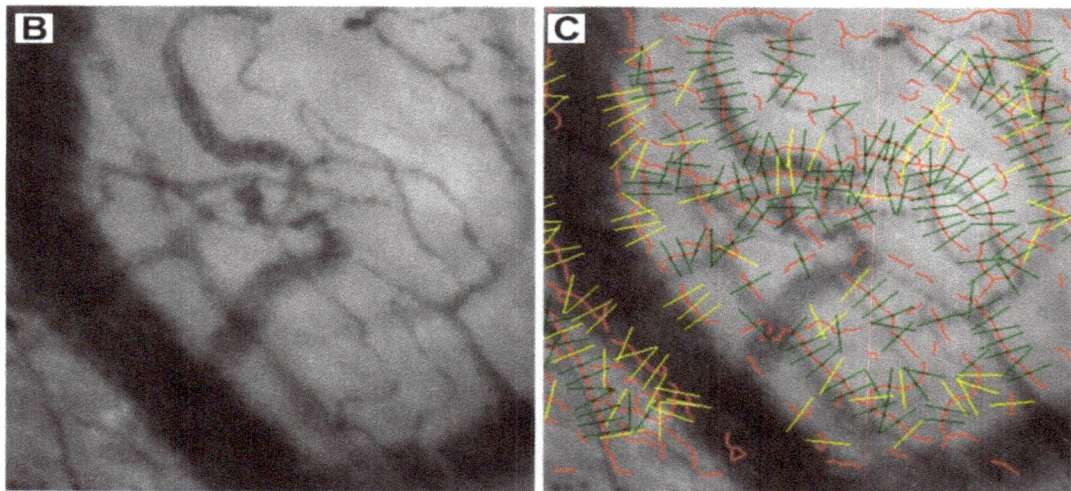

Figure 2. (**A**): Boxplots of PBR values of patients with a high C/D ratio (white) and low C/D ratio (grey) based on the different microvascular diameter ranges. No difference was detected between the groups. (**B**): Representative image of the sublingual mucosa acquired with the SDF camera in a kidney transplant patient. (**C**): Exemplary picture of a video recording showing the automatic identification of all available micro-vessels with a diameter between 5 to 25 μm. Vascular segments are marked every 10 μm along the assessed microvasculature (red lines) by the GlycoCheck software (green lines: valid segments for further analysis, yellow lines: discarded by quality check).

2.3. Cell Culture

Tubular epithelial cells (NRK-52E; ATCC) were cultivated in Dulbecco's modified Eagle medium (DMEM) (Invitrogen, Darmstadt, Germany) supplemented with 10% fetal calf serum (FCS) (Biochrom, Berlin, Germany), 1% antibiotics (Pen/Strep) and L-Glutamine (PAA; Cölbe, Germany), and were cultured at 37 °C and 5% CO_2. NRK-52E cells were grown in 12-well or 96-well plates until 80% confluence followed by treatment with tacrolimus (Prograf®i.v., Astellas, Munich, Germany) diluted in 0.9% sodium chloride) or medium only as a control over 12 h. Tac working solutions were freshly prepared by appropriate dilution of stock solution in the culture medium. Due to the inherent robustness of rat cells, titration series were conducted to determine the optimal tacrolimus concentrations that induce an appropriate reduction in cell viability. Culture medium was changed every hour using the indicated Tac concentrations between 6 and 20 µg/mL that were based on our titration studies and previous studies by Lamoureux et al. (Figure S1) [22]. After the incubation period of 12 h, the culture medium was removed and cells were washed three times with PBS and then prepared for quantitative Western blot analysis or MTT assay as described below. All samples were tested in triplicate wells. Data are representative of three different experiments.

2.4. Lysate Preparation and Western Blot Analysis

As fibroblast growth factor-inducible 14 (Fn14) is involved in the pathogenesis of CNIT we analyzed its expression in Tac-treated NRK cells using primary antibodies against α-actinin 4 and Fn14, respectively [3].

Preparation and quantitative Western blot analysis of cell lysates have been described previously [23]. Briefly, for quantitative Western blotting, cells were grown on dishes and then scraped into 1x LaemmLi (4% SDS, 5% 2-mercaptoethanol, 10% glycerol, 0.002% bromophenol blue, 0.0625 M Tris-HCl; pH 6.8). Samples were shaken at 1000 rpm for 2 h and then subjected to ultrasound bath treatment for 15 min. After being boiled for 5 min, equal volumes of cell lysates were separated onto 10% SDS-PAGE gels (Bio-Rad). Proteins were transferred to a PVDF membrane (Millipore) and incubated for 1 h at room temperature in blocking buffer (5% skim milk powder dissolved in TBS containing 0.05% Tween-20). A primary antibody against Fn14 (Cell Signaling, Danvers, MA, USA) was used in a 1:1000 dilution in TBS–Tween-20 and incubated at 4 °C overnight. After being washed three times with TBS–Tween-20, the membrane was incubated with horseradish peroxidase–coupled secondary antibodies (Jackson Immunoresearch, via Dianova, Hamburg, Germany) diluted 1:5000 in blocking buffer for 45 min at room temperature. After three washes, the Western blot was developed using a chemiluminescence detection reagent (Roche). For normalization of band density following chemiluminescence detection the samples were equalized using α-actinin (Enzo, Loerrach, Germany) as the loading control. All samples were tested in triplicate wells and three different experiments.

2.5. MTT Test

Cell viability was assessed by a colorimetric assay, which is based on the conversion of dissolved yellow 3-[4,5-dimethylthiazol-2-yl]-2,5-diphenyltetrazolium bromide (MTT) to insoluble purple formazan by cleavage of the tetrazolium ring by mitochondrial dehydrogenases of living cells as previously described [24,25]. Therefore, this MTT assay offers precise quantification of cell viability in mammalian cell cultures. Briefly, after Tac treatment for 12 h, the medium was carefully removed and replaced by 200 µL of fresh complete cell culture medium. 10 µL of MTT solution containing 5 mg/mL of the dye were added to each well, and the cells were again incubated for 3 h. The medium was then removed and 100 µL of lysis buffer containing 10% (w/v) sodium dodecyl sulfate and 40% (v/v) dimethylformamide was added to each well. The plates were shaken for 10 min to destroy the cell structure and dissolve the blue formazan dye. Finally, the absorbance was measured at 590 nm using an automated microtiter plate reader (Infinite M200; Tecan, Männedorf, Switzerland). The percentage of viable cells in the untreated controls was compared to that for the respective Tac treatments.

2.6. Statistical Analysis

Statistical analysis were performed using IBM SPSS®Statistics 25 for Windows (IBM Corporation, Somers, NY, USA) or GraphPad Prism version 4.0 (GraphPad Sofware, La Jolla, CA, USA). Normally distributed continuous variables are shown as mean ± standard deviation (SD) or as mean ± SEM and non-normally distributed continuous variables as median and first and third quartiles (interquartile range, IQR). Absolute and relative frequencies have been given for categorical variables. Pairs of independent groups were compared using the Student's t-test for normally distributed data,

Mann–Whitney U test for non-normal data, and Fisher's exact test for categorical variables. To compare paired data, we used the Wilcoxon test for continuous variables and the McNemar test for categorical variables. Comparison among groups in Western blot experiments was performed by one-way ANOVA along with post-hoc Tukey test. p-values < 0.05 were considered as statistically noticeable.

3. Results

3.1. Histology

The histological re-analysis of 55 consecutive kidney transplant biopsy samples from patients (low C/D ratio, $n = 27$) with evidence of CNIT indicated by the presence of the characteristic isometric vacuolization of the tubular epithelial cells in $< 10\%$ ($n = 20$), 10–24% ($n = 15$), 25–49% ($n = 12$) and eight biopsies $\geq 50\%$ of affected tubular cells. For further comparison, samples were regrouped according to $< 25\%$ ($n = 35$) or $\geq 25\%$ ($n = 20$) tubular isometric vacuolization (Figure 3, Table 1).

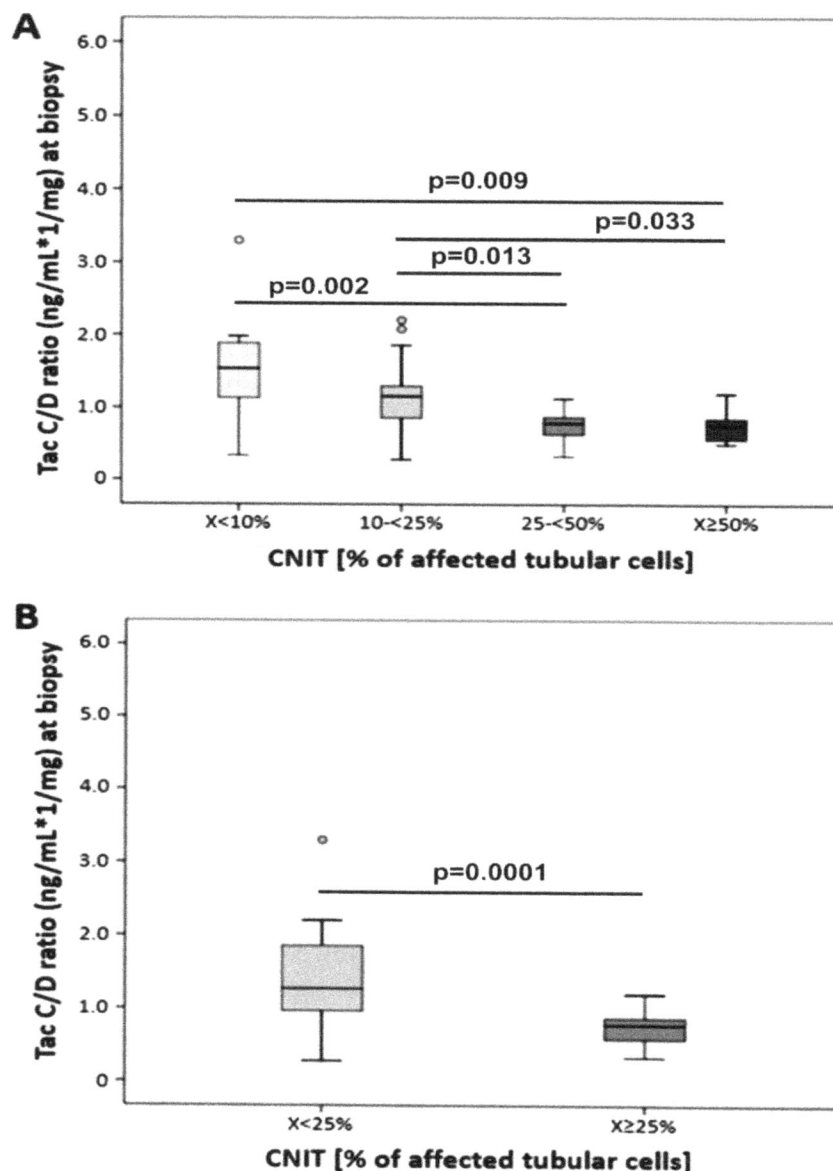

Figure 3. Histological analysis of calcineurin inhibitor-induced nephrotoxicity (CNIT) in kidney transplant biopsies, assessing the degree percentage of tubular cells with isometric vacuolization of the cytoplasm. The C/D ratio indicated a strong negative association with the severity of CNIT.

Although the trough levels at the time of biopsy were similar for both groups (Table 2), the degree of CNIT indicated a strong negative association to the C/D ratio values (Figure 3). Trough levels in 56 additional patients were comparable between patients with a low and high C/D ratio (6.3 ± 2.4 µg/L vs. 6.6 ± 2.2 µg/L respectively; $p = 0.669$). However, patients with a low C/D ratio displayed significantly higher C2 levels (19.2 ± 8.7 µg/L vs. 12.2 ± 5.2 µg/L, respectively; $p = 0.001$, Figure 4A). In a subgroup of 25 patients, C0 levels (6.3 ± 3.2 µg/L vs. 6.2 ± 2.3 µg/L, respectively; $p = 0.620$) and C4 (11.3 ± 5.8 µg/L vs. 9.0 ± 2.7 µg/L, respectively; $p = 0.466$) were comparable between groups. However, C2 levels of patients with a low C/D ratio were increased (20.2 ± 10.3 µg/L vs. 9.8 ± 4.2 µg/L, respectively; $p = 0.004$, Figure 4B).

Table 2. Tac trough level and dose of two calcineurin inhibitor toxicity groups.

	x < 25% (n = 35)	x ≥ 25% (n = 20)	p-Value
Tac trough level (ng/mL ± SD)	6.0 (3.1–15.1)	5.8 (2.4–12.5)	0.431
Tac dose (mg, mean ± SD)	5.0 (1.0–18.0)	8.0 (3.0–16.0)	0.009
C/D ratio, ng/mL×1/mg, median (min-max)	1.27 (0.28–5.03)	0.78 (0.33–1.20)	< 0.001

Tac, tacrolimus; Mann–Whitney U test.

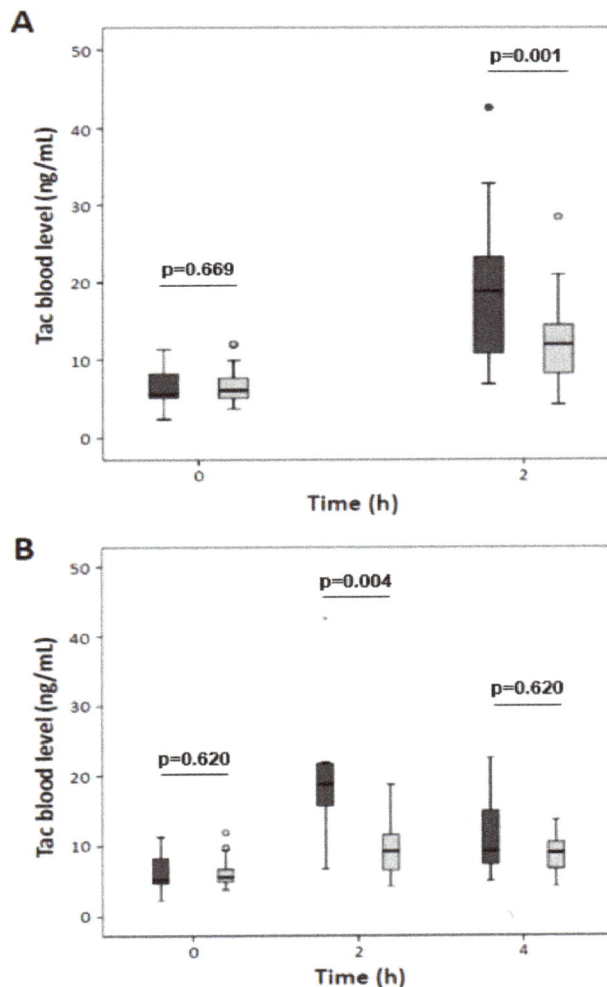

Figure 4. Presented are C0, C2 (n = 56) (**A**), and C4 (n = 25) (**B**) Tac levels in stable kidney transplanted patients. While the trough level (C0) and the C4 level were comparable between patients with a high (dark grey bars) and low (light grey bars) C/D ratio, C2 levels were significantly increased in patients with a low C/D ratio.

3.2. Pulse Wave Velocity Analysis

PWV correlated with age and systolic blood pressure (SBP) but not with the C/D ratio (Table S1, Figure 5).

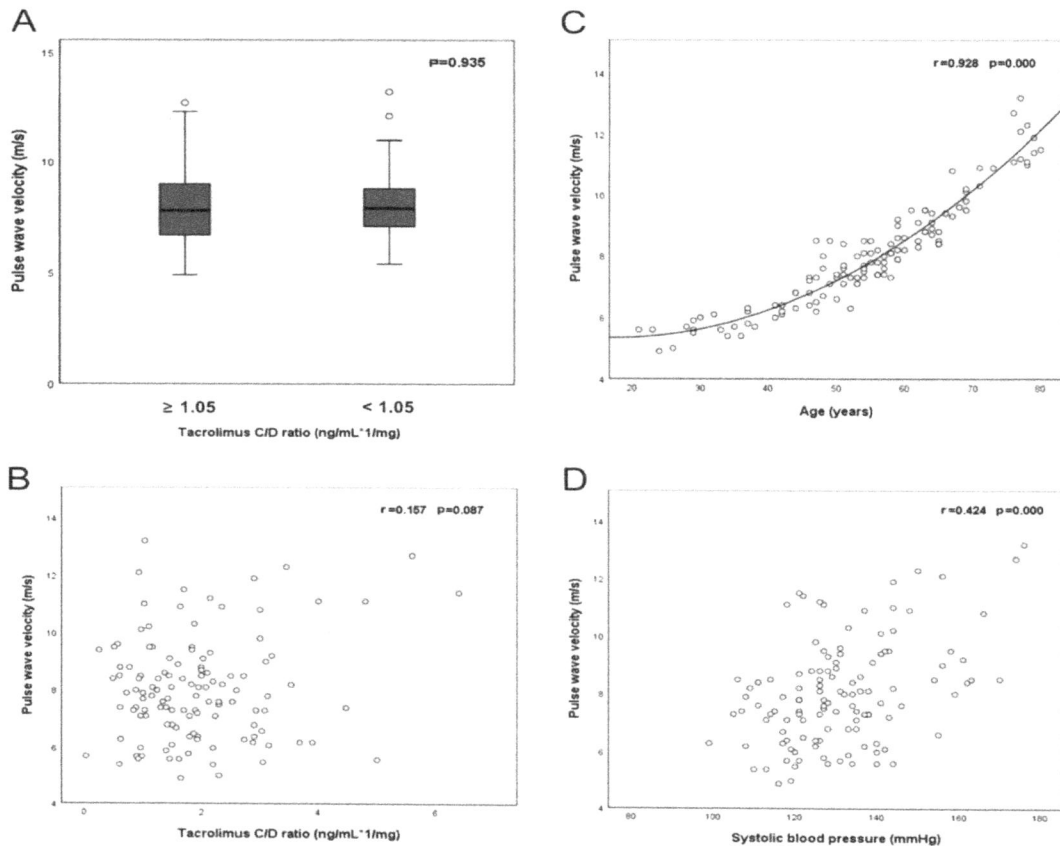

Figure 5. Pulse wave analysis of kidney transplanted patients. No correlation was observed between the C/D ratio and pulse wave velocity (**A,B**). The scatter plot in (**C**) indicates a strong quadratic relation of age and pulse wave velocity. Systolic blood pressure showed a moderately strong correlation to pulse wave velocity (**D**). R: Pearson correlation coefficient.

3.3. Glycocalyx Analysis

The PBR, an inverse parameter of endothelial glycocalyx dimensions in sublingual vessels, was comparable between the patients with a low and a high C/D ratio (Figure 2).

3.4. Cell Culture

Titration series revealed a tacrolimus concentration between 6 µg/mL and 20 µg/mL to induce an appropriate reduction of NRK cell viability in MTT assays. Tac exposure decreased the viability of NRK cells (Figure 6A) the most in cells that were treated with Tac corresponding to the PK profiles of fast metabolizers (6 µg/mL to 19 µg/mL) (77.3%) compared to cells that were exposed to continuous Tac treatment (8.5 µg/mL) or to Tac corresponding to the PK profiles of slow metabolizers (6 µg/mL to 12 µg/mL, respectively (81.3% vs. 84.7%, Figure 6A). Accordingly, these cells showed the highest Fn14 expression (Figure 6B).

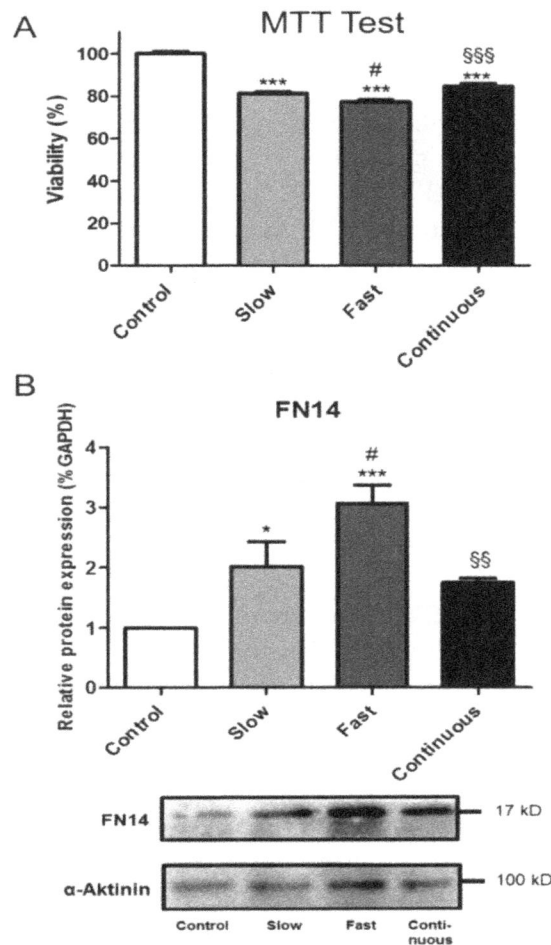

Figure 6. The viability of tubular epithelial cells (NRK-52E; ATCC) assessed by 3-[4,5-dimethylthiazol-2-yl]-2,5-diphenyltetrazolium bromide (MTT) test (**A**). Cells treated for 12 h with Tac according to the pharmakokinetic profile of fast metabolizers (Fast) showed the most reduced viability (*** $p < 0.001$ vs. Control, # $p < 0.05$ vs. Tac slow, §§§ $p < 0.001$ vs. Tac fast. Western blot analysis of Fn14 expression in NRK cells (**B**), showed higher Fn14 expression levels in NRK cells when compared to the other groups (* $p < 0.05$ vs. Control, *** $p < 0.001$ vs. Control, # $p < 0.05$ vs. Tac slow. §§ $p < 0.01$ vs. Tac fast). An exemplary Western blot is presented below.

4. Discussion

CNIT is a frequent complication of Tac exposure and is associated with reduced renal function and kidney graft loss. So far, no specific treatment of CNIT is available. Therefore, approaches to minimize its occurrence and identify the patients at risk are required.

The C/D ratio is a simple estimate of the Tac metabolism rate and is therefore useful to stratify patients' risk [1]. Since we identified a strong negative association between the C/D ratio and degree of acute CNIT observed in RTx biopsies, we describe in this study for the first time that a low C/D ratio (defined as a C/D ratio < 1.05 µg/L×1/mg) is linked to CNIT severity (Figure 3).

We previously observed that a low C/D ratio is associated with an inferior renal function after transplantation [1]. This effect persisted in a five-year follow-up, and a low C/D ratio was identified as an independent risk factor for a decreased graft and patient survival [16]. In an earlier study, the indication biopsy rate, that histologically showed more frequently CNIT in patients with a low C/D ratio, was higher than in patients with a high C/D ratio [9]. However, the sample size in this study was low and no information was available on the severity of the CNIT lesions. To fill these gaps, we performed the presented combined retro- and prospective studies to further investigate the influence of fast Tac metabolism on CNIT occurrence and severity.

Despite higher daily Tac dosages, patients with a low C/D ratio do not usually display higher trough concentrations, AUCs, and Tac metabolites compared to patients with a high C/D ratio (Table 2) [5–7,9,26]. Patients' PK profiles, including the peak level concentration, must consequently differ—a finding that we can confirm (Figure 4) [27]. In a study on the PK Tac profiles of stable RTx patients, Miura et al. presented in Figure 1 12 h PK profiles from their patients whose Tac concentration sharply increases to an early, high peak after Tac intake followed by a rapid decrease of the Tac blood level (suggestive of a low C/D ratio). In contrast, other patients exhibited a slow increase of Tac levels to a lower peak level after Tac intake that was followed by a slower decrease of Tac concentration to the trough level (suggestive of a high C/D ratio) [28]. In this regard, a randomized, prospective crossover study that assessed 24 h Tac PK profiles in genotyped, kidney transplanted African Americans provided informative insights [29]. African Americans, who are predominantly CYP3A5 expressors and therefore fast metabolizers, required double doses of weight-normalized immediate release (IR) Tac as compared to CYP3A5 non-expressors. Despite comparable Tac AUCs and a similar total exposure of fast and slow metabolizers to the compound, PK profiles and the exposure to Tac at different time points after intake differ. This is important because peak level concentrations that presumably cause temporary Tac overexposure are linked, e.g., to neurotoxicity [30].

In our cell culture model, the viability of NRK tubular epithelial cells significantly decreased when cells were incubated with Tac according to the PK profiles of fast metabolizers (Figure 6). These most affected cells notably expressed the highest amount of Fn14, a receptor protein known to be involved in the pathogenesis of CNIT [3]. It has to be considered that due to the robustness of NRK cells we applied Tac concentrations that are supra-therapeutic compared to Tac blood concentrations that are observed in patients and a direct translation into clinical practice and exact modelling of patients' Tac exposure, which is much more complex and influenced by many factors in vivo, is limited. However, by using this rather simple in vitro system we herein provide insights into the pathophysiologic effects of the different Tac PK profiles. Since endothelial dysfunction is essentially involved in the pathogenesis of acute CNIT, we exemplarily analyzed the functioning of the glycocalyx and the PWV; such analysis has been recently shown to be of additive value for the assessment of vessel function [2,31]. However, no differences were observed between the matched patients with low and high C/D ratios. The underlying causes for this could be the small sample size or a relatively small impact of Tac on the vessels [19]. Tac, in contrast to cyclosporine, does not reduce renal plasma flow, GFR, or blood pressure—at least not in healthy subjects [32].

Our study has limitations. First, Tac metabolites have not been measured and the analysis of Tac peak levels was not performed in the same group of RTx patients in whom the association of C/D ratio and histological CNIT was investigated since this part of the study was of a retrospective nature and could therefore only be hypothesis generating. Assessment of Tac metabolism is complex as it includes different processes such as uptake, metabolism in the intestine, liver, blood, and kidneys as well as its elimination. All these steps underlie many influencing factors (e.g., genetics, albumin level, hematocrit, differences in absorption and compliance). As we did not assess Tac metabolites, the C/D ratio can only serve as an estimate (sum of all effects that affect Tac metabolism in vivo) of the true Tac metabolism rate. Rather, the C/D ratio constitutes a simple tool to describe the stable condition between uptake and elimination of Tac in the blood. Nevertheless, a correlation between the C/D ratio and several CYP3A subtypes has already been shown by others (e.g. Reference [33]). To note, in terms of clinical outcomes it has been very recently demonstrated by Jouve et al. that e.g., genetics, were in contrast to the C/D ratio not suitable to predict the outcome of patients [13]. Despite the aforementioned limitations, the C/D ratio can serve as a simple estimate of the metabolism rate which is practical, cost-effective and can assist physicians in the daily routine for risk assessment and to individualize their patients' immunosuppressive therapy. Second, the vascular parameters PBR and PWV have not been analyzed directly in the kidney but are usually extrapolated from measures at other body sides. Therefore, local effects of Tac on the renal endothelial might have been missed using our approach. Moreover, there are further parameters that can impact on the glycocalyx and the vascular stiffness such as diabetes or hypertension (frequently present in RTx patients and also potentially related to Tac) which have not been investigated in our study. Third, the sample size of our single center study is limited.

Despite these limitations, we demonstrated that a low C/D ratio is associated with significantly higher Tac C2 levels and more severe CNIT. We also showed that systemic markers of endothelial (dys-)function were not associated with the C/D ratio and NRK tubular epithelial cells in vitro were most affected when exposed to Tac according to a fast metabolism PK profile. The C/D ratio may, therefore, be an appropriate tool for identifying patients at risk of developing CNIT.

Author Contributions: Conceptualization, G.T. and S.R.; methodology, A.R., M.D., V.V.M., B.H., G.T., K.S.-N. and S.R.; formal analysis, A.R., J.B., U.J., K.S.-N., G.T. and J.S.; data curation, A.R., M.D., U.J., K.S.-N. and J.S.; writing—original draft preparation, S.R., K.S.-N. and G.T.; writing—review and editing, A.R., V.V.M., B.H., H.P. and B.S.; supervision, H.P., B.S. and S.R.; project administration, H.P., B.S. and S.R.; funding acquisition, K.S.-N. and S.R.

Acknowledgments: The authors would like to express their gratitude to Birgit Jaxy, Ute Neugebauer, and Rita Schröter for their excellent technical assistance.

References

1. Schütte-Nütgen, K.; Thölking, G.; Suwelack, B.; Reuter, S. Tacrolimus-Pharmacokinetic Considerations for Clinicians. *Curr. Drug Metab.* **2018**, *19*, 342–350. [CrossRef] [PubMed]
2. Naesens, M.; Kuypers, D.R.; Sarwal, M. Calcineurin inhibitor nephrotoxicity. *Clin. J. Am. Soc. Nephrol.* **2009**, *4*, 481–508. [CrossRef] [PubMed]
3. Claus, M.; Herro, R.; Wolf, D.; Buscher, K.; Rudloff, S.; Huynh-Do, U.; Burkly, L.; Croft, M.; Sidler, D. The TWEAK/Fn14 pathway is required for calcineurin inhibitor toxicity of the kidneys. *Am. J. Transplant.* **2018**, *18*, 1636–1645. [CrossRef]
4. Egeland, E.J.; Reisaeter, A.V.; Robertsen, I.; Midtvedt, K.; Strom, E.H.; Holdaas, H.; Hartmann, A.; Asberg, A. High tacrolimus clearance—A risk factor for development of interstitial fibrosis and tubular atrophy in the transplanted kidney: A retrospective single-center cohort study. *Transpl. Int.* **2019**, *32*, 257–269. [CrossRef] [PubMed]
5. Gwinner, W.; Hinzmann, K.; Erdbruegger, U.; Scheffner, I.; Broecker, V.; Vaske, B.; Kreipe, H.; Haller, H.; Schwarz, A.; Mengel, M. Acute tubular injury in protocol biopsies of renal grafts: Prevalence, associated factors and effect on long-term function. *Am. J. Transplant.* **2008**, *8*, 1684–1693. [CrossRef] [PubMed]
6. Kershner, R.P.; Fitzsimmons, W.E. Relationship of FK506 whole blood concentrations and efficacy and toxicity after liver and kidney transplantation. *Transplantation* **1996**, *62*, 920–926. [CrossRef] [PubMed]
7. Kuypers, D.R.; Naesens, M.; De Jonge, H.; Lerut, E.; Verbeke, K.; Vanrenterghem, Y. Tacrolimus dose requirements and CYP3A5 genotype and the development of calcineurin inhibitor-associated nephrotoxicity in renal allograft recipients. *Ther. Drug Monit.* **2010**, *32*, 394–404. [CrossRef] [PubMed]
8. Shimizu, T.; Tanabe, K.; Tokumoto, T.; Ishikawa, N.; Shinmura, H.; Oshima, T.; Toma, H.; Yamaguchi, Y. Clinical and histological analysis of acute tacrolimus (TAC) nephrotoxicity in renal allografts. *Clin. Transplant.* **1999**, *13* (Suppl. 1), 48–53.
9. Thölking, G.; Fortmann, C.; Koch, R.; Gerth, H.U.; Pabst, D.; Pavenstädt, H.; Kabar, I.; Hüsing, A.; Wolters, H.; Reuter, S.; et al. The tacrolimus metabolism rate influences renal function after kidney transplantation. *PLoS ONE* **2014**, *9*, e111128. [CrossRef]
10. Bardou, F.N.; Guillaud, O.; Erard-Poinsot, D.; Chambon-Augoyard, C.; Thimonier, E.; Vallin, M.; Boillot, O.; Dumortier, J. Tacrolimus exposure after liver transplantation for alcohol-related liver disease: Impact on complications. *Transpl. Immunol.* **2019**, *56*, 101227. [CrossRef]
11. Genvigir, F.D.; Salgado, P.C.; Felipe, C.R.; Luo, E.Y.; Alves, C.; Cerda, A.; Tedesco-Silva, H., Jr.; Medina-Pestana, J.O.; Oliveira, N.; Rodrigues, A.C.; et al. Influence of the CYP3A4/5 genetic score and ABCB1 polymorphisms on tacrolimus exposure and renal function in Brazilian kidney transplant

patients. *Pharmacogenet. Genom.* **2016**, *26*, 462–472. [CrossRef] [PubMed]

12. Thölking, G.; Siats, L.; Fortmann, C.; Koch, R.; Hüsing, A.; Cicinnati, V.R.; Gerth, H.U.; Wolters, H.H.; Anthoni, C.; Pavenstädt, H.; et al. Tacrolimus Concentration/Dose Ratio is Associated with Renal Function After Liver Transplantation. *Ann. Transplant.* **2016**, *21*, 167–179. [CrossRef] [PubMed]

13. Jouve, T.; Fonrose, X.; Noble, J.; Janbon, B.; Fiard, G.; Malvezzi, P.; Stanke-Labesque, F.; Rostaing, L. The TOMATO study (TacrOlimus MetabolizAtion in kidney TransplantatiOn): Impact of the concentration-dose ratio on death-censored graft survival. *Transplantation* **2019**. [CrossRef] [PubMed]

14. Nowicka, M.; Gorska, M.; Nowicka, Z.; Edyko, K.; Edyko, P.; Wislicki, S.; Zawiasa-Bryszewska, A.; Strzelczyk, J.; Matych, J.; Kurnatowska, I. Tacrolimus: Influence of the Posttransplant Concentration/Dose Ratio on Kidney Graft Function in a Two-Year Follow-Up. *Kidney Blood Press Res.* **2019**, 1–14. [CrossRef] [PubMed]

15. Bartlett, F.E.; Carthon, C.E.; Hagopian, J.C.; Horwedel, T.A.; January, S.E.; Malone, A. Tacrolimus Concentration-to-Dose Ratios in Kidney Transplant Recipients and Relationship to Clinical Outcomes. *Pharmacotherapy* **2019**, *39*, 827–836. [CrossRef] [PubMed]

16. Schütte-Nütgen, K.; Tholking, G.; Steinke, J.; Pavenstädt, H.; Schmidt, R.; Suwelack, B.; Reuter, S. Fast Tac Metabolizers at Risk (-) It is Time for a C/D Ratio Calculation. *J. Clin. Med.* **2019**, *8*, 587. [CrossRef] [PubMed]

17. Thölking, G.; Schmidt, C.; Koch, R.; Schütte-Nütgen, K.; Pabst, D.; Wolters, H.; Kabar, I.; Hüsing, A.; Pavenstädt, H.; Reuter, S.; et al. Influence of tacrolimus metabolism rate on BKV infection after kidney transplantation. *Sci. Rep.* **2016**, *6*, 32273. [CrossRef] [PubMed]

18. Milan, A.; Zocaro, G.; Leone, D.; Tosello, F.; Buraioli, I.; Schiavone, D.; Veglio, F. Current assessment of pulse wave velocity: Comprehensive review of validation studies. *J. Hypertens.* **2019**, *37*, 1547–1557. [CrossRef]

19. Seibert, F.; Behrendt, C.; Schmidt, S.; Van der Giet, M.; Zidek, W.; Westhoff, T.H. Differential effects of cyclosporine and tacrolimus on arterial function. *Transpl. Int.* **2011**, *24*, 708–715. [CrossRef]

20. Van Bortel, L.M.; Laurent, S.; Boutouyrie, P.; Chowienczyk, P.; Cruickshank, J.K.; De, B.T.; Filipovsky, J.; Huybrechts, S.; Mattace-Raso, F.U.; Protogerou, A.D.; et al. Expert consensus document on the measurement of aortic stiffness in daily practice using carotid-femoral pulse wave velocity. *J. Hypertens.* **2012**, *30*, 445–448. [CrossRef]

21. Rovas, A.; Lukasz, A.H.; Vink, H.; Urban, M.; Sackarnd, J.; Pavenstädt, H.; Kümpers, P. Bedside analysis of the sublingual microvascular glycocalyx in the emergency room and intensive care unit-The GlycoNurse study. *Scand. J. Trauma Resusc. Emerg. Med.* **2018**, *26*, 16. [CrossRef] [PubMed]

22. Lamoureux, F.; Mestre, E.; Essig, M.; Sauvage, F.L.; Marquet, P.; Gastinel, L.N. Quantitative proteomic analysis of cyclosporine-induced toxicity in a human kidney cell line and comparison with tacrolimus. *J. Proteom.* **2011**, *75*, 677–694. [CrossRef] [PubMed]

23. Schütte-Nütgen, K.; Edeling, M.; Mendl, G.; Krahn, M.P.; Edemir, B.; Weide, T.; Kremerskothen, J.; Michgehl, U.; Pavenstadt, H. Getting a Notch closer to renal dysfunction: Activated Notch suppresses expression of the adaptor protein Disabled-2 in tubular epithelial cells. *FASEB J.* **2019**, *33*, 821–832. [CrossRef] [PubMed]

24. Ciarimboli, G.; Holle, S.K.; Vollenbrocker, B.; Hagos, Y.; Reuter, S.; Burckhardt, G.; Bierer, S.; Herrmann, E.; Pavenstädt, H.; Rossi, R.; et al. New clues for nephrotoxicity induced by ifosfamide: Preferential renal uptake via the human organic cation transporter 2. *Mol. Pharm.* **2011**, *8*, 270–279. [CrossRef] [PubMed]

25. Mosmann, T. Rapid colorimetric assay for cellular growth and survival: Application to proliferation and cytotoxicity assays. *J. Immunol. Methods* **1983**, *65*, 55–63. [CrossRef]

26. Hryniewiecka, E.; Zegarska, J.; Zochowska, D.; Samborowska, E.; Jazwiec, R.; Kosieradzki, M.; Nazarewski, S.; Dadlez, M.; Pa, C.L. Dose-adjusted and dose/kg-adjusted concentrations of mycophenolic acid precursors reflect metabolic ratios of their metabolites in contrast to tacrolimus and cyclosporine. *Biosci. Rep.* **2019**, *39*, BSR20182031. [CrossRef]

27. Tremblay, S.; Nigro, V.; Weinberg, J.; Woodle, E.S.; Alloway, R.R. A Steady-State Head-to-Head Pharmacokinetic Comparison of All FK-506 (Tacrolimus) Formulations (ASTCOFF): An Open-Label, Prospective, Randomized, Two-Arm, Three-Period Crossover Study. *Am. J. Transplant.* **2017**, *17*, 432–442. [CrossRef]

28. Miura, M.; Satoh, S.; Niioka, T.; Kagaya, H.; Saito, M.; Hayakari, M.; Habuchi, T.; Suzuki, T. Early phase limited sampling strategy characterizing tacrolimus and mycophenolic acid pharmacokinetics adapted to

the maintenance phase of renal transplant patients. *Ther. Drug Monit.* **2009**, *31*, 467–474. [CrossRef]

29. Trofe-Clark, J.; Brennan, D.C.; West-Thielke, P.; Milone, M.C.; Lim, M.A.; Neubauer, R.; Nigro, V.; Bloom, R.D. Results of ASERTAA, a Randomized Prospective Crossover Pharmacogenetic Study of Immediate-Release Versus Extended-Release Tacrolimus in African American Kidney Transplant Recipients. *Am. J. Kidney Dis.* **2018**, *71*, 315–326. [CrossRef]

30. Langone, A.; Steinberg, S.M.; Gedaly, R.; Chan, L.K.; Shah, T.; Sethi, K.D.; Nigro, V.; Morgan, J.C. Switching STudy of Kidney TRansplant PAtients with Tremor to LCP-TacrO (STRATO): An open-label, multicenter, prospective phase 3b study. *Clin. Transplant.* **2015**, *29*, 796–805. [CrossRef]

31. Ikonomidis, I.; Voumvourakis, A.; Makavos, G.; Triantafyllidi, H.; Pavlidis, G.; Katogiannis, K.; Benas, D.; Vlastos, D.; Trivilou, P.; Varoudi, M.; et al. Association of impaired endothelial glycocalyx with arterial stiffness, coronary microcirculatory dysfunction, and abnormal myocardial deformation in untreated hypertensives. *J. Clin. Hypertens. (Greenwich.)* **2018**, *20*, 672–679. [CrossRef] [PubMed]

32. Zaltzman, J.S. A comparison of short-term exposure of once-daily extended release tacrolimus and twice-daily cyclosporine on renal function in healthy volunteers. *Transplantation* **2010**, *90*, 1185–1191. [CrossRef] [PubMed]

33. Goto, M.; Masuda, S.; Kiuchi, T.; Ogura, Y.; Oike, F.; Okuda, M.; Tanaka, K.; Inui, K. CYP3A5*1-carrying graft liver reduces the concentration/oral dose ratio of tacrolimus in recipients of living-donor liver transplantation. *Pharmacogenetics* **2004**, *14*, 471–478. [CrossRef] [PubMed]

4

Should we Perform Old-For-Old Kidney Transplantation during the COVID-19 Pandemic? The Risk for Post-Operative Intensive Stay

Philip Zeuschner [1], Urban Sester [2], Michael Stöckle [1], Matthias Saar [1], Ilias Zompolas [3], Nasrin El-Bandar [3], Lutz Liefeldt [4], Klemens Budde [4], Robert Öllinger [5], Paul Ritschl [5], Thorsten Schlomm [3], Janine Mihm [2,†] and Frank Friedersdorff [3,*,†]

[1] Department of Urology and Pediatric Urology, Saarland University, Kirrberger Street 100, 66421 Homburg/Saar, Germany; philip.zeuschner@uks.eu (P.Z.); michael.stoeckle@uks.eu (M.S.); matthias.saar@uks.eu (M.S.)

[2] Department of Nephrology and Hypertension, Internal Medicine IV, Saarland University, Kirrberger Street 100, 66421 Homburg/Saar, Germany; urban.sester@uks.eu (U.S.); janine.mihm@uks.eu (J.M.)

[3] Department of Urology, Charité-Universitätsmedizin Berlin, Corporate Member of Freie Universität Berlin, Humbold-Universität zu Berlin, and Berlin Institute of Health, Charitéplatz 1, 10117 Berlin, Germany; ilias.zompolas@charite.de (I.Z.); nasrin.el-bandar@charite.de (N.E.-B.); thorsten.schlomm@charite.de (T.S.)

[4] Department of Nephrology, Charité-Universitätsmedizin Berlin, Corporate Member of Freie Universität Berlin, Humbold-Universität zu Berlin, and Berlin Institute of Health, Charitéplatz 1, 10117 Berlin, Germany; lutz.liefeldt@charite.de (L.L.); klemens.budde@charite.de (K.B.)

[5] Department of Surgery, Campus Charité Mitte/Campus Virchow-Klinikum CCM/CVK, Charité-Universitätsmedizin Berlin, Corporate Member of Freie Universität Berlin, Humbold-Universität zu Berlin, and Berlin Institute of Health, Charitéplatz 1, 10117 Berlin, Germany; robert.oellinger@charite.de (R.Ö.); paul.ritschl@charite.de (P.R.)

* Correspondence: frank.friedersdorff@charite.de

† Both authors contributed equally.

Abstract: Health care systems worldwide have been facing major challenges since the outbreak of the SARS-CoV-2 pandemic. Kidney transplantation (KT) has been tremendously affected due to limited personal protective equipment (PPE) and intensive care unit (ICU) capacities. To provide valid information on risk factors for ICU admission in a high-risk cohort of old kidney recipients from old donors in the Eurotransplant Senior Program (ESP), we retrospectively conducted a bi-centric analysis. Overall, 17 (16.2%) patients out of 105 KTs were admitted to the ICU. They had a lower BMI, and both coronary artery disease (CAD) and hypertensive nephropathy were more frequent. A risk model combining BMI, CAD and hypertensive nephropathy gained a sensitivity of 94.1% and a negative predictive value of 97.8%, rendering it a valuable search test, but with low specificity (51.1%). ICU admission also proved to be an excellent parameter identifying patients at risk for short patient and graft survivals. Patients admitted to the ICU had shorter patient (1-year 57% vs. 90%) and graft (5-year 49% vs. 77%) survival. To conclude, potential kidney recipients with a low BMI, CAD and hypertensive nephropathy should only be transplanted in the ESP in times of SARS-CoV-2 pandemic if the local health situation can provide sufficient ICU capacities.

Keywords: kidney transplantation; organ donation; deceased donor; Eurotransplant Senior Program; risk stratification; intensive care

1. Introduction

Health care systems all over the world have been facing major and unprecedented challenges since the outbreak of Coronavirus Disease 2019 (COVID-19). Extensive restrictions and nation-wide lockdowns were implemented to contain the spread of the novel coronavirus SARS-CoV-2. Its special features contributed to its fast and widespread transmission, including (1) being highly contagious, (2) the possible transmission from asymptomatic individuals and (3) causing mild symptoms in most of the infected patients [1,2]. Some countries were unexpectedly overwhelmed by a considerable increase in patients admitted to hospitals in need of intensive care [3]. Meanwhile, a worldwide shortage of personal protective equipment (PPE) in conjunction with limited bed capacities at intensive care units (ICU) resulted in suspension of elective surgeries. PPE and ICU beds were urgently needed as scarce medical resources for the management of COVID-19 cases and for the protection of the medical staff [4,5]. Another reason for postponing elective surgeries was the fear that patients admitted to hospital for elective surgery would become vectors for the transmission of a nosocomial infection with SARS-CoV-2 [3,4].

The outbreak of the pandemic also resulted in restrictions and cancellations in terms of kidney transplantation (KT) [6–9]. In Italy, a notable decrease in solid organ transplantation and procurement has already been observed in the first four weeks of the pandemic [10]. Currently, decisions on prioritizing certain procedures—including KT—are based on expert opinions rather than on evidence, contributing to different spread-dependent restrictions between regions [7]. In addition, it is unclear which immunosuppressive induction regimen can be administered safely. Especially, the administration of thymoglobulins causing long-lasting lymphopenia has been discussed critically, as a low lymphocyte count has been negatively associated with the disease severity of SARS-CoV-2 infection [1,11,12]. Even planned immunosuppression in living donation has been questioned [1]. The American Society of Transplantation and the European Association of Urology currently recommend to defer non-urgent KTs with living donors, but to perform urgent KTs—depending on the local situation [13,14]. However, the main aim should be rationing scarce medical resources, especially PPE, ventilators and ICU beds, while providing the best possible medical care to our patients [4].

The costs and benefits of a kidney transplantation during a pandemic should be counterbalanced [2]. We know that KT is the best treatment option for patients suffering from end-stage kidney disease (ESKD), with an improved survival rate and quality of life [15]. On the other hand, we lack information about the risk for admission to ICU after KT. In the context of scarce ICU resources, knowing about risk factors for ICU admission is crucial. Especially, older patients with comorbidities could have a higher risk for admission to ICU. The Eurotransplant Senior Program (ESP) is a special kidney transplant program which was initiated in 1999 to reduce waiting times by allocating kidneys from deceased donors aged ≥65 years to old recipients aged ≥65 years. Before that date, only 3% of patients aged 65 years or older actually received a KT offer within the Eurotransplant region, because younger patients with more favorable outcomes were prioritized [16]. In ESP, organ allocation is not based on immunological compatibility, but on local, regional or national allocation and AB0-compatibility, in order to reduce cold ischemia time (CIT). For this reason, risk assessment scores such as the Kidney Donor Risk Index (KDRI) are not integrated into the standard allocation protocols [17]. Double kidney allocation is not allowed at the beginning of the allocation procedure. Within the regular Eurotransplant Kidney Allocation System (ETKAS), kidneys can be allocated for donation after brain death (DCB) and, if allowed by national law, donation after cardiocirculatory death (DCD). Within the first 10 years, ESP has significantly increased the number of old kidney recipients. Local allocation resulted in shorter CITs and lower delayed graft function (DGF) rates compared to old kidney recipients in the regular Eurotransplant Kidney Allocation System (ETKAS) [18,19].

We lately had to decide whether or not to accept an allocated kidney from a 66 year old donor with a negative SARS-CoV-2 test result, allocated within ESP. The recipient was a 70 year old male with a solitary kidney who had an underlying hypertensive nephropathy. He had been on dialysis for 36 months and additionally suffered from coronary artery disease (CAD). This was the first organ offer within the ESP program at our department since the beginning of the SARS-CoV-2 pandemic. To provide valid information and thereby help decision-making in times of SARS-CoV-2, we conducted the first risk assessment for post-operative ICU stay among patients in the ESP so far. Additionally, the impact of an ICU admission on further outcome was assessed in this bi-center study.

2. Materials and Methods

In total, 105 KTs in the ESP performed at two tertiary referral centers were retrospectively analyzed. From 2010 to 2020, 40 (38.1%) and 65 (61.9%) kidneys were locally allocated to two transplant centers. In accordance with local law, all donors were brain-dead. No double kidney transplantations were included. All KTs were conducted in an open fashion by experienced transplant surgeons. After KT, the patients were admitted to an intermediate care unit by default. Only in the case of severe complications which could not be treated in an intermediate care unit, patients were admitted to the ICU. All kidney recipients received basiliximab as an induction treatment in combination with tacrolimus, mycophenolate mofetil and (methyl)prednisolone as the standard immunosuppressive regimen in both transplant centers.

This entire analysis was conducted in adherence with the correct scientific research work terms of the Charité Medical University of Berlin and Saarland University. Patients provided written informed consent and patient data was fully anonymized.

2.1. Data Collection and Outcome Measures

For the recipient characteristics, age, gender, BMI (kg/m^2) and relevant health-conditions (arterial hypertension, CAD, diabetes mellitus, history of smoking) were obtained. The underlying cause for ESKD, duration and type of dialysis, and number of prior kidney transplantations characterized recipient's nephrological history. For the graft characteristics, donor age, number of HLA-mismatches and cold ischemia time (CIT) were obtained. Regarding KT, operating time, warm ischemia time (WIT) and intraoperative complications served as surgical outcomes. Admission to ICU, length of ICU stay, complications based on Clavien Dindo within 30 days after surgery (major complications defined as ≥grade 3a) and length of hospital stay characterized the recipient's postoperative course. The graft function was assessed by DGF rates, defined as the need for dialysis within 7 days after transplantation, and serum creatinine during follow-up. Over 10 years, graft and patient survival were compared.

As the primary outcome, risk factors for ICU admission after KT in ESP were identified. Therefore, patients with ICU admission were compared with patients without an ICU stay. To assess the influence of recipient and donor age on ICU admission, age-dependent comparisons were conducted, considering very old donors ≥75 years (very old-for-old vs. old-for-old) and very old recipients ≥70 years (old-for-very old vs. old-for-old). A multivariate binary logistic regression analysis identified significant risk predictors for ICU stay, which were used to create a risk model.

As the secondary outcome, the impact of ICU admission on further outcome was assessed. For this objective, survival and regression analyses identifying factors impacting graft and overall survival were calculated. Graft survival was always censored for death with functioning graft (DWFG).

2.2. Statistical Analysis

Categorical variables were reported as frequencies and proportions, and continuous data as the median and range. Fisher's exact test and Mann-Whitney U test were conducted to compare between the groups. Kaplan Meier analyses compared graft and patient survival between groups by log-rank test. For binary logistic and cox regression analyses, covariates were included in multivariate regression analysis only if the respective effect was significant in the univariate analysis. For multivariate regression analyses, forward Wald selection was applied. The best cut-off for predicted probability of ICU stay in the multivariate risk model was estimated via ROC-analysis and Youden index. Statistical analyses were performed by SPSS version 25 with Fix pack 2 installed (IBM, Armonk, NY, USA). All tests were two-sided, and p-values < 0.05 were considered significant.

3. Results

3.1. Overall Results Regarding ICU Admission

Overall, 17 (16.2%) patients were admitted to the ICU for a median length of 2 days (range 1–27). The main reason for ICU admission was significant hypotension requiring catecholamines in the absence of acute bleeding in five (29.4%) patients. Three (17.6%) patients were admitted for respiratory insufficiency, three (17.6%) for sepsis with multiple organ failure, and two (11.7%) for cardiac infarction. One (5.9%) patient had hyperkalemia, another a compartment syndrome due to occlusion of iliac arteries. One (5.9%) patient had a significant bleeding requiring surgical re-exploration, another had his graft surgically removed because of arterial stenosis and consecutive graft necrosis, and required intensive care thereafter. The median time between KT and ICU admission was 0 days, as 10 (58.8%) patients were admitted to the ICU immediately after KT. In total, 4 (23.5%) patients were admitted on postoperative day (POD) 2 to 4, and 2 (11.7%) patients on POD 8 and 9. One (5.9%) patient was admitted to the ICU on POD 36; he suffered from a late-onset sepsis. The admission rate to the ICU did not differ between the two transplant centers.

Patients admitted to the ICU were insignificantly older than patients without an ICU stay (71 vs. 69 years, n.s.) (see Table 1). They had a lower BMI (24.2 vs. 26.7, $p < 0.05$) and CAD twice as often (64.7% vs. 35.2%, $p < 0.05$). Regarding the underlying renal disease, hypertensive nephropathy was more common in patients admitted to the ICU (35.3% vs. 10.2%, $p < 0.05$). In both groups, the median number of HLA-mismatches was four (range 1–6, n.s.). There was a tendency towards longer CIT for patients admitted to the ICU (667.8 vs. 552.3 min), but it was not significant.

Table 1. Comparison of patient characteristics with or without ICU stay after kidney transplantation in the ESP program.

	$\sum$ (n = 105)	ICU Yes (n = 17)	ICU No (n = 88)	p
Recipient				
age (year)	69 (65; 82)	71 (65; 80)	69 (65; 82)	n.s.
male gender	68 (64.8%)	10 (58.8%)	58 (65.9%)	n.s.
BMI (kg/m^2)	26.3 (19.2; 37.9)	24.2 (19.3; 31)	26.7 (19.2; 37.9)	0.014
Pre-transplant				
hypertension	101 (96.2%)	17 (100%)	84 (95.5%)	n.s.
CAD	42 (40%)	11 (64.7%)	31 (35.2%)	0.031
diabetes	41 (39%)	6 (35.3%)	35 (39.8%)	n.s.
history of smoking	18 (17.1%)	2 (11.8%)	16 (18.2%)	n.s.
Cause for ESKD				
chronic GN	23 (18.9%)	1 (5.9%)	22 (25%)	n.s.
diabetic NP	17 (13.9%)	2 (11.8%)	15 (17%)	n.s.
hypertensive NP	15 (12.3%)	6 (35.3%)	9 (10.2%)	0.015
other *	50 (47.6%)	9 (52.9%)	46 (52.2%)	n.s.
time on dialysis (d)	918.5 (2; 3830)	1384 (484; 3830)	855.5 (12; 3302)	n.s.
hemodialysis	84 (80%)	16 (94.1%)	68 (77.3%)	n.s.
first Tx	101 (96.2%)	17 (100%)	84 (95.5%)	n.s.
Graft				
donor age (year)	71 (65; 85)	71 (66; 82)	71 (65; 85)	n.s.
HLA-mismatches	4 (1; 6)	4 (1; 6)	4 (1; 6)	n.s.
CIT (min)	571.8 (181.2; 1236)	667.8 (228; 1166.4)	552.3 (181.2; 1236)	0.053

* see Appendix A Table A3 for further information.

Regarding KTs, patients admitted to the ICU had slightly longer operating times (212 vs. 180 min, $p = 0.053$), and neither WIT nor intraoperative complication rates differed (see Table 2). During the postoperative course, patients with an ICU stay suffered from more frequent and higher complications based on Clavien Dindo, although this was not significant. Although there were fewer minor complications, 9 (52.9%) patients admitted to the ICU had more complications at grade 5 (17.6% vs. 0, $p < 0.01$). Patients with an ICU stay were discharged insignificantly later (21.5 vs. 18 days, n.s.).

Table 2. Perioperative outcome.

	$\sum$ ($n = 105$)	ICU Yes ($n = 17$)	ICU No ($n = 88$)	p-Value
Transplantation				
operating time (min)	184 (116; 436)	212 (129; 268)	180 (116; 436)	n.s.
WIT (min)	46.5 (21; 126)	47 (35; 70)	46 (21; 126)	n.s.
complications	12 (11.4%)	2 (11.8%)	10 (11.4%)	n.s.
Postoperative				
complications				n.s.
none	42 (40%)	5 (29.4%)	37 (42%)	n.s.
minor	28 (26.7%)	3 (17.6%)	25 (28.4%)	n.s.
major	35 (33.3%)	9 (52.9%)	26 (29.5%)	n.s.
length of stay	19 (8–66)	21.5 (12–66)	18 (8–62)	n.s.
Graft Function				
DGF rate	42 (40%)	9 (52.9%)	33 (37.5%)	n.s.

DGF rates were higher for patients admitted to the ICU (52.9% vs. 37.5%, n.s.) (see Table 2). Serum creatinine significantly declined after KT ($p < 0.05$) and did not differ between patients with or without ICU stay (see Figure 1).

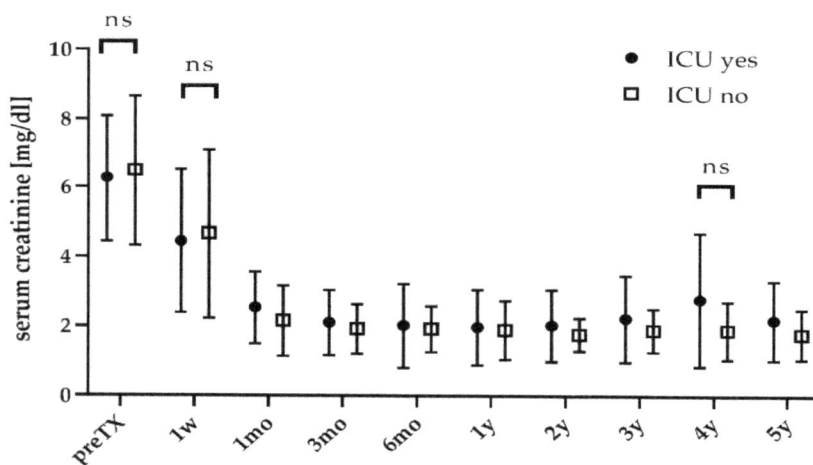

Figure 1. Graft function during follow-up. w: week; mo: month; y: year.

3.2. Donor- and Recipient-Age-Dependent Comparison

In total, 28 (26.7%) patients received a graft from very old donors ≥75 years, compared to 77 (73.3%) old donors ('old-for-old') (see Table 3). When stratifying for donor age (very old-for-old vs. old-for-old), neither recipient nor graft characteristics differed. Grafts from very old donors had a tendency towards a longer CIT, which was not significant (677.1 vs. 540.6 min). Kidney recipients of very old donors had a tendency to be admitted to the ICU more frequently (21.4% vs. 14.3%, n.s.), but were discharged significantly earlier (16 vs. 20 days, $p < 0.05$). Neither DGF rates nor the kidney function differed during follow-up.

When stratifying for recipient age (old-for-very old vs. old-for-old), 47 (44.7%) recipients were ≥70 years old, and thereby were considered as very old (see Table 3). Regarding recipient characteristics, only the history of smoking differed, as fewer very old recipients had a history of smoking (8.5% vs. 24.1%, $p < 0.05$). Neither graft nor transplantation-specific factors were different. Very old recipients were admitted to the ICU insignificantly more often (21.3% vs. 12.1%). Graft function one week after KT was the only parameter that differed when comparing very old to old recipients, as very old recipients had a lower serum creatinine than old recipients (3.35 vs. 5.36, $p < 0.01$). During follow-up, the kidney function became equivalent.

Table 3. Age-dependent comparison stratifying for donor age (very old donors ≥75 years vs. old donors) or recipient age (very old recipients ≥70 years vs. old recipients).

	Donors: *Very Old*-For-Old vs. Old-For-Old			Recipients: Old-For-*Very* Old vs. Old-For-Old		
	Very Old (*n* = 28)	Old (*n* = 77)	*p*	Very Old (*n* = 47)	Old (*n* = 58)	*p*
Transplantation						
operating time	180 (120; 281)	188 (116; 436)	n.s.	190 (128; 268)	181 (116; 436)	n.s.
WIT (min)	46 (21; 126)	49.5 (32; 85)	n.s.	48 (32; 104)	46 (21; 126)	n.s.
complications	4 (14.3%)	8 (10.4%)	n.s.	6 (12.8%)	6 (10.3%)	n.s.
Postoperative						
ICU admission	6 (21.4%)	11 (14.3%)	n.s.	10 (21.3%)	7 (12.1%)	n.s.
Clavien–Dindo			n.s.			n.s.
none	13 (46.4%)	29 (37.7%)		16 (34%)	26 (44.8%)	
minor	10 (35.7%)	18 (23.4%)		13 (27.7%)	15 (25.9%)	
major	5 (17.9%)	30 (39%)		18 (38.3%)	17 (29.3%)	
length of stay	16 (12; 46)	20 (8; 66)	0.028	20 (10; 66)	18.5 (8; 65)	
Graft Function						
DGF	14 (50%)	28 (36.4%)	n.s.	19 (40.4%)	23 (39.7%)	n.s.

3.3. Risk Model for ICU Stay

Among recipient and graft characteristics as well as transplantation-specific outcomes, the BMI of the recipient, an underlying hypertensive nephropathy and CAD were the only significant predictors for ICU admission in univariate and multivariate analysis (see Table 4). A higher BMI lowered the OR for ICU admission (OR 0.8, $p < 0.01$), but a hypertensive nephropathy (OR 4.0, $p < 0.05$) and CAD (OR 4.46, $p < 0.05$) significantly increased the OR for ICU admission during the hospital stay. Donor or recipient age did not impact the risk for ICU admission.

Table 4. Multivariate regression analysis to predict an ICU admission during the hospital stay.

Variable	OR (95% CI)	*p*-Value
BMI	0.80 (0.68; 0.94)	0.008
hypertensive nephropathy	4 (1.02; 15.67)	0.046
coronary artery disease	4.46 (1.32; 15.07)	0.016

When combining these three factors in a risk model to estimate the probability for ICU admission, the c-index reached 0.789 ($p < 0.001$) (see Figure A1). When setting the cut-off for the predicted probability of ICU admission to 0.08, which had highest Youden-index, the risk model reached a sensitivity of 94.1%, specificity of 51.1%, false positive rate (FPR) of 48.9%, false negative rate (FNR) of 5.9%, positive predictive value (PPV) of 27.1% and negative predictive value (NPV) of 97.8% (see Table A1).

3.4. Survival Analysis

For all 105 patients, the median length of follow-up was 49.5 months. The overall graft survival at 1, 5 and 9 years was 84%, 73% and 42%, respectively, with a median death-censored graft survival of 113.9 months. Median patient survival was 108.2 months, with a 1-, 5- and 9-year survival of 85%, 62% and 38%, respectively.

When stratifying for ICU admission, patients admitted to the ICU had a significantly shorter graft survival (59.1 vs. 115.7 months, $p = 0.049$) (see Figure 2a). Their 1- and 5-year graft survivals were 75% and 49%, and thereby worse compared to patients without an ICU stay (86% and 77%). Over the whole study period, the death-rate for patients with an ICU stay was almost three times higher compared to patients without an ICU stay (70.6% vs. 26.1%, $p < 0.001$). Consequently, the median patient survival for patients admitted to the ICU was significantly shorter (ICU 36.9 vs. 114.9 months, $p < 0.001$) (see Figure 2b). 1- and 5-year patient survival for patients admitted to an ICU was 57% and 0% and for patients without an ICU stay 90% (1 year), 72% (5 years) and 44% after 9 years, respectively. In total, 17 (48.6%) patients died with a functioning graft, and the DWFG rate did not differ between groups (ICU 50% vs. 47.8%, n.s.). Neither the age of the donor nor the recipient affected graft or patient survival (see Table A2).

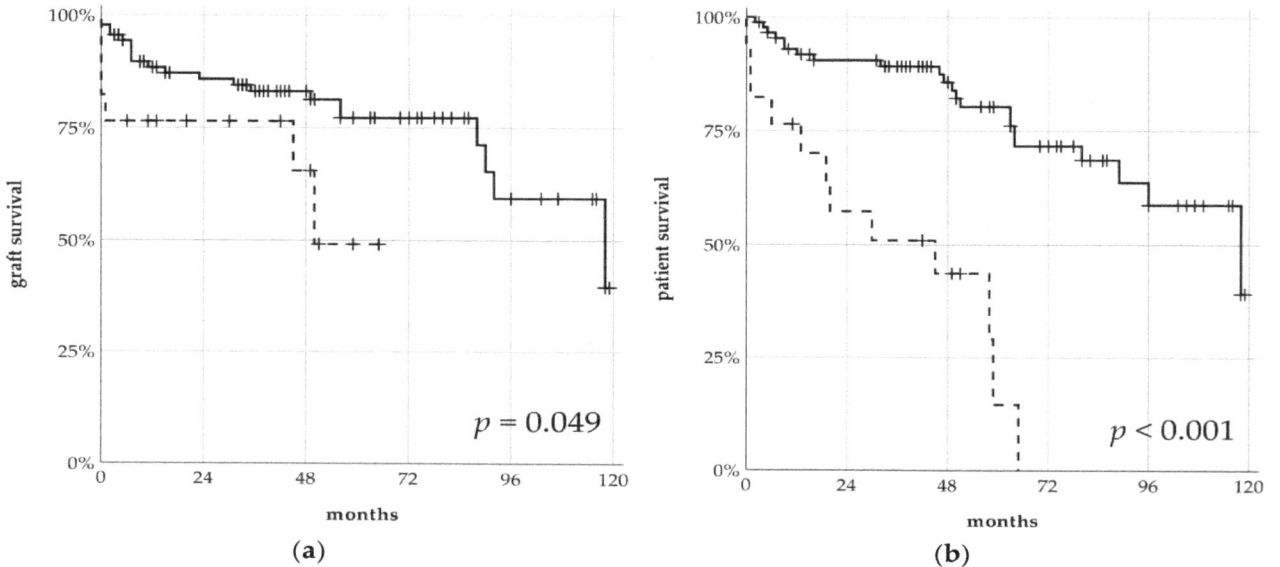

Figure 2. Death-censored graft survival (**a**) and patient survival (**b**) comparing patients admitted to the ICU (**dashed line**) vs. patients not admitted to the ICU (**solid line**) after kidney transplantation in the ESP program.

In a multivariate cox regression, higher numbers of prior KTs and HLA-mismatches significantly shortened graft survival (hazard ratio (HR) for graft loss 9.66, $p = 0.001$; HR 1.53, $p < 0.05$) (see Table 5). Additionally, higher serum creatinine 1 month after KT was associated with worse graft survival (HR 1.37, $p < 0.05$). ICU admission during the hospital stay after KT did not affect graft survival. Regarding patient survival, a pre-transplant diabetes mellitus and an ICU admission during the hospital stay were significant predictors for worse outcomes in the multivariate analysis (HR for patient death 2.22, $p < 0.05$, HR 4.7, $p < 0.001$). Major complications during the hospital stay and the serum creatinine 1 month after KT were only associated with patient survival in univariate analysis.

Table 5. Significant impact factors on graft loss and patient death in multivariate cox regression.

Variable	HR (95% CI)	p-Value
Graft Loss		
number of Tx	9.66 (2.48; 37.69)	0.001
HLA-mismatches	1.53 (1.03; 2.27)	0.033
serum creatinine 1 mo	1.37 (1.01; 1.87)	0.04
Patient Death		
pre-transplant diabetes	2.22 (1.02; 4.86)	0.046
ICU admission	4.72 (2.02; 11.03)	<0.001

4. Discussion

In this bi-centric study, an analysis of 105 kidney transplantations of deceased donors, allocated within the Eurotransplant Senior Program, was conducted. We aimed to identify risk factors for ICU admission after KT during a hospital stay in times of shortened PPE and ICU capacities because of the SARS-CoV-2 pandemic.

Overall, recipient and graft characteristics were comparable with other cohorts [19–22]. CIT was lower, lasting on average 9.5 h, while most other ESP programs have CITs averaging 10 to 12 h [19,20]. ESP aims to reduce CIT by prioritizing local organ allocation, as longer CITs have been clearly linked with higher DGF rates. Nonetheless, our DGF rate of 40% is higher than that of one of the largest ESP cohorts so far, with 1406 KTs, by Frei et al. They reported a median DGF rate of 29.7% [19]. In contrast, other groups have comparable DGF rates ranging between 34.7 to 41.1% in their ESP cohorts [22,23]. Chavalitdhamrong et al. even stated a DGF rate of 60.4% for 601 KTs, but for organs allocated by ECD (extended criteria donors) for donors aged 50–69 years, and 63.9% for donors aged $\geq$70 years [24].

In a high-risk cohort like ESP recipients, complications are common. There were 11.4% intraoperative complications, and 26.7% minor and 33.3% major complications occurred postoperatively, according to Clavien–Dindo. Reports on complication rates state highly variable results, mainly due to inconsistent definitions. Bentas et al. have "surgical complications" in 47% of cases in their ESP program, whereas Bahde et al. reported 15.7% intraoperative and 22.5% post-operative surgical complications among their recipients [23,25]. Only Gallinat et al. defined postoperative complications according to Clavien–Dindo. In their comparison of very old donors in the ECD program, the rate for major complications was 48%, defined as $\geq$grade 3b [26].

During follow-up, death-censored graft survival (1- and 5-year: 84% and 73%) and patient survival (1- and 5-year: 85% and 62%) were superior to Frei et al. and comparable with Quast et al., who retrospectively analyzed 217 ESP transplantations at their department from 1998 to 2014, considering donor age [19,20] (see Table 6). In accordance with Boesmueller and Giessing et al., the main reason for graft loss was death with functioning graft [18,22]. Our analysis comprises one of the longest follow-ups in ESP so far. Overall, graft-survival after 9 years was 42%, and patient survival was 38%. Quast et al. reported a 10-year patient survival of 40% for old donors, and 35% for very old donors, whereas graft survival was 30% and 10%, respectively.

Table 6. Comparison of death-censored graft and patient survival in ESP programs.

	Frei [19] $n = 1406$	Quast [20] $n = 217$	Bahde [23] $n = 89$	Jacobi [21] $n = 89$	Our Results $n = 105$
Graft Survival					
1-year	75%	76.4% [1]	n.a.	87%	84%
5-year	47%	57.3% [1]	77%	63%	73%
Patient Survival					
1-year	86%	88.2% [1]	n.a.	87%	85%
5-year	60%	71.8% [1]	69.8%	63%	62%

[1] Only considering old, but not very old, donors.

Based on this data, we have identified risk factors for ICU admission during a hospital stay in the ESP. In times of the SARS-CoV-2 pandemic with a shortage of ICU capacities, risk stratification is crucial to identify patients at high risk for ICU admission (after KT). This aspect has rarely been addressed so far. To the best of our knowledge, only three working groups have stratified their data for ICU admission [27–29]. Two working groups focused on ICU admission at any time after KT, even years after KT, which clearly does not help when trying to decide whether or not to perform a KT during the present SARS-CoV-2 pandemic. Abrol et al. retrospectively analyzed 1527 kidney transplantations between 2007 and 2016 and found higher age, increasing BMI, pre-transplant dialysis and deceased donor transplantation to be associated with ICU admission in their multivariate analysis. Living donor KT and preemptive KT were associated with a lower risk [27]. Nonetheless, 82.8% of the included KTs were living kidney transplantations. As such, we are the first to report on the risk for ICU admission immediately after kidney transplantation in the ESP.

17 (16.2%) patients in our cohort were admitted to the ICU for a mean time of 2 days. More than 80% of patients were admitted directly postoperatively or within four days after KT. The main cause for ICU admission was significant hypotension requiring catecholamines. Overall, patients admitted to the ICU had a lower BMI, and CAD as well as hypertensive nephropathy were more common. Graft characteristics and surgical outcomes during transplantation did not differ. The DGF rate of patients admitted to the ICU was high, with 52.9%, but did not significantly differ from patients without an ICU stay (37.5%).

As stated elsewhere, neither the donor nor the recipient's age had an impact on the postoperative course [18,20]. Therefore, age did not affect ICU admission rates in the regression analysis. We assume that within this (very) old patient cohort, age differences were not as important as in younger patient cohorts due to preselection during the workup for listing. As patients admitted to the ICU had a lower BMI, an increasing BMI lowered the risk for ICU admission (OR 0.8, see Table 4). This is an interesting finding, referring to the 'obesity paradox', which describes the association of obesity with higher mortality in the general population on the one hand, but with a survival advantage among obese patients with several diseases on the other hand. In this regard, meta-analyses have shown that patients with a higher BMI might have (i) a reduced risk of ICU admission or death when suffering from pneumonia, (ii) a reduced adjusted mortality when admitted to the ICU with sepsis, severe sepsis or shock, and (iii) a lower mortality on mechanical ventilation in an ICU [30–32]. Although the concept of the obesity paradox has been questioned, there is also convincing evidence for underlying molecular mechanisms, i.e., that a lower energy reservoir in underweight patients cannot equally counteract the adverse influence of increased catabolic stress [33,34].

As further variables, hypertensive nephropathy and CAD increased the OR for ICU admission by 4 and 4.5, respectively. Most patients were admitted to the ICU because of hypotension as a major symptom for cardiac insufficiency, which is more likely in patients with CAD. In addition, hypertensive nephropathy has been linked with a higher risk for cardiovascular events and death [35]. When combining these three independent risk factors in a risk model, it gained a c-index of 0.789 with a sensitivity of 94.1%, a FNR of 5.9% and a NPV of 97.8% (see Table A1). For this reason, our risk model is highly valuable for the identification of patients at high risk for ICU admission. When applied to our cohort, the risk model was false negative in only one case. We are aware that it has a rather low specificity and PPV, whereas the FPR is high. Furthermore, the confidence intervals for the corresponding odds ratios are large, because only 17 (16.2%) patients were admitted to the ICU and not all of them suffered from hypertensive nephropathy or CAD (see Table 1). However, the high sensitivity and NPV of more than 94% render our risk model an ideal search test.

Our patient who had an organ offer in ESP during the SARS-CoV-2 pandemic had a probability of 92.8% to be admitted to the ICU according to our risk model, with a hypertensive nephropathy, CAD and BMI of 29.4 kg/m^2 (see A1 for further explanation). Of note, this patient was not included within the analyzed cohort. Indeed, after transplantation, he had to be admitted to the ICU on postoperative day seven due to urosepsis and suspected cardiac infarction. Infectious complications are common among old kidney recipients and have been shown to be their second most frequent cause for DWFG [16]. In our cohort, 3 out of 17 (17.6%) patients had to be admitted to the ICU because of sepsis. Especially in the context of the ongoing SARS-CoV-2 pandemic, the question of how to manage immunosuppression for KT recipients is still a matter of debate [11,12].

As standard, all patients were administered tacrolimus, mycophenolate mofetil, (methyl)prednisolone and basiliximab for induction therapy. Consequently, the regimen did not affect ICU admission rates. Since lymphopenia has been associated both with a higher risk for SARS-CoV-2 infection and for severe forms of Covid-19, the questions (i) whether or not to perform the transplantation at all and (ii) whether the induction therapy should be reduced were intensively discussed at the transplant center which had an organ offer in ESP during the SARS-CoV-2 pandemic [11]. Finally, the patient was transplanted and received an induction therapy with basiliximab, and unfortunately suffered from sepsis and neutropenia. For this reason, mycophenolate mofetil was stopped and the dose of prednisolone reduced. Of note, SARS-CoV-2 had been ruled out prior to transplantation and after the onset of sepsis again; as we have not experienced a major shortage of ICU capacities, we could guarantee maximum care for this patient at all times. However, we might decide differently if we receive another organ offer in the ESP program during the ongoing SARS-CoV-2 pandemic again.

Interestingly, ICU admission also proved to be an excellent indicator for the identification of patients at risk for short graft and patient survival. In Kaplan–Meier analysis, patients admitted to the ICU had a significantly shorter graft survival of 59.1 months; all of them died within five years (see Figure 2). Consequently, ICU admission impacted patient survival with a HR of 4.72, but did not impact graft survival in Cox regression (see Table 5). Diabetes mellitus was the only other covariate impacting patient survival. Other studies were inconclusive about the effect of pre-transplant diabetes mellitus or new-onset diabetes mellitus (NODAT) on patient survival. Some studies have found associations with NODAT, but not pre-transplant diabetes, with mortality and graft failure, and others the inverse [36–38]. By contrast, ICU admission did not impact death-censored graft survival in Cox regression. The individual number of kidney transplantations per patient (HR 9.66), number of HLA-mismatches (HR 1.53) and the serum creatinine one month after transplantation (HR 1.37) were significant. The negative impact of increasing HLA-mismatches on graft survival was reported more than two decades ago [39]. To shorten waiting times for old recipients, ESP does not integrate HLA-matching in the allocation algorithm.

This analysis is not devoid of limitation. To exclude center-specific factors and enlarge cohort size, we performed a bicentric analysis and included 105 patients. This is a rather low sample size, but big sample sizes in ESP programs are rare. Due to its retrospective nature, we could not test our new risk model for ICU admission in a prospective, independent manner. Before extrapolating our results to other centers, an external validation of our risk model will be needed. For this reason, we encourage other transplantation centers to test our risk model to further enhance its validity. With a bigger cohort size, the confidence intervals for the risk factors BMI, CAD and hypertensive nephropathy will potentially be reduced. Currently, our risk model is an excellent search test, but has a rather low PPV and therefore cannot replace individual and local risk assessment in times of reduced ICU capacities during the SARS-CoV-2 pandemic.

5. Conclusions

The SARS-CoV-2 pandemic has impacted health care systems tremendously worldwide, making the deferral of elective and non-urgent surgical interventions necessary due to limited PPE and ICU capacities. To provide a valid risk assessment tool concerning the risk of ICU admission for old patients in the Eurotransplant Senior Program, we have identified a low BMI, coronary artery disease and hypertensive nephropathy as significant predictors for ICU admission. For this reason, each transplant center should always carefully discuss whether local ICU capacities allow high-risk KT or not.

Author Contributions: Conceptualization, P.Z., J.M., F.F.; methodology, P.Z.; software, P.Z.; validation, P.Z., J.M., F.F.; formal analysis, P.Z.; investigation, P.Z. and F.F.; data curation, P.Z., J.M., F.F.; writing—original draft preparation, P.Z.; writing—review and editing, all authors, P.Z., U.S., M.S. (Michael Stöckle), M.S. (Matthias Saar), I.Z., N.E.-B., L.L., K.B., R.Ö., P.R., T.S., J.M. and F.F.; visualization, P.Z.; supervision, F.F., All authors have read and agreed to the published version of the manuscript.

Appendix A

Appendix A.1. Risk Model for ICU Admission

In a multivariate binary logistic regression analysis, BMI, hypertensive nephropathy and coronary artery disease had significant impact on ICU admission. The prediction probability (P) of an ICU stay for each individual patient was calculated with the equation

$$P = \frac{1}{1 + e^{-z}}$$

in which the logit z is

$$z = 3.557 + 4.004 \times HN + 1.495 \times CAD - 0.221 \times BMI$$

- HN: presence of hypertensive nephropathy (binary: no = 0, yes = 1)
- CAD: presence of coronary artery disease (binary: no = 0, yes = 1)
- BMI: body-mass-index in kg/m^2 (continuous)

The optimal cut-off for the predicted probability of ICU admission was calculated via ROC analysis by using a Youden index (see Figure A1). By setting the cut-off to 0.08, this risk model gained a sensitivity of 94.1%, specificity of 51.1%, false positive rate of 48.9%, false negative rate of 5.9%, positive predictive value of 27.1% and negative predictive value of 97.8% (see Table A1).

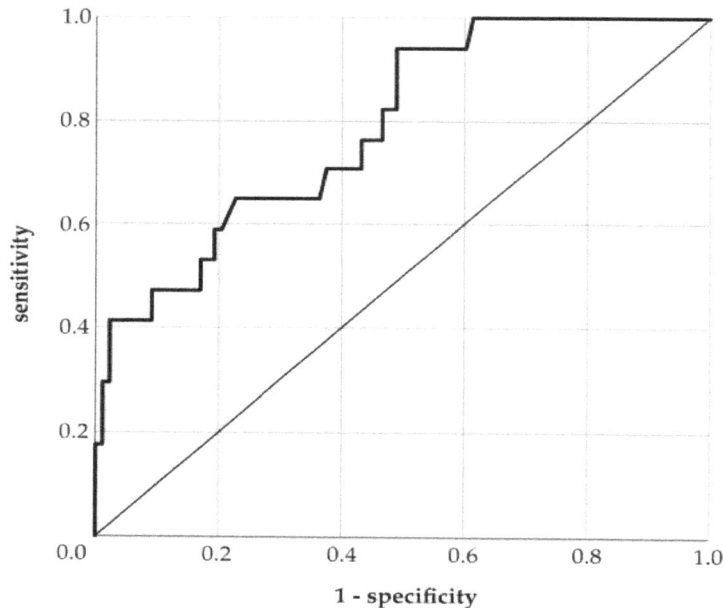

Figure A1. ROC analysis examining the relationship between the predicted probability of ICU stay and actual ICU admission.

Table A1. Crosstabulation illustrating case assignment in our cohort by risk model.

	ICU Yes	ICU No	Σ
risk model: ICU yes	16	43	59
risk model: ICU no	1	45	46
Σ	17	88	105

Appendix A.2. Graft and Patient Survival Stratified for Donor and Recipient Age

Table A2. Mortality table with age-dependent comparison stratified for donor age (very old donors ≥75 vs. old donors) or recipient age (very old recipients ≥70 years vs. old recipients).

	Donors: *Very* Old-For-Old vs. Old-For-Old			Recipients: Old-For-*Very* Old vs. Old-For-Old		
	Very Old (*n* = 28)	Old (*n* = 77)	*p*	Very Old (*n* = 47)	Old (*n* = 58)	*p*
Graft Survival			n.s.			n.s.
1 year	22 (78%)	61 (86%)		37 (87%)	46 (82%)	
5 years	11 (78%)	25 (72%)		18 (73%)	18 (75%)	
9 years	2 (58%)	6 (41%)		108 (60%)	4 (35%)	
Patient Survival			n.s.			n.s.
1 year	25 (78%)	63 (90%)		39 (82%)	49 (87%)	
5 years	12 (74%)	28 (59%)		21 (60%)	19 (63%)	
9 years	1 (36%)	6 (54%)		2 (55%)	5 (33%)	

Appendix A.3. Underlying Renal Diseases

Table A3. Underlying renal diseases for patients with or without ICU stay after KT.

	∑ (*n* = 105)	ICU Yes (*n* = 17)	ICU No (*n* = 88)	*p*-Value
ADPKD	11 (10.5%)	2 (11.8%)	9 (10.2%)	n.s.
amyloidosis	3 (2.9%)	-	3 (3.4%)	n.s.
analgesic nephropathy	3 (2.9%)	1 (5.9%)	2 (2.3%)	n.s.
chronic glomerulonephritis	23 (21.9%)	1 (5.9%)	22 (25%)	n.s.
cardiac cirrhosis	1 (1%)		1 (1.1%)	n.s.
diabetic nephropathy	17 (16.2%)	2 (11.8%)	15 (17%)	n.s.
FSGS	2 (1.9%)	-	2 (2.3%)	n.s.
goodpasture syndrome	2 (1.9%)	-	2 (2.3%)	n.s.
hypertensive nephropathy	15 (14.3%)	6 (35.3%)	9 (10.2%)	<0.05
IgA nephropathy	3 (2.9%)	-	3 (3.4%)	n.s.
kidney cirrhosis	8 (7.6%)	2 (11.8%)	6 (6.8%)	n.s.
nephrosclerosis	7 (6.7%)	2 (11.8%)	5 (5.7%)	n.s.
other cystic disease	3 (2.9%)	1 (5.9%)	2 (2.2%)	n.s.
renal cell carcinoma	2 (1.9%)	1 (5.9%)	1 (1.1%)	n.s.
vascular nephropathy	7 (6.7%)	3 (17.6%)	4 (4.5%)	n.s.
vasculitis	2 (1.9%)	1 (5.9%)	1 (1.1%)	n.s.
not known	13 (12.5%)	-	13 (14.8%)	n.s.

References

1. Kumar, D.; Manuel, O.; Natori, Y.; Egawa, H.; Grossi, P.; Han, S.-H.; Fernández-Ruiz, M.; Humar, A. COVID-19: A global transplant perspective on successfully navigating a pandemic. *Arab. Archaeol. Epigr.* **2020**. [CrossRef]
2. Gori, A.; Dondossola, D.; Antonelli, B.; Mangioni, D.; Alagna, L.; Reggiani, P.; Bandera, A.; Rossi, G. Coronavirus disease 2019 and transplantation: A view from the inside. *Am. J. Transplant. Off. J. Am. Soc. Transplant. Am. Soc. Transpl. Surg.* **2020**. [CrossRef]
3. Nacoti, M.; Ciocca, A.; Giupponi, A.; Brambillasca, P.; Lussana, F.; Pisano, M.; Goisis, G.; Bonacina, D.; Fazzi, F.; Naspro, R.; et al. *At the Epicenter of the Covid-19 Pandemic and Humanitarian Crises in Italy: Changing Perspectives on Preparation and Mitigation*; NEJM Catalyst: Waltham, MA, USA, 2020.
4. Stahel, P.F. How to risk-stratify elective surgery during the COVID-19 pandemic? *Patient Saf. Surg.* **2020**, *14*, 1–4. [CrossRef] [PubMed]

5. Phua, J.; Weng, L.; Ling, L.; Egi, M.; Lim, C.-M.; Divatia, J.V.; Shrestha, B.R.; Arabi, Y.M.; Ng, J.; Gomersall, C.D.; et al. Intensive care management of coronavirus disease 2019 (COVID-19): Challenges and recommendations. *Lancet Respir. Med.* **2020**, *8*, 506–517. [CrossRef]

6. Stensland, K.D.; Morgan, T.M.; Moinzadeh, A.; Lee, C.T.; Briganti, A.; Catto, J.W.; Canes, D. Considerations in the Triage of Urologic Surgeries During the COVID-19 Pandemic. *Eur. Urol.* **2020**, *77*, 663–666. [CrossRef]

7. Boyarsky, B.J.; Chiang, T.P.-Y.; Werbel, W.A.; Durand, C.M.; Avery, R.; Getsin, S.N.; Jackson, K.R.; Kernodle, A.B.; Rasmussen, S.E.V.P.; Massie, A.B.; et al. Early impact of COVID-19 on transplant center practices and policies in the United States. *Arab. Archaeol. Epigr.* **2020**. [CrossRef] [PubMed]

8. Akalin, E.; Azzi, Y.; Bartash, R.; Seethamraju, H.; Parides, M.; Hemmige, V.; Ross, M.; Forest, S.; Goldstein, Y.D.; Ajaimy, M.; et al. Covid-19 and Kidney Transplantation. *N. Engl. J. Med.* **2020**. [CrossRef] [PubMed]

9. Ritschl, P.; Nevermann, N.; Wiering, L.; Wu, H.H.; Morodor, P.; Brandl, A.; Hillebrandt, K.; Tacke, F.; Friedersdorff, F.; Schlomm, T.; et al. Solid organ transplantation programs facing lack of empiric evidence in the COVID-19 pandemic: A By-proxy Society Recommendation Consensus approach. *Arab. Archaeol. Epigr.* **2020**. [CrossRef]

10. Angelico, R.; Trapani, S.; Manzia, T.M.; Lombardini, L.; Tisone, G.; Cardillo, M. The COVID-19 outbreak in Italy: Initial implications for organ transplantation programs. *Arab. Archaeol. Epigr.* **2020**. [CrossRef]

11. Kronbichler, A.; Gauckler, P.; Windpessl, M.; Shin, J.I.; Jha, V.; Rovin, B.H.; Oberbauer, R. COVID-19: implications for immunosuppression in kidney disease and transplantation. *Nat. Rev. Nephrol.* **2020**, 1–3. [CrossRef]

12. Maggiore, U.; Abramowicz, D.; Crespo, M.; Mariat, C.; Mjoen, G.; Peruzzi, L.; Sever, M.S.; Oniscu, G.C.; Hilbrands, L.; Watschinger, B. How should I manage immunosuppression in a kidney transplant patient with COVID-19? An Era-Edta Descartes expert opinion. *Nephrol. Dial. Transplant. Off. Publ. Eur. Dial. Transpl. Assoc. Eur. Ren. Assoc.* **2020**. [CrossRef] [PubMed]

13. American Society of, T. FAQs for Organ Transplantation. Available online: https://www.myast.org/sites/default/files/internal/COVID19%20FAQ%20Tx%20Centers%2005.11.2020.pdf (accessed on 18 May 2020).

14. Ribal, M.J.; Cornford, P.; Briganti, A.; Knoll, T.; Gravas, S.; Babjuk, M.; Harding, C.; Breda, A.; Bex, A.; Rassweiler, J.J.; et al. European Association of Urology Guidelines Office Rapid Reaction Group: An Organisation-wide Collaborative Effort to Adapt the European Association of Urology Guidelines Recommendations to the Coronavirus Disease 2019 Era. *Eur. Urol.* **2020**. [CrossRef] [PubMed]

15. Garcia, G.G.; World Kidney Day Steering Committee 2012; Harden, P.; Chapman, J. The global role of kidney transplantation. *J. Nephrol.* **2012**, *25*, 1–6. [CrossRef] [PubMed]

16. Dreyer, G.J.; De Fijter, J.W. Transplanting the Elderly: Mandatory Age- and Minimal Histocompatibility Matching. *Front. Immunol.* **2020**, *11*, 359. [CrossRef]

17. Lehner, L.J.; Kleinsteuber, A.; Halleck, F.; Khadzhynov, D.; Schrezenmeier, E.; Duerr, M.; Eckardt, K.-U.; Budde, K.; Staeck, O. Assessment of the Kidney Donor Profile Index in a European cohort. *Nephrol. Dial. Transplant.* **2018**, *33*, 1465–1472. [CrossRef]

18. Giessing, M.; Fuller, T.F.; Friedersdorff, F.; Deger, S.; Wille, A.; Neumayer, H.-H.; Schmidt, D.; Budde, K.; Liefeldt, L. Outcomes of transplanting deceased-donor kidneys between elderly donors and recipients. *J. Am. Soc. Nephrol.* **2008**, *20*, 37–40. [CrossRef] [PubMed]

19. Frei, U.; Noeldeke, J.; Machold-Fabrizii, V.; Arbogast, H.; Margreiter, R.; Fricke, L.; Voiculescu, A.; Kliem, V.; Ebel, H.; Albert, U.; et al. Prospective Age-Matching in Elderly Kidney Transplant Recipients—A 5-Year Analysis of the Eurotransplant Senior Program. *Arab. Archaeol. Epigr.* **2007**, *8*, 50. [CrossRef]

20. Quast, L.S.; Grzella, S.; Lengenfeld, T.; Pillokeit, N.; Hummels, M.; Zgoura, P.; Westhoff, T.H.; Viebahn, R.; Schenker, P. Outcome of Kidney Transplantation Using Organs From Brain-dead Donors Older Than 75 Years. *Transplant. Proc.* **2020**, *52*, 119–126. [CrossRef]

21. Jacobi, J.; Beckmann, S.; Heller, K.; Hilgers, K.F.; Apel, H.; Spriewald, B.; Eckardt, K.-U.; Amann, K.U. Deceased Donor Kidney Transplantation in the Eurotransplant Senior Program (ESP): A Single-Center Experience from 2008 to 2013. *Ann. Transplant.* **2016**, *21*, 94–104. [CrossRef]

22. Boesmueller, C.; Biebl, M.; Scheidl, S.; Öllinger, R.; Margreiter, C.; Pratschke, J.; Margreiter, R.; Schneeberger, S. Long-Term Outcome in Kidney Transplant Recipients Over 70 Years in the Eurotransplant Senior Kidney Transplant Program: A Single Center Experience. *Transplantation* **2011**, *92*, 210–216. [CrossRef]

23. Wolters, H.; Bahde, R.; Vowinkel, T.; Unser, J.; Anthoni, C.; Hölzen, J.P.; Suwelack, B.; Senninger, N. Prognostic factors for kidney allograft survival in the Eurotransplant Senior Program. *Ann. Transplant.* **2014**, *19*, 201–209. [CrossRef]

24. Chavalitdhamrong, D.; Gill, J.; Takemoto, S.; Madhira, B.R.; Cho, Y.W.; Shah, T.; Bunnapradist, S. Patient and Graft Outcomes from Deceased Kidney Donors Age 70 Years and Older: An Analysis of the Organ Procurement Transplant Network/United Network of Organ Sharing Database. *Transplantation* **2008**, *85*, 1573–1579. [CrossRef]

25. Bentas, W.; Jones, J.; Karaoguz, A.; Tilp, U.; Probst, M.; Scheuermann, E.; Hauser, I.A.; Jonas, D.; Gossmann, J. Renal transplantation in the elderly: surgical complications and outcome with special emphasis on the Eurotransplant Senior Programme. *Nephrol. Dial. Transplant.* **2008**, *23*, 2043–2051. [CrossRef] [PubMed]

26. Gallinat, A.; Feldkamp, T.; Schaffer, R.; Radunz, S.; Treckmann, J.W.; Minor, T.; Witzke, O.; Paul, A.; Sotiropoulos, G.C. Single-Center Experience With Kidney Transplantation Using Deceased Donors Older Than 75 Years. *Transplantation* **2011**, *92*, 76–81. [CrossRef] [PubMed]

27. Abrol, N.; Kashyap, R.; Frank, R.D.; Iyer, V.N.; Dean, P.G.; Stegall, M.D.; Prieto, M.; Kashani, K.B.; Taner, T. Preoperative Factors Predicting Admission to the Intensive Care Unit After Kidney Transplantation. *Mayo Clin. Proc. Innov. Qual. Outcomes* **2019**, *3*, 285–293. [CrossRef] [PubMed]

28. De Freitas, F.G.R.; Lombardi, F.; Pacheco, E.S.; De Sandes-Freitas, T.V.; Viana, L.A.; Junior, H.T.-S.; Medina-Pestana, J.O.; Bafi, A.T.; Machado, F.R. Clinical Features of Kidney Transplant Recipients Admitted to the Intensive Care Unit. *Prog. Transplant.* **2017**, *28*, 56–62. [CrossRef]

29. Marques, I.; Caires, R.A.; Machado, D.; Goldenstein, P.; Rodrigues, C.; Pegas, J.; De Paula, F.; David-Neto, E.; Costa, M. Outcomes and Mortality in Renal Transplant Recipients Admitted to the Intensive Care Unit. *Transplant. Proc.* **2015**, *47*, 2694–2699. [CrossRef]

30. Cai, F.; Wang, M.; Wu, X.D.; Xu, X.M.; Su, X.; Shi, Y. Body mass index is associated with the risk of ICU admission and death among patients with pneumonia: A systematic review and meta-analysis. *Int. J. Clin. Exp. Med.* **2016**, *9*, 5269–5278.

31. Pepper, D.J.; Sun, J.; Welsh, J.; Cui, X.; Suffredini, A.F.; Eichacker, P.Q. Increased body mass index and adjusted mortality in ICU patients with sepsis or septic shock: A systematic review and meta-analysis. *Crit. Care* **2016**, *20*, 181. [CrossRef]

32. Zhao, Y.; Li, Z.; Yang, T.; Wang, M.; Xi, X. Is body mass index associated with outcomes of mechanically ventilated adult patients in intensive critical units? A systematic review and meta-analysis. *PLoS ONE* **2018**, *13*, e0198669. [CrossRef]

33. Banack, H.R.; Stokes, A. The 'obesity paradox' may not be a paradox at all. *Int. J. Obes.* **2017**, *41*, 1162–1163. [CrossRef] [PubMed]

34. Antonopoulos, A.S.; Tousoulis, D. The molecular mechanisms of obesity paradox. *Cardiovasc. Res.* **2017**, *113*, 1074–1086. [CrossRef] [PubMed]

35. Nakayama, M.; Sato, T.; Miyazaki, M.; Matsushima, M.; Sato, H.; Taguma, Y.; Ito, S. Increased risk of cardiovascular events and mortality among non-diabetic chronic kidney disease patients with hypertensive nephropathy: The Gonryo study. *Hypertens. Res.* **2011**, *34*, 1106–1110. [CrossRef] [PubMed]

36. Kasiske, B.L.; Snyder, J.J.; Gilbertson, D.; Matas, A.J. Diabetes mellitus after kidney transplantation in the United States. *Arab. Archaeol. Epigr.* **2003**, *3*, 178–185. [CrossRef]

37. Cosio, F.G.; Pesavento, T.E.; Kim, S.; Osei, K.; Henry, M.; Ferguson, R.M. Patient survival after renal transplantation: IV. Impact of post-transplant diabetes. *Kidney Int.* **2002**, *62*, 1440–1446. [CrossRef]

38. Kuo, H.-T.; Sampaio, M.S.; Vincenti, F.; Bunnapradist, S. Associations of Pretransplant Diabetes Mellitus, New-Onset Diabetes After Transplant, and Acute Rejection With Transplant Outcomes: An Analysis of the Organ Procurement and Transplant Network/United Network for Organ Sharing (OPTN/UNOS) Database. *Am. J. Kidney Dis.* **2010**, *56*, 1127–1139. [CrossRef]

39. Held, P.J.; Kahan, B.D.; Hunsicker, L.G.; Liska, D.; Wolfe, R.A.; Port, F.K.; Gaylin, D.S.; García, J.R.; Agodoa, L.; Krakauer, H. The Impact of HLA Mismatches on the Survival of First Cadaveric Kidney Transplants. *N. Engl. J. Med.* **1994**, *331*, 765–770. [CrossRef]

5

Validation of Identified Susceptible Gene Variants for New-Onset Diabetes in Renal Transplant Recipients

Hyeon Seok Hwang [1], Kyung-Won Hong [2], Jin Sug Kim [1], Yang Gyun Kim [1], Ju Young Moon [1], Kyung Hwan Jeong [1], Sang Ho Lee [1,*] and The Korean Organ Transplantation Registry Study Group

[1] Division of Nephrology, Department of Internal Medicine, College of Medicine, Kyung Hee University, Seoul 130-702, Korea; hwanghsne@gmail.com (H.S.H.); jinsuk0902@hanmail.net (J.S.K.); apple8840@hanmail.net (Y.G.K.); kidmjy@hanmail.net (J.Y.M.); aprilhwan@naver.com (K.H.J.)
[2] Division of Healthcare Innovation, TheragenEtex Bio Institute Co., Ltd., Suwon 443-721, Korea; kyungwon.hong@therabio.kr
* Correspondence: lshkidney@khu.ac.kr

Abstract: Genome-wide association studies (GWAS) and candidate gene approaches have identified single nucleotide polymorphisms (SNPs) associated with new-onset diabetes after renal transplantation (NODAT). We evaluated associations between NODAT and SNPs identified in previous studies. We genotyped 1102 renal transplant recipients from the Korean Organ Transplantation Registry (KOTRY) database; 13 SNPs were assessed for associations with NODAT (occurring in 254 patients; 23.0%), within one year after transplantation. The frequency of the T allele at *KCNQ1* rs2237892 was significantly lower in patients with NODAT compared to control patients (0.30 vs. 0.39; $p = 8.5 \times 10^{-5}$). The T allele at rs2237892 was significantly associated with decreased risk of NODAT after adjusting for multiple variables, compared to the C allele (OR 0.63, 95% CI 0.51–0.79; $p = 5.5 \times 10^{-5}$). Dominant inheritance modeling showed that CT/TT genotypes were associated with a lower risk for development of NODAT (OR 0.56, 95% CI 0.42–0.76; $p = 2.0 \times 10^{-4}$) compared to the CC genotype. No other SNPs were associated with NODAT. Our study validated the protective effect of T allele at *KCNQ1* rs2237892 on the development of NODAT in a large cohort of renal transplant recipients. Our findings on susceptibility variants might be a useful tool to predict NODAT development after renal transplantation.

Keywords: new onset diabetes after renal transplantation; single nucleotide polymorphisms; renal transplantation

1. Introduction

Development of new-onset diabetes after renal transplantation (NODAT) is a common complication in patients that have undergone transplantation. The cumulative incidence of NODAT is approximately 15%–30% at 1-year post-transplantation, and the annual incidence of NODAT is approximately 4%–6% [1–3]. This metabolic disorder induces a worse cardiovascular risk profile and results in a three-fold risk of cardiovascular morbidity [4,5]. In addition, NODAT is associated with a 1.5- to 3-fold risk of allograft loss and results in a 10%–20% reduction in long-term patient survival [1,6,7]. The accumulated health-care cost is also considerable, with an estimated cost of US $21,500 per new patient with diabetes in the second year after transplantation [8]. Therefore, NODAT is a critical burden of recipient care and a major clinical challenge for the longevity and survival of renal allograft patients.

The risk of developing NODAT is associated with several clinical factors, including the recipient age, BMI, use of tacrolimus and corticosteroid, acute rejection, hepatitis C virus, cytomegalovirus infection, autosomal dominant polycystic kidney disease, and hypomagnesemia [1,9–15]. However, evidence suggests an increased incidence of NODAT despite the identification of clinical risk factors and the effort to mitigate the risk [16]. As current strategies have limited effectiveness in preventing NODAT, genetic risk stratification emerges as a key approach to address this problem.

Several studies have shown genetic predisposition as a risk factor for the development of NODAT. Genetic polymorphism studies on NODAT led to the identification of several candidate genes, derived from genome-wide association studies (GWAS) for type 2 diabetes [17,18]. Commonly evaluated genetic determinants included genes involving carbohydrate metabolism, insulin secretion, and insulin resistance [19]. In addition, genes that encode inflammatory cytokines correlated with type 2 diabetes and were also associated significantly with NODAT [20]. More recently, GWAS showed that genes involved in β-cell apoptosis are associated with the development of NODAT [21,22]. However, candidate gene approaches included only a few individuals with NODAT, leading to inconsistent results, and the significant genes identified in GWAS are not replicated in independent cohorts. Therefore, these limitations severely interrupt the development of prevention strategies against NODAT.

This study aimed to verify the association of previously identified genetic polymorphisms with NODAT in a large nationwide prospective cohort. We selected 17 single nucleotide polymorphisms (SNPs) on susceptibility loci and evaluated the effects of these independent SNPs on the risk of developing NODAT.

2. Materials and Methods

2.1. Study Population

The study population was selected from the Korean Organ Transplantation Registry (KOTRY), which is a prospective, multicenter, nationwide cohort study that includes transplantation information in Korea. Thirty-two representative national hospitals and transplantation centers participated in KOTRY. Recipients were enrolled consecutively upon undergoing a transplantation procedure and followed up accordingly from July 2014 to December 2018. The registry accumulated data on individual patients including demographics, comorbidities, laboratory data, induction and maintenance of the immunosuppressive regimen, and several other types of events. Our study was reviewed and approved by the Institutional Review Board of each transplantation center. All patients provided written informed consent before enrollment in the study.

Blood samples from 1826 patients were stored for genotyping and screened using the KOTRY database. The following patients were excluded: Renal transplant recipients with established diabetes ($n = 503$), patients followed up for less than one year ($n = 107$), non-functioning graft at one-year follow-up ($n = 32$), incomplete record of medical or laboratory findings ($n = 65$), missing information on human leukocyte antigen (HLA) typing ($n = 2$), and others ($n = 15$). In total, finally, 1102 patients were enrolled for this study.

2.2. Selection of SNPs and Genotyping

We conducted an extensive literature review for published variants that were significantly associated with NODAT in renal transplant recipients. We evaluated SNPs, which showed top-ranked associations with NODAT in individual studies. We selected seventeen SNPs that were significantly associated with NODAT from GWAS or well-established association studies of NODAT [18,20–22].

Blood samples (3 mL each) were collected in tubes containing RBC lysis solution. The blood sample from each study participant was centrifuged to obtain white blood cells. Genomic DNA was extracted from white blood cells using a DEX^{TM} II genomic DNA extraction kit (Intron, Sungnam, Korea). DNA samples were stored at -80 °C before analysis. Quality of stored DNA samples was evaluated using agarose gel electrophoresis to confirm sample integrity. SNPs were genotyped from these DNA samples using TaqMan-based QuantStudio OpenArray® (Life Technologies, Carlsbad, CA, USA). DNA from patients and controls was randomly transferred into 96-well plates and genotyped using a blinded method. The call rates for genotyping of the SNPs were >98%.

2.3. Data Collection and Definition

We collected the following baseline patient characteristics at the time of transplantation: Age, gender, body mass index (BMI), relevant comorbid conditions, information on human leukocyte antigen (HLA), blood typing, desensitization, and induction and maintenance of the immunosuppressive regimen. Laboratory data were collected at baseline and regularly followed up. Clinical events were identified, including diabetes, the occurrence of biopsy-proven acute rejection, all-cause graft loss, and patient death or follow-up loss.

The primary outcome was the evaluation of SNP impact on the risk of developing NODAT within the first year after transplantation. Based on the definition of the American Diabetes Association, NODAT was diagnosed when fasting blood sugar was higher than 126 mg/dL six months after transplantation, or when insulin or oral hypoglycemic agents were required for treatment [23]. The control group consisted of renal transplant recipients who did not meet NODAT criteria during the follow-up period.

2.4. Statistical Analysis

Continuous variables were presented as the mean ± standard deviation. Allelic frequencies were analyzed using a chi-squared test between the two groups. Student's t-tests and chi-squared tests were used to evaluate between-group differences for continuous and categorical variables, respectively. For all SNPs, minor allele frequency (MAF), compliance with Hardy-Weinberg equilibrium (HWE), linkage disequilibrium analysis, and the association between rs2237892 and NODAT in different genetic models were assessed using SNPstats software (https://www.snpstats.net/start.htm). A multivariate logistic regression model was used to investigate the confounding effects of clinical variables significantly associated with NODAT and SNP associations. We included clinical covariates according to their weights in univariate testing, and we included clinically fundamental parameters. The confounders used in this analysis were recipient age, recipient sex, BMI, HLA mismatch number, desensitization in HLA incompatibility, ABO incompatibility, use of tacrolimus, use of steroids, biopsy-proven acute rejection, donor age, and deceased donor. Bonferroni correction was used in the association analysis when multiple comparisons were performed. We used multiple inheritance models, including codominant (major allele homozygotes vs. heterozygotes vs. minor allele homozygotes), dominant (major allele homozygotes vs. minor allele homozygotes plus heterozygotes), recessive (major allele homozygotes plus heterozygotes vs. minor allele homozygotes), and log-additive (major allele homozygotes vs. heterozygotes vs. minor allele homozygotes) models. Statistical analyses were performed using SPSS for Windows software (version 20.0; SPSS, Chicago, IL, USA). The significance level was set at $p < 0.05$.

3. Results

3.1. Baseline Clinical Characteristics and SNP Information

The incidence of NODAT in this study population was 23.0% (254/1102 patients). Baseline characteristics of recipients are summarized in Table 1. Transplant recipients who developed NODAT were significantly older, tended to be male, and had higher BMI scores than those who did not develop NODAT. Donor age in the NODAT group was significantly higher than in the control group. Desensitization treatment for HLA incompatibility was used more frequently in the control group. There was no difference between the two groups in the incidence of biopsy-proven acute rejection, or the use of tacrolimus or steroids as maintenance immunosuppressant treatments.

We excluded *AGMAT* rs11580170 from further analysis because it was in strong linkage disequilibrium with *DNAJC16* rs7533125 ($r^2 = 0.99$). Of rs1494558 and rs2172749 in *IL7R*, only rs2172749 was analyzed, because these SNPs were also in linkage disequilibrium ($r^2 = 0.98$). Of the 15 SNPs tested, 14 were consistent with HWE ($p > 0.05$). While *DNAJC16* rs7533125 violated HWE in the control group ($p = 0.037$), minor allele frequency (MAF) did not deviate from that of the East Asian population [24]. Therefore, we included *DNAJC16* rs7533125 in the genetic association test. We additionally excluded *TCF7L2* rs7903146 and *NPPA* rs198372 in the association test, because MAF was less than 0.05 (frequency of T allele at *TCF7L2* rs7903146, 0.02; and frequency of A allele at *NPPA* rs198372, 0.01).

Table 1. Baseline demographics and characteristics of the study population.

	NODAT ($n = 254$)	Controls ($n = 848$)	p
Recipient			
Age (years)	52.2 ± 10.4	45.1 ± 12.0	<0.001
Male (%)	152 (59.8)	445 (52.5)	0.039
Dialysis duration (months)	63.7 ± 72.0	59.1 ± 67.0	0.384
BMI	23.2 ± 3.3	22.3 ± 3.2	<0.001
Donor			
Age (years)	48.6 ± 12.5	45.7 ± 12.9	0.001
Male (%)	136 (53.5)	467 (55.1)	0.668
Deceased (%)	108 (42.5)	310 (36.6)	0.086
HLA mismatch number	3.4 ± 1.7	3.2 ± 1.7	0.083
Desensitization for HLA incompatibility (%)	42 (16.5)	189 (22.3)	0.048
ABO incompatibility (%)	18 (7.1)	75 (8.8)	0.377
Anti-thymocyte globulin induction (%)	64 (25.2)	196 (23.1)	0.493
Tacrolimus (%)	252 (99.2)	831 (98.0)	0.191
Steroid (%)	252 (99.2)	845 (99.6)	0.367
Biopsy-proven acute rejection (%)	35 (13.8)	96 (11.3)	0.288

BMI = body mass index; and NODAT = new-onset diabetes after renal transplantation.

3.2. Allelic Frequency and Association between SNPs and NODAT

The allele frequencies of the genetic polymorphisms in the NODAT and control groups are summarized in Table 2. The allelic frequency of the T allele at *KCNQ1* rs2237892 was significantly lower in patients with NODAT compared to that in the control group (0.30 vs. 0.39; $p = 8.5 \times 10^{-5}$). The C allele at *CDKAL1* rs10946398 had a higher frequency in the NODAT group, with marginal statistical significance (0.52 vs. 0.47; $p = 0.080$).

We examined the genetic association between SNPs and NODAT in an allele-specific pattern (Table 3). Univariate analyses showed that the T allele at *KCNQ1* rs2237892 was significantly associated with decreased risk of NODAT (odds ratio (OR) 0.66, 95% confidence interval (CI) 0.53–0.82; $p = 1.3 \times 10^{-4}$). The C allele at *CDKAL1* rs10946398 was associated with a 1.2-fold higher risk for development of NODAT (95% CI 0.98–1.46; $p = 0.078$). However, none of the other SNPs evaluated in this study (*ATP5F1P6* rs10484821, *DNAJC16* rs7533125, *CELA2B* rs2861484, *CASP9* rs2020902, *NOX4* rs1836882, *INPP5A* rs4394754, *IL7R* rs2172749, *IL17R* rs4819554, *IL17RB* rs1025689, *IL17RB* rs1043261, and *PLXDC1* rs72823322) were significantly associated with NODAT. The association between *KCNQ1* rs2237892 and NODAT was enhanced when evaluated using multivariate logistic regression analysis (OR 0.63, 95% CI 0.51–0.79; $p = 5.5 \times 10^{-5}$). However, no other SNPs were significantly associated with NODAT in the multivariate logistic regression analysis.

Table 2. Allele frequencies of polymorphisms previously associated with NODAT.

Gene	SNP	Chr: Position	Minor Allele	MAF			
				All	NODAT	Control	p
CDKAL1	rs10946398	6:20660803	C	0.48	0.52	0.47	0.080
KCNQ1	rs2237892	11:2818521	T	0.37	0.30	0.39	8.5×10^{-5}
ATP5F1P6	rs10484821	6:139547773	C	0.33	0.32	0.33	0.583
DNAJC16	rs7533125	1:15557249	C	0.07	0.07	0.07	0.747
CELA2B	rs2861484	1:15486170	T	0.07	0.07	0.06	0.599
CASP9	rs2020902	1:15507865	G	0.04	0.04	0.04	0.930
NOX4	rs1836882	11:89498993	C	0.27	0.28	0.27	0.587
INPP5A	rs4394754	10:132529558	T	0.09	0.10	0.09	0.632
IL7R	rs2172749	5:3585516	C	0.40	0.40	0.40	0.976
IL17R	rs4819554	22:17084145	G	0.43	0.45	0.42	0.256
IL17RB	rs1025689	3:53849695	C	0.45	0.47	0.44	0.226
IL17RB	rs1043261	3:53865249	T	0.10	0.11	0.10	0.256
PLXDC1	rs72823322	17:39130161	G	0.21	0.22	0.21	0.185

NODAT = new onset diabetes after renal transplantation; Chr = chromosome; MAF = minor allele frequency; and SNP = single nucleotide polymorphism.

Table 3. Allele-based incidence and risk of NODAT.

Gene	SNP	Allele	Crude		Adjusted *	
			OR (95% CI)	p	OR (95% CI)	p
CDKAL1	rs10946398	C (vs. A)	1.20 (0.98, 1.46)	0.078	1.22 (0.98, 1.50)	0.070
KCNQ1	rs2237892	T (vs. C)	0.66 (0.53, 0.82)	1.3×10^{-4}	0.63 (0.51, 0.79)	5.5×10^{-5}
ATP5F1P6	rs10484821	C (vs. T)	0.94 (0.76, 1.17)	0.583	0.96 (0.77, 1.20)	0.726
DNAJC16	rs7533125	C (vs. T)	0.94 (0.65, 1.37)	0.756	0.96 (0.65, 1.43)	0.855
CELA2B	rs2861484	T (vs. G)	1.11 (0.76, 1.62)	0.607	1.07 (0.71, 1.60)	0.751
CASP9	rs2020902	G (vs. A)	0.98 (0.61, 1.56)	0.933	0.92 (0.56, 1.50)	0.733
NOX4	rs1836882	C (vs. T)	1.06 (0.85, 1.33)	0.588	1.02 (0.80, 1.29)	0.904
INPP5A	rs4394754	T (vs. C)	1.08 (0.78, 1.51)	0.635	1.08 (0.76, 1.54)	0.657
IL7R	rs2172749	C (vs. G)	1.00 (0.81, 1.22)	0.976	1.07 (0.86, 1.33)	0.535
IL17R	rs4819554	G (vs. A)	1.12 (0.92, 1.37)	0.255	1.09 (0.88, 1.35)	0.415
IL17RB	rs1025689	C (vs. G)	1.13 (0.93, 1.38)	0.226	1.15 (0.93, 1.41)	0.204
IL17RB	rs1043261	T (vs. C)	1.21 (0.87, 1.67)	0.252	1.21 (0.86, 1.71)	0.265
PLXDC1	rs72823322	G (vs. A)	0.85 (0.66, 1.09)	0.190	0.84 (0.65, 1.10)	0.199

NODAT = new onset diabetes after renal transplantation; CI = 95% confidence interval; OR = odds ratio; and SNP = single nucleotide polymorphism. * Adjusted for recipient age, recipient sex, BMI, HLA mismatch number, desensitization in HLA incompatibility, ABO incompatibility, use of tacrolimus, use of steroids, biopsy-proven acute rejection, donor age, and deceased donor.

3.3. Genotype Distribution and Association between KCNQ1 rs2237892 and NODAT

We tested the effect of *KCNQ1* rs2237892 genotype on NODAT using a multiple inheritance model as shown in Table 4). In the codominant model, the TT genotype at rs2237892 was associated with the lowest risk for development of NODAT, compared to the CC genotype (OR 0.41, 95% CI 0.25–0.67; $p = 4.7 \times 10^{-4}$). In the dominant model, the CT/TT genotype was also associated with a reduced risk for development of NODAT (OR 0.56, 95% CI 0.42–0.76; $p = 2.0 \times 10^{-4}$). The T allele significantly reduced the risk of NODAT compared to the CC genotype in the log-additive model. However, no significant differences were observed in the recessive model with Bonferroni correction.

Table 4. NODAT incidence and risk of *KCNQ1* rs2237892 in multiple inheritance models.

Model	Type	N (%)		OR (95% CI) *	p
		NODAT	**Control**		
Codominant	CC	128 (50.4)	317 (37.4)	Reference	
	CT	101 (39.8)	395 (46.6)	0.62 (0.45, 0.85)	2.8×10^{-3}
	TT	25 (9.8)	136 (16.0)	0.41 (0.25, 0.67)	4.7×10^{-4}
Dominant	CC	128 (50.4)	317 (37.4)	Reference	
	CT/TT	126 (49.6)	531 (62.6)	0.56 (0.42, 0.76)	2.0×10^{-4}
Recessive	CC/CT	229 (90.2)	712 (84.0)	Reference	
	TT	25 (9.8)	136 (16.0)	0.53 (0.33, 0.84)	0.0051
Log-additive	-			0.63 (0.51, 0.79)	$<1.0 \times 10^{-4}$

NODAT = new onset diabetes after renal transplantation; CI = 95% confidence interval; and OR = odds ratio. *Adjusted for recipient age, recipient sex, BMI, HLA mismatch number, desensitization in HLA incompatibility, ABO incompatibility, use of tacrolimus, use of steroids, biopsy-proven acute rejection, donor age, and deceased donor.

4. Discussion

In the present study, using samples from a large cohort of renal transplant recipients, we examined the association of 13 SNP pairs and candidate genes for risk of NODAT development. Of the studied variants, there was a significant difference in the frequency of the T allele at *KCNQ1* rs2237892 between the NODAT and control groups, and this allele showed an independent association with NODAT. The TT and CT genotypes of *KCNQ1* rs2237892 were associated with a significantly reduced risk for development of NODAT in codominant, dominant, and log-additive models. These findings suggested that the genetic variant of *KCNQ1* is a significant contributor to the development of NODAT in renal transplant recipients.

Although NODAT results from the combined effect of insulin resistance and β-cell dysfunction, several recent studies have shown that β-cell dysfunction is the main contributing factor for the development of NODAT [3,25,26]. *KCNQ1* rs2237892 and *CDKAL1* rs10946398 were identified as a susceptibility gene for type 2 diabetes in GWAS, and each of these genes is associated with β-cell dysfunction [27–31]. Previous studies with type 2 diabetes risk genes suggested an association between *KCNQ1* rs2237892 and NODAT [19]. Our study also validated that variant rs2237892 of the T allele was associated with decreased risk for development of NODAT compared to the C allele. Similarly, *CDKAL1* rs10946398 was also associated with NODAT, as reported in a study that used a candidate gene approach in patients who underwent transplantation [18,19]. However, our data did not confirm this association. These findings suggested that *KCNQ1* is a more robust and influential indicator of β-cell dysfunction in renal transplant recipients.

KCNQ1 encodes a subunit of the voltage-gated K$^+$ channel, which is expressed in pancreatic islets [32]. In the *KCNQ1*-overexpressing pancreatic β-cell line, the density of the K+ current increased significantly and affected the pancreatic cell membrane action potential [33]. Therefore, *KCNQ1* overexpression contributes to impairment of glucose-stimulated insulin secretion, and a specific *KCNQ1* blocker also stimulates insulin secretion [34]. In addition, allelic mutation of *KCNQ1* results in up-regulation of the neighboring gene, cyclin-dependent kinase inhibitor 1C, which encodes a cell cycle inhibitor and leads to reduction in pancreatic β-cell mass [35]. Therefore, we suggest that variant *KCNQ1* induces impaired β-cell function and reduced β-cell mass, and this biological function could be a potential underlying mechanism for the association between *KCNQ1* variants and increased risk for NODAT development.

Three types of *KCNQ1* SNPs were evaluated as potential risk factors for the development of NODAT in Spanish patients who received kidney transplants from deceased donors [17]. *KCNQ1* rs2237895, rs2237892, and rs8234 were genotyped, and SNP rs2237895, but not rs2237892, was found to be associated with an increased risk for development of NODAT in the first year after transplantation. This apparent discrepancy could be due to the allele frequencies of these SNPs. The T allele frequency at rs2237892 was reported to be 0.34–0.36 in the East Asian population, but only 0.04–0.08 in the European population [36]. Consequently, lower MAF at rs2237892 was not significantly associated with NODAT in Spanish transplant recipients. Therefore, we suggest that different genetic backgrounds should be considered when attempting to determine the risk of development of NODAT using *KCNQ1* genetic variants as indicators.

In a recent GWAS, numerous variants were found to be associated with risk for the development of NODAT [21]. *ATP5F1P6, CELA2B, CASP9, NOX4,* and *INPP5A* were identified as risk genes in Caucasian renal transplant recipients. These genetic variants were implicated in β-cell apoptotic pathways, but not insulin resistance, suggesting that β-cell apoptosis was a critical component of NODAT pathogenesis. However, our study did not find a significant association between NODAT and any SNPs from this GWAS. Three possible factors might explain this inconsistency: First, the β-cell apoptotic pathways could be a weak contributor to the development of NODAT in Asian compared to Caucasian recipients of a renal transplant. Second, a different definition of NODAT phenotype might have resulted in dissimilar findings in the two studies. Third, the limited sample size in the GWAS may have less power to detect significant associations [37].

Inflammatory cytokines are involved in insulin action and insulin secretion. An SNP within the gene encoding the IL-7R chain was found to be associated with type 1 diabetes mellitus [38,39]. Moreover, our previous study showed that genetic variants of *IL-7R, IL-17R,* and *IL-17RB* were associated significantly with NODAT [14]. However, the relevant SNPs of these interleukin genes were not associated with NODAT in the exploratory GWAS analysis or the secondary verification analysis [17]. Furthermore, our validation study also showed no meaningful differences in allele frequencies. These findings suggested that the effects of interleukin gene polymorphisms on the risk for development of NODAT were inconclusive, and further studies are necessary to obtain precise results.

The present study had a few limitations. As data regarding family history of type 2 diabetes were not available, the association between family history and the development of NODAT could not be evaluated. In addition, the effect of BMI and weight gain after transplantation was not included in our analysis. Finally, we did not perform an oral glucose tolerance test or HbA1c estimation before kidney transplantation. Therefore, patients with prediabetes might have been included in our study.

In conclusion, our validation study showed a significant association between *KCNQ1* rs2237892 and development of NODAT in a large cohort. Our results suggest that *KCNQ1* might play a crucial role in the pathogenesis of NODAT following renal transplantation. *KCNQ1* variants might be a useful tool to predict NODAT development in renal transplant recipients, and help screen for patients at a higher risk for NODAT.

Author Contributions: Conceptualization, S.H.L.; methodology, H.S.H.; software, K.-W.H.; validation, all authors; formal analysis, H.S.H.; investigation, J.S.K., Y.G.K., J.Y.M., K.H.J.; resources, J.S.K., Y.G.K., J.Y.M., K.H.J.; data curation, H.S.H.; writing—original draft preparation, H.S.H.; writing—review and editing, S.H.L.; visualization, H.S.H.; supervision, S.H.L.; project administration, J.S.K., Y.G.K., J.Y.M., K.H.J., S.H.L.; funding acquisition, S.H.L.

Acknowledgments: The authors appreciate the support and cooperation of Korean Organ Transplantation Registry Study Group: Jin Min Kong [1], Oh Jung Kwon [2], Myung-Gyu Kim [3], Sung Hoon Kim [4], Yeong Hoon Kim [5], Joong Kyung Kim [6], Chan-Duck Kim [7], Ji Won Min [8], Sung Kwang Park[9], Yeon Ho Park [10], Inwhee Park [11], Park Jae Berm [12], Jung Hwan Park [13], Jong-Won Park [14], Tae Hyun Ban [15], Sang Heon Song [16], Seung Hwan Song [17], Ho Sik Shin [18], Chul Woo Yang [19], Hye Eun Yoon [20], Kang Wook Lee [21], Dong Ryeol Lee [22], Dong Won Lee [23], Sam Yeol Lee [24], Sang-Ho Lee [25], Jung Jun Lee [26], Lee Jung Pyo [27], Jeong-Hoon Lee [28], Jin Seok Jeon [29], Heungman Jun [30], Kyung Hwang Jeong [31], Ku Yong Chung [32], Hong Rae Cho [33], Ju Man Ki [34], Dong-Wan Chae [35], Soo Jin Na Choi [36], Duck Jong Han [37], Seungyeup Han [38], Kyu Ha Huh [39], Jaeseok Yang [40], Curie Ahn [41]; [1] Department of Nephrology, BHS Hanseo Hospital, [2] Department of Surgery, College of Medicine, Han Yang University, [3] Department of Internal Medicine, Korea University Anam Hospital, [4] Department of Surgery, Yonsei University Wonju College of Medicine, Wonju Severance Christian Hospital, [5] Department of Internal Medicine, Inje University Busan Paik Hospital, [6] Department of Internal Medicine, Bongseng Memorial Hospital, [7] Department of Internal Medicine, School of Medicine, Kyungpook National University

Hospital, [8] Division of Nephrology, Department of Internal Medicine, Bucheon St. Mary's Hospital, [9] Department of Internal Medicine, Chonbuk National University Medical School, [10] Department of Surgery, Gil Medical Center, Gachon University College of Medicine, [11] Department of Nephrology, Ajou University School of Medicine, [12] Department of Surgery, Samsung Medical Center, [13] Konkuk University School of Medicine, Department of Nephrology, [14] Department of Nephrology, Yeungnam University Hospital, [15] Division of Nephrology, Department of Internal Medicine, Eunpyeong St. Mary's hospital, [16] Organ Transplantation Center and Department of Internal Medicine, Pusan National University Hospital, [17] Department of Surgery, Ewha Womans University Medical Center, [18] Kosin University College of Medicine, Department of Internal Medicine, Division of Nephrology, [19] Division of Nephrology, Department of Internal Medicine, Seoul St. Mary's hospital, [20] Department of Internal Medicine, Incheon St. Mary's Hospital, [21] Department of Nephrology, Chungnam National University Hospital, [22] Division of Nephrology, Department of Internal Medicine, Maryknoll Medical Center, [23] Division of Nephrology, Department of Internal Medicine, Pusan National University School of Medicine, [24] Department of Surgery, Kangdong Sacred Heart Hospital, [25] Department of Nephrology, Kyung Hee University Hospital at Gangdong, [26] Department of Surgery, CHA Bundang Medical Center, [27] Department of Nephrology, SNU Boramae Medical Center, [28] Department of Surgery, Myongji Hospital, [29] Department of Internal Medicine, Soonchunhyang University Seoul Hospital, [30] Department of Surgery, Inje University Ilsan Paik Hospital, [31] Department of Internal Medicine, Kyung Hee University College of Medicine, [32] Department of Surgery, Ewha Womans University Mokdong Hospital, [33] Department of Surgery, Ulsan University Hospital, [34] Department of Surgery, Gangnam Severance Hospital, Yonsei University College of Medicine, [35] Division of Nephrology, Seoul National University Bundang Hospital, [36] Department of Surgery, Chonnam National University Medical School, [37] Department of Surgery, Asan Medical Center, [38] Department of Internal Medicine, Keimyung University School of Medicine, [39] Department of Transplantation Surgery, Severance Hospital, [40] Department of Surgery, Seoul National University Hospital, [41] Department of Nephrology, Seoul National University Hospital.

References

1. Kasiske, B.L.; Snyder, J.J.; Gilbertson, D.; Matas, A.J. Diabetes mellitus after kidney transplantation in the United States. *Am. J. Transplant.* **2003**, *3*, 178–185. [CrossRef]
2. Choi, Y.K.; Kim, Y.; Choi, N.; Kim, M.Y.; Baek, N.N.; Youm, J.Y.; Lee, J.E.; Kim, D.J.; Kim, Y.; Oh, H.Y.; et al. Risk Factors for New Onset Diabetes after Transplantation among Renal Transplant Recipients Treated with Tacrolimus. *Kidney Res. Clin. Pract.* **2010**, *29*, 761–767.
3. Chakkera, H.A.; Weil, E.J.; Pham, P.T.; Pomeroy, J.; Knowler, W.C. Can new-onset diabetes after kidney transplant be prevented? *Diabetes Care* **2013**, *36*, 1406–1412. [CrossRef]
4. González-Posada, J.M.; Hernández, D.; Genís, B.B.; Tamajón, L.P.; Pérez, J.G.; Maceira, B.; Sánchez, M.R.; Serón, D.; Spanish Chronic Allograft Nephropathy Study Group. Increased cardiovascular risk profile and mortality in kidney allograft recipients with post-transplant diabetes mellitus in Spain. *Clin. Transplant.* **2006**, *20*, 650–658.
5. Hjelmesaeth, J.; Hartmann, A.; Leivestad, T.; Holdaas, H.; Sagedal, S.; Olstad, M.; Jenssen, T. The impact of early-diagnosed new-onset post-transplantation diabetes mellitus on survival and major cardiac events. *Kidney Int.* **2006**, *69*, 588–595. [CrossRef]
6. Cosio, F.G.; Pesavento, T.E.; Kim, S.; Osei, K.; Henry, M.; Ferguson, R.M. Patient survival after renal transplantation: IV. Impact of post-transplant diabetes. *Kidney Int.* **2002**, *62*, 1440–1446. [CrossRef]
7. Miles, A.M.; Sumrani, N.; Horowitz, R.; Homel, P.; Maursky, V.; Markell, M.S.; Distant, D.A.; Hong, J.H.; Sommer, B.G.; Friedman, E.A. Diabetes mellitus after renal transplantation: As deleterious as non-transplant-associated diabetes? *Transplantation* **1998**, *65*, 380–384. [CrossRef]
8. Woodward, R.S.; Schnitzler, M.A.; Baty, J.; Lowell, J.A.; Lopez-Rocafort, L.; Haider, S.; Woodworth, T.G.; Brennan, D.C. Incidence and cost of new onset diabetes mellitus among U.S. wait-listed and transplanted renal allograft recipients. *Am. J. Transplant.* **2003**, *3*, 590–598. [CrossRef]
9. Rodrigo, E.; Fernández-Fresnedo, G.; Valero, R.; Ruiz, J.C.; Piñera, C.; Palomar, R.; González-Cotorruelo, J.; Gómez-Alamillo, C.; Arias, M. New-onset diabetes after kidney transplantation: Risk factors. *J. Am. Soc. Nephrol.* **2006**, *17*, S291–S295. [CrossRef]
10. Israni, A.K.; Snyder, J.J.; Skeans, M.A.; Kasiske, B.L.; PORT Investigators. Clinical diagnosis of metabolic syndrome: Predicting new-onset diabetes, coronary heart disease, and allograft failure late after kidney transplant. *Transpl. Int.* **2012**, *25*, 748–757. [CrossRef]

11. Fabrizi, F.; Martin, P.; Dixit, V.; Bunnapradist, S.; Kanwal, F.; Dulai, G. Post-transplant diabetes mellitus and HCV seropositive status after renal transplantation: Meta-analysis of clinical studies. *Am. J. Transplant.* **2005**, *5*, 2433–2440. [CrossRef] [PubMed]

12. Hjelmesaeth, J.; Sagedal, S.; Hartmann, A.; Rollag, H.; Egeland, T.; Hagen, M.; Nordal, K.P.; Jenssen, T. Asymptomatic cytomegalovirus infection is associated with increased risk of new-onset diabetes mellitus and impaired insulin release after renal transplantation. *Diabetologia* **2004**, *47*, 1550–1556. [CrossRef] [PubMed]

13. Räkel, A.; Karelis, A.D. New-onset diabetes after transplantation: Risk factors and clinical impact. *Diabetes Metab.* **2011**, *37*, 1–14. [CrossRef] [PubMed]

14. Cheungpasitporn, W.; Thongprayoon, C.; Vijayvargiya, P.; Anthanont, P.; Erickson, S.B. The Risk for New-Onset Diabetes Mellitus after Kidney Transplantation in Patients with Autosomal Dominant Polycystic Kidney Disease: A Systematic Review and Meta-Analysis. *Can. J. Diabetes* **2016**, *40*, 521–528. [CrossRef]

15. Cheungpasitporn, W.; Thongprayoon, C.; Harindhanavudhi, T.; Edmonds, P.J.; Erickson, S.B. Hypomagnesemia linked to new-onset diabetes mellitus after kidney transplantation: A systematic review and meta-analysis. *Endocr. Res.* **2016**, *41*, 142–147. [CrossRef]

16. Cole, E.H.; Johnston, O.; Rose, C.L.; Gill, J.S. Impact of acute rejection and new-onset diabetes on long-term transplant graft and patient survival. *Clin. J. Am. Soc. Nephrol.* **2008**, *3*, 814–821. [CrossRef]

17. Tavira, B.; Coto, E.; Díaz-Corte, C.; Ortega, F.; Arias, M.; Torres, A.; Díaz, J.M.; Selgas, R.; López-Larrea, C.; Campistol, J.M.; et al. *KCNQ1* gene variants and risk of new-onset diabetes in tacrolimus-treated renal-transplanted patients. *Clin. Transplant.* **2011**, *25*, E284–E291. [CrossRef]

18. Benson, K.A.; Maxwell, A.P.; McKnight, A.J. A HuGE Review and Meta-Analyses of Genetic Associations in New Onset Diabetes after Kidney Transplantation. *PLoS ONE* **2016**, *11*, e0147323. [CrossRef]

19. Kang, E.S.; Kim, M.S.; Kim, C.H.; Nam, C.M.; Han, S.J.; Hur, K.Y.; Ahn, C.W.; Cha, B.S.; Kim, S.I.; Lee, H.C.; et al. Association of common type 2 diabetes risk gene variants and posttransplantation diabetes mellitus in renal allograft recipients in Korea. *Transplantation* **2009**, *88*, 693–698. [CrossRef]

20. Kim, Y.G.; Ihm, C.G.; Lee, T.W.; Lee, S.H.; Jeong, K.H.; Moon, J.Y.; Chung, J.H.; Kim, S.K.; Kim, Y.H. Association of genetic polymorphisms of interleukins with new-onset diabetes after transplantation in renal transplantation. *Transplantation* **2012**, *93*, 900–907. [CrossRef]

21. McCaughan, J.A.; McKnight, A.J.; Maxwell, A.P. Genetics of new-onset diabetes after transplantation. *J. Am. Soc. Nephrol.* **2014**, *25*, 1037–1049. [CrossRef] [PubMed]

22. Giri, A.; Sanders, M.; Velez Edwards, D.; Ikizler, T.; Roden, D.; Birdwell, K. A Genome Wide Association Study of New Onset Diabetes after Transplant in Kidney Transplantation. *Am. J. Transplant.* **2016**, *16*, 578–579.

23. American Diabetes Association. Diagnosis and classification of diabetes mellitus. *Diabetes Care* **2004**, *27*, S5–S10. [CrossRef] [PubMed]

24. Ensembl. Available online: https://asia.ensembl.org/Homo_sapiens/Variation/Population?db=core;r=1:15556749-15557749;v=rs7533125;vdb=variation;vf=502267474 (accessed on 30 August 2019).

25. Hur, K.Y.; Kim, M.S.; Kim, Y.S.; Kang, E.S.; Nam, J.H.; Kim, S.H.; Nam, C.M.; Ahn, C.W.; Cha, B.S.; Kim, S.I.; et al. Risk factors associated with the onset and progression of posttransplantation diabetes in renal allograft recipients. *Diabetes Care* **2007**, *30*, 609–615. [CrossRef] [PubMed]

26. Nam, J.H.; Mun, J.I.; Kim, S.I.; Kang, S.W.; Choi, K.H.; Park, K.; Ahn, C.W.; Cha, B.S.; Song, Y.D.; Lim, S.K.; et al. beta-Cell dysfunction rather than insulin resistance is the main contributing factor for the development of postrenal transplantation diabetes mellitus. *Transplantation* **2001**, *71*, 1417–1423. [CrossRef] [PubMed]

27. Yasuda, K.; Miyake, K.; Horikawa, Y.; Hara, K.; Osawa, H.; Furuta, H.; Hirota, Y.; Mori, H.; Jonsson, A.; Sato, Y.; et al. Variants in KCNQ1 are associated with susceptibility to type 2 diabetes mellitus. *Nat. Genet.* **2008**, *40*, 1092–1097. [CrossRef] [PubMed]

28. Unoki, H.; Takahashi, A.; Kawaguchi, T.; Hara, K.; Horikoshi, M.; Andersen, G.; Ng, D.P.; Holmkvist, J.; Borch-Johnsen, K.; Jørgensen, T.; et al. SNPs in KCNQ1 are associated with susceptibility to type 2 diabetes in East Asian and European populations. *Nat. Genet.* **2008**, *40*, 1098–1102. [CrossRef]

29. Sladek, R.; Rocheleau, G.; Rung, J.; Dina, C.; Shen, L.; Serre, D.; Boutin, P.; Vincent, D.; Belisle, A.; Hadjadj, S.; et al. A genome-wide association study identifies novel risk loci for type 2 diabetes. *Nature* **2007**, *445*, 881–885. [CrossRef]

30. Saxena, R.; Voight, B.F.; Lyssenko, V.; Burtt, N.P.; de Bakker, P.I.; Chen, H.; Roix, J.J.; Kathiresan, S.; Hirschhorn, J.N.; Daly, M.J.; et al. Genome-wide association analysis identifies loci for type 2 diabetes and triglyceride levels. *Science* **2007**, *316*, 1331–1336.

31. Brambillasca, S.; Altkrueger, A.; Colombo, S.F.; Friederich, A.; Eickelmann, P.; Mark, M.; Borgese, N.; Solimena, M. CDK5 regulatory subunit-associated protein 1-like 1 (CDKAL1) is a tail-anchored protein in the endoplasmic reticulum (ER) of insulinoma cells. *J. Biol. Chem.* **2012**, *287*, 41808–41819. [CrossRef]

32. Nakajo, K. Gating modulation of the KCNQ1 channel by KCNE proteins studied by voltage-clamp fluorometry. *Biophys. Physicobiol.* **2019**, *16*, 121–126. [CrossRef] [PubMed]

33. Yamagata, K.; Senokuchi, T.; Lu, M.; Takemoto, M.; Fazlul Karim, M.; Go, C.; Sato, Y.; Hatta, M.; Yoshizawa, T.; Araki, E.; et al. Voltage-gated K+ channel KCNQ1 regulates insulin secretion in MIN6 β-cell line. *Biochem. Biophys. Res. Commun.* **2011**, *407*, 620–625. [CrossRef] [PubMed]

34. Liu, L.; Wang, F.; Lu, H.; Ren, X.; Zou, J. Chromanol 293B, an inhibitor of KCNQ1 channels, enhances glucose-stimulated insulin secretion and increases glucagon-like peptide-1 level in mice. *Islets* **2014**, *6*, e962386. [CrossRef] [PubMed]

35. Asahara, S.; Etoh, H.; Inoue, H.; Teruyama, K.; Shibutani, Y.; Ihara, Y.; Kawada, Y.; Bartolome, A.; Hashimoto, N.; Matsuda, T.; et al. Paternal allelic mutation at the Kcnq1 locus reduces pancreatic β-cell mass by epigenetic modification of Cdkn1c. *Proc. Natl. Acad. Sci. USA* **2015**, *112*, 8332–8337. [CrossRef] [PubMed]

36. Ensembl. Available online: http://asia.ensembl.org/Homo_sapiens/Variation/Population?db=core;v=rs2237892;vdb=variation#population_freq_EUR (accessed on 30 August 2019).

37. International Genetics & Translational Research in Transplantation Network (iGeneTRAiN). Design and Implementation of the International Genetics and Translational Research in Transplantation Network. *Transplantation* **2015**, *99*, 2401–2412. [CrossRef] [PubMed]

38. Todd, J.A.; Walker, N.M.; Cooper, J.D.; Smyth, D.J.; Downes, K.; Plagnol, V.; Bailey, R.; Nejentsev, S.; Field, S.F.; Payne, F.; et al. Robust associations of four new chromosome regions from genome-wide analyses of type 1 diabetes. *Nat. Genet.* **2007**, *39*, 857–864. [CrossRef]

39. Santiago, J.L.; Alizadeh, B.Z.; Martínez, A.; Espino, L.; de la Calle, H.; Fernández-Arquero, M.; Figueredo, M.A.; de la Concha, E.G.; Roep, B.O.; Koeleman, B.P.; et al. Study of the association between the CAPSL-IL7R locus and type 1 diabetes. *Diabetologia* **2008**, *51*, 1653–1658. [CrossRef]

6

Robot-Assisted versus Laparoscopic Donor Nephrectomy: A Comparison of 250 Cases

Philip Zeuschner [1], Linda Hennig [2], Robert Peters [2], Matthias Saar [1], Johannes Linxweiler [1], Stefan Siemer [1], Ahmed Magheli [3], Jürgen Kramer [3], Lutz Liefeldt [4], Klemens Budde [4], Thorsten Schlomm [2], Michael Stöckle [1,†] and Frank Friedersdorff [2,*,†]

[1] Department of Urology and Pediatric Urology, Saarland University, Kirrberger Street 100, 66421 Homburg/Saar, Germany; philip.zeuschner@uks.eu (P.Z.); matthias.saar@uks.eu (M.S.); johannes.linxweiler@uks.eu (J.L.); stefan.siemer@uks.eu (S.S.); michael.stoeckle@uks.eu (M.S.)

[2] Department of Urology, Charité-Universitätsmedizin Berlin, Corporate Member of Freie Universität Berlin, Humbold-Universität zu Berlin, and Berlin Institute of Health, Charitéplatz 1, 10117 Berlin, Germany; linda.hennig@charite.de (L.H.); robert.peters@charite.de (R.P.); thorsten.schlomm@charite.de (T.S.)

[3] Department of Urology, Klinikum am Urban, 10967 Berlin, Germany; ahmed.magheli@vivantes.de (A.M.); juergen.kramer@vivantes.de (J.K.)

[4] Department of Nephrology, Charité-Universitätsmedizin Berlin, Corporate Member of Freie Universität Berlin, Humbold-Universität zu Berlin, and Berlin Institute of Health, Charitéplatz 1, 10117 Berlin, Germany; lutz.liefeldt@charite.de (L.L.); klemens.budde@charite.de (K.B.)

* Correspondence: frank.friedersdorff@charite.de

† These authors contributed equally.

Abstract: Living kidney donation is the best treatment for end-stage renal disease, however, the best surgical approach for minimally-invasive donor nephrectomy (DN) is still a matter of debate. This bi-centric study aimed to retrospectively compare perioperative outcomes and postoperative kidney function after 257 transperitoneal DNs including 52 robot-assisted (RDN) and 205 laparoscopic DNs (LDN). As primary outcomes, the intraoperative (operating time, warm ischemia time (WIT), major complications) and postoperative (length of stay, complications) results were compared. As secondary outcomes, postoperative kidney and graft function were analyzed including delayed graft function (DGF) rates, and the impact of the surgical approach was assessed. Overall, the type of minimally-invasive donor nephrectomy (RDN vs. LDN) did not affect primary outcomes, especially not operating time and WIT; and major complication and DGF rates were low in both groups. A history of smoking and preoperative kidney function, but not the surgical approach, were predictive for postoperative serum creatinine of the donor and recipient. To conclude, RDN and LDN have equivalent perioperative results in experienced centers. For this reason, not the surgical approach, but rather the graft- (preoperative kidney function) and patient-specific (history of smoking) aspects impacted postoperative kidney function.

Keywords: minimally-invasive donor nephrectomy; robot-assisted surgery; laparoscopic surgery; kidney transplantation; organ donation; living kidney donation

1. Introduction

Living kidney donation is the ultimate treatment for end-stage renal disease (ESRD) [1]. Since the first successful living kidney donation in 1955 was carried out by Murray et al., many advances in surgical techniques and immunosuppressive therapy have led to substantial improvements in life expectancy and quality of life, not only for kidney recipients, but also for kidney donors [2]. In particular, minimally-invasive approaches for donor nephrectomy (DN) have increased the incidence of living kidney donation since the first laparoscopic DN (LDN) in 1995 and the first robot-assisted DN (RDN) in 2000 [3–5]. Unfortunately, higher donation rates have not been able to compensate for higher demand, which has led to at least 120,000 patients worldwide waiting for a kidney transplant today.

Many variations of minimally-invasive DN techniques have been described so far. Apart from hand-assisted methods as a bridge to open surgery, DN has also been performed in a retroperitoneoscopic (hand-assisted) manner [6,7]. In line with shorter flank incisions for open DN ("minimally invasive" open DN), Gill et al. conducted the first LDN via a LESS approach (laparoendoscopic single site surgery) in 2008 and inserted all trocars through the umbilicus [8,9]. Others have even tried to perform DN as a NOTES (natural orifice transluminal endoscopic surgery), and Pietrabissa et al. were the first to report a transvaginal extraction of the kidney after RDN in 2010 [10]. Today, some high-volume centers have performed more than 100 RDNs or LESS single-port RDNs, and employ specialized robotic single-site platforms [11,12]. However, the robotic approach still accounts for less than 5% of all minimally-invasive DNs, with increasing incidence compared to conventional transperitoneal LDN at more than 50% [13].

Irrespective of this magnitude of variations, minimally-invasive approaches for donor nephrectomy represent the standard of care, and are recommended as "the preferential technique", according to the current guidelines for renal transplantation of the European Association of Urology (EAU) [14,15]. Multiple studies have shown that LDN is superior to open DN (ODN) in terms of hospital stay or postoperative pain, but the operating and warm ischemia time (WIT) are longer [16]. Importantly, LDN is not inferior in terms of complication rates, short- and long-term graft function. On the other hand, when comparing LDN with the robotic approach, RDN appears to have even less postoperative pain and less blood loss, but a longer WIT and operating time [17]. Nonetheless, analyses of cohorts with big sample sizes are still lacking, and the high variability of minimally-invasive DN renders it difficult to draw direct conclusions.

With this in mind, we conducted a retrospective bi-centric comparison of transperitoneal LDN with RDN and included more than 250 interventions. We aimed to compare perioperative outcomes as well as short- and mid-term kidney function of the donor and recipient up to four years after surgery. Alongside sub-analyses controlling for inherent learning, regression analyses to predict postoperative kidney and graft function were performed. All LDNs were conducted at the largest German kidney transplant program run by a urologic department that has been performing LDNs since 1999. All RDNs including the very first RDN in Germany in 2007, were performed at a urologic department highly specialized in robotic surgery [18].

2. Materials and Methods

In total, 257 DNs performed at two tertiary referral centers were retrospectively analyzed. All 205 LDNs were conducted by 11 surgeons with a median caseload of 11 (range 2–43) at a urologic department specialized in laparoscopic kidney surgery including LDNs. The 52 RDNs were performed at another urologic department, which is specialized in robotic surgery in general. All RDNs were conducted by five surgeons with a median caseload of 10 (range 2–29). The interventions were performed in a transperitoneal fashion between 2007–2020 (RDN) and 2011–2016 (LDN).

At the robotic department, the very first RDN in Germany was conducted [18]. Before 2007, all donor nephrectomies had been held in an open fashion, so none of the robotic surgeons had prior expertise in LDN, but in a large variety of other robotic interventions. Thereafter, DN was standardized to a robot-assisted approach. The other department in this study has been performing LDNs since 1999. Both departments always conducted DNs in a minimally-invasive fashion during the study period, unless the donor had a significant amount of prior abdominal surgeries and consequently high risk for conversion. The corresponding kidney transplantations were held in an open fashion, except for the last 18 (34.6%) cases at the robotic department. As a part of the EAU-RAKT working group (European Association of Urology working group for robotic kidney transplantation), the first RAKT in Germany was performed there in June 2016 [19,20]. From then, all RDNs were followed by RAKTs.

This entire analysis was conducted in adherence with the correct scientific research work terms of the Charité Medical University of Berlin and Saarland University including full anonymization of patient data. All the patients included in the analysis provided written informed consent.

2.1. Surgical Technique

All RDNs were performed using a transperitoneal approach, with either a DaVinci® Si or X system with four arms. The ports were placed pararectally. For the first RDNs, the graft was removed in a hand-assisted manner without a specimen bag via a Pfannenstiel incision, and later on via a periumbilically placed GelPOINT® trocar (Applied Medical, Los Angeles, CA, USA). For LDN, the approach was purely laparoscopic, without the hand-assisted technique, which has been described previously [21,22]. In brief, four ports were used, and the kidney was extracted through an enlarged lateral trocar incision measuring 5 to 6 cm.

2.2. Data Collection and Outcome Measures

For the donor characteristics, age, gender, body mass index (BMI, kg/m^2), pre-existing arterial hypertension, diabetes, and history of smoking were obtained. The graft's side, scintigraphic split-renal function (DTPA), and number of arteries and veins served as organ-specific factors. For the recipient characteristics, age, gender, BMI, implantation side, and individual number of prior kidney transplantations were obtained.

Intraoperative (operating time, WIT, complications) and postoperative (length of stay, major postoperative complications based on Clavien–Dindo grade ≥3 within 30 days after surgery) results were analyzed as *primary outcomes*. The comparison and prediction of postoperative kidney function of the donor and of the recipient up to four years after transplantation served as *secondary outcomes*. Delayed graft function (DGF), defined as dialysis within one week after transplantation or insufficient serum creatinine decline not below 2 mg/dL, was analyzed as a further kidney-related secondary outcome.

2.3. Statistical Analysis

Primary and secondary outcomes were compared between the LDN and RDN group. To assess whether perioperative outcome was affected by an inherent learning curve, both groups were split in half and the outcomes were compared within each group. The first 34 (65.4%) RDNs were followed by an open transplantation, but the last 18 (34.6%) were followed by a robot-assisted kidney transplantation. To ensure that RAKT did not affect the perioperative results of RDN, the last 18 RDNs were excluded in another sub-analysis. The impact of patient-, graft- or surgery-specific factors on postoperative kidney function of the donor at discharge was assessed by linear regression analysis. To predict kidney function of the recipient one week after surgery, donor and recipient characteristics, DN, and transplantation-specific aspects were included in another uni- and multivariate regression analysis.

Categorical variables were reported as frequencies and proportions, and continuous data as the median and range. Fisher's exact test and the Mann–Whitney U test were used to compare between groups. Covariates were included in the multiple regression analysis only if their respective effect was significant in the univariate analysis. The statistical analysis was performed by SPSS version 25 with Fix pack 2 installed (IBM, Armonk, NY, USA). All tests were two-sided, and p-values < 0.05 were considered significant.

3. Results

3.1. Overall Results: Primary Outcomes

In the RDN and LDN groups, most kidney donors were female (63–68%), 51–54 years old, and had a BMI of 25.4–25.9 (see Table 1). Donor characteristics only differed concerning the individual history of smoking, as there were more smokers in the LDN group (52.7 vs. 9.6%, $p < 0.001$). Donor organs were 20% right-sided and had a split-renal function of 50%. The number of organs with multiple arteries was no different between RDN and LDN (11.5% vs. 18.5%), but significantly more grafts in the LDN group had multiple veins (12.7% vs. none, $p < 0.01$). The groups did not differ regarding recipient characteristics. Most were male (67–70%), 42–45 years old, and had a BMI of 24.7–25.3. For more than 90% of recipients, it was their first kidney transplantation.

Table 1. Comparison of donor, graft, and recipient characteristics.

	RDN ($n = 52$)	LDN ($n = 205$)	p-Value
donor			
age (yr)	54 (20; 70)	51 (21; 78)	n.s.
male gender	16 (30.8%)	75 (36.6%)	n.s.
BMI (kg/m^2)	25.4 (17.6; 36.7)	25.9 (17.6; 36.1)	n.s.
pre-existing hypertension	15 (28.8%)	44 (21.5%)	n.s.
diabetes	1 (1.9%)	3 (1.5%)	n.s.
history of smoking	5 (9.6%)	108 (52.7%)	<0.001
graft			
right side	11 (21.2%)	45 (22%)	n.s.
multiple arteries	6 (11.5%)	38 (18.5%)	n.s.
multiple veins	0	26 (12.7%)	<0.01
scintigraphic function	50% (39; 57)	50% (38; 58)	n.s.
recipient			
age (yr)	42 (18; 66)	45 (6; 76)	n.s.
male gender	35 (67.3%)	144 (70.2%)	n.s.
BMI (kg/m^2)	25.1 (17.6; 37)	24.7 (16.8; 40.8)	n.s.
side left	8 (15.4%)	46 (22.4%)	n.s.
first transplantation	48 (92.3%)	187 (91.2%)	n.s.

Concerning primary outcomes, neither the median operating time (RDN 223.5 vs. LDN 213 min), WIT (3 vs. 2.45 min), nor intraoperative complication rate (5.7 vs. 2.9%) were significantly different between groups (see Table 2). One RDN had to be converted to open surgery because of massive obesity and multiple trocar dislocations. In two other cases, a malfunction of the stapler and a lumbal vein caused bleeding, which could be managed robotically without the need for blood transfusions. In the LDN group, in one case, bleeding from a dorsal branch of the renal vein could not be controlled laparoscopically, leading to a conversion to open surgery. In another LDN case, the renal vein was torn during kidney removal, but could be reconstructed. Once, the donor's spleen and the renal parenchyma were accidentally cut, and a small hole in the descending colon had to be sutured. A previously undetected obstructed ureteropelvic junction made one pyelovesicostomy necessary for a recipient in the LDN group.

The median length of stay of five days was no different between the LDN and RDN groups, nor was the postoperative major complication rate. In the RDN group, one patient had an ileus that dissolved after gastroscopy. In the LDN group, a bronchoscopy had to be performed because of dyspnea, and a retention of chylous ascites had to be punctured. In another case, continuous arterial bleeding from the abdominal internal oblique muscle made electrocoagulation necessary in the LDN group.

3.2. Learning Curve

When comparing the first half of the RDNs with the second half to analyze for inherent learning effects, the WIT, intra- and postoperative complication rate, and length of stay remained unchanged (see Table 3). Operating time significantly increased from 185 to 265 min in the RDN group ($p < 0.001$). This difference no longer remained significant when the last 18 RDN cases were excluded; in these cases, RDN was followed by robot-assisted kidney transplantation (185 vs. 226 min, n.s.). In the LDN group, the surgical results remained unchanged over time.

Table 2. Outcomes of 257 donor nephrectomies.

	RDN (*n* = 52)	LDN (*n* = 205)	*p*-Value
Intraoperative			
operating time (min)	223.5 (127; 363)	213 (120; 392)	n.s.
WIT (min)	3 (0.5; 1)	2.45 (0.4; 5.27)	n.s.
complications	3 (5.7%)	6 (2.9%)	n.s.
conversions	1 (1.9%)	1 (0.5%)	n.s.
postoperative			
length of stay (d)	5 (2; 12)	5 (3; 18)	n.s.
Clavien–Dindo			n.s.
grade 3	1 (1.9%)	1 (0.5%)	n.s.
grade 4	-	2 (1%)	n.s.
grade 5	-	-	n.s.
recipient			
DGF	6 (11.5%)	13 (6.3%)	n.s.

Table 3. Assessment for the inherent learning curves in RDN and LDN by comparing the first with the second half of cases within each group.

	RDN			LDN		
	1st half (*n* = 26)	2nd half (*n* = 26)	*p*	1st half (*n* = 102)	2nd half (*n* = 103)	*p*
Intraoperative						
operating time	185 (148; 284)	265 (127; 363)	<0.001 [1]	213 (135; 392)	216 (120; 363)	n.s.
WIT (min)	3 (0.5; 9)	2 (1; 10)	n.s.	2.4 (0.4; 5)	2.5 (0.5; 5.2)	n.s.
complications	2 (7.7%)	1 (3.8%)	n.s.	3 (2.9%)	3 (2.9%)	n.s.
conversions	1 (3.8%)	-	n.s.	-	1 (0.9%)	n.s.
postoperative						
length of stay (d)	5 (3–12)	5 (2–7)	n.s.	5 (3; 18)	5 (3; 11)	n.s.
Clavien–Dindo	0 (0; 2)	0 (0)	n.s.	0 (0; 4)	0 (0; 4)	n.s.
grade 3	1 (3.8%)	-	n.s.	1 (1%)	-	n.s.
grade 4	-	-	n.s.	1 (1%)	1 (1%)	n.s.
grade 5	-	-	n.s.	-	-	n.s.
recipient						
DGF	4 (15.4%)	2 (7.7%)	n.s.	6 (5.9%)	7 (6.8%)	n.s.

[1] When excluding the last 18 cases, where RDN was followed by robot-assisted kidney transplantation, the difference was no longer significant (185 vs. 226 min, n.s.).

3.3. Kidney Function of the Donor and Recipient: Secondary Outcomes

The type of surgical approach of DN did not impact the postoperative kidney function either of the donor or the recipient (see Figure 1). Among the donors, kidney function did not differ preoperatively or at discharge between groups. For recipients, kidney function significantly improved after transplantation, irrespective of the type of DN, and stayed stable thereafter.

DGF rates were 6.3 to 11.5% (LDN vs. RDN), and did not significantly differ between groups and did not change over time (see Tables 2 and 3). In the RDN group, DGF was caused by three (5.7%) suspected transplant renal artery stenoses, one (1.9%) perirenal hematoma due to double anticoagulation of the mechanic aortic valve and prolonged serum creatinine decline (no dialysis needed), one (1.9%) prolonged CIT (cold ischemia time) due to vascular complications during transplantation, and one (1.9%) insufficient serum creatinine decline without other cause. In the LDN group, DGF resulted from seven (3.4%) acute rejections, one (0.5%) lesion of the arterial anastomosis after the Fogarty maneuver, and one (0.5%) case of donor-related pre-existing vascular damage. One (0.5%) patient needed dialysis for depletion of potassium only, and in three (1.5%) other cases, the cause for DGF in the LDN group was unknown.

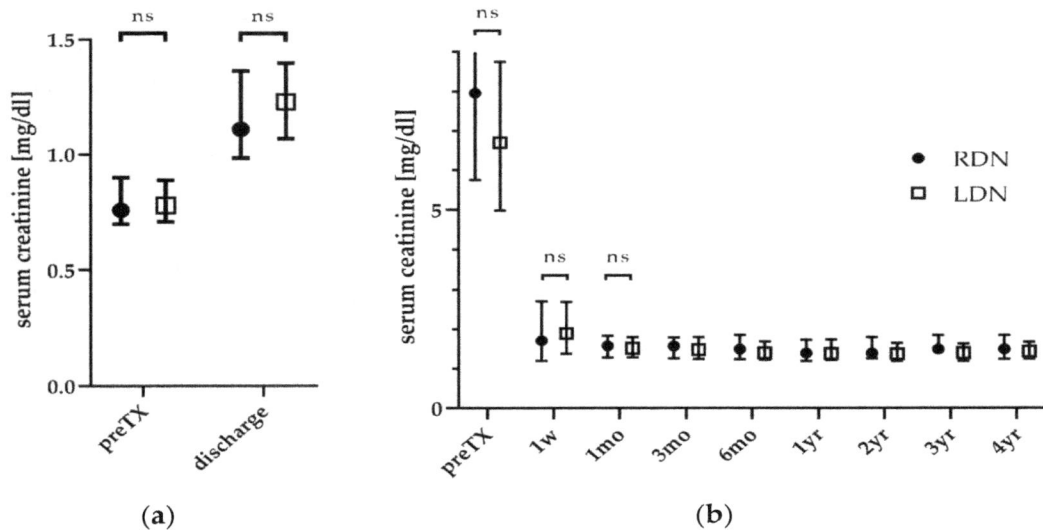

Figure 1. Follow-up of kidney function of the donor (**a**) and graft (**b**). The kidney function did not differ between robot-assisted (RDN) and laparoscopic donor nephrectomy (LDN).

In the multivariate regression analysis, only patient-specific factors were found to have an impact on postoperative kidney function, but not surgical factors (see Table 4). Concerning the kidney function of the donor at discharge, male patient gender was predictive for worse kidney function (*B*-value 0.14, $p < 0.001$). Furthermore, worse preoperative kidney function was associated with worse postoperative function (*B*-value 1.0, $p < 0.001$). A history of smoking only had an impact on postoperative kidney function in the univariate analysis. No other (surgical) factors such as approach (LDN vs. RDN), operating time, intraoperative complications, WIT, kidney side, or number of arteries or veins, had an impact on the kidney function of the donor at discharge.

Table 4. Multivariable regression analysis to predict the serum creatinine (1) of the donor at discharge ("donor kidney function") or (2) of the recipient one week after transplantation ("graft function").

Variable	*B*-Value	*p*-Value
donor kidney function		
gender	0.14 (0.09; 0.19)	<0.001
preTX serum creatinine	1.00 (0.82; 1.18)	<0.001
surgical approach	-	n.s.
graft function		
smoking donor	0.63 (1.21; 0.05)	<0.05
preemptive Tx	-	n.s.
preTX serum creatinine	0.22 (0.12; 0.31)	<0.001
surgical approach	-	n.s.

A history of donor smoking also had a significant impact on the kidney function of the recipient in the multivariate regression analysis: a kidney donor with a history of smoking caused worse graft function one week after transplantation (*B*-value 0.63, $p < 0.05$, see Table 4). Again, the preoperative kidney function of the recipient was predictive for their postoperative graft function (*B*-value 0.22, $p < 0.001$). In the univariate, but not the multivariate analysis, a preemptive kidney transplantation predicted better graft function (*B*-value −0.72, *p* < 0.05). Again, no surgical factors, either the type of donor nephrectomy (LDN vs. RDN) or the type of transplantation (open vs. robot-assisted), had an impact on graft function one week after transplantation.

4. Discussion

In this bi-centric study, a comparison of 257 minimally-invasive donor nephrectomies with 205 laparoscopic and 52 robot-assisted DNs was conducted. Of note, this analysis included the very first RDN in Germany, and all LDNs were performed at a urologic department where LDNs have been conducted since 1999 [18].

Concerning the primary outcomes, operating time was no different between RDN and LDN (223.5 vs. 213 min, see Table 1). Most studies describe shorter operating times for LDNs, but report highly variable results [17]. Mean operating times for RDNs range from 144 to 306 min [23,24], and for LDNs between 178 and 270 min [25,26], even when only studies with cohorts larger than 100 patients are included. These differences could result from inherent learning curves: Horgan et al. and Janki et al. have shown that operating times in RDN shorten with growing expertise [27,28]. Interestingly, our data do not show an inherent learning effect, either in the RDN or in the LDN cohort. Outcomes remained unchanged over time (see Table 3). Conversely, operating time became significantly longer within the second half of the RDNs (185 vs. 265 min, *p* < 0.001).

This counterintuitive development resulted from the way transplantations were organized, as both institutions perform DNs and transplantations in different operating rooms simultaneously, but not sequentially. Two surgical teams work in parallel, but the graft is not removed unless the transplantation team is ready, to avoid long cold ischemia times. The RDN cohort not only comprised the first RDN, but also the first robot-assisted kidney transplantation in Germany (procedure #35) [18,20]. Operating times in the RDN cohort became longer from that point, as the learning curve for RAKTs had not yet been passed. Naturally, the RDN team started more than 30 min before the transplantation team, but RAKT proved to be much more challenging and time-consuming. When excluding the last 18 cases, when RDN was followed by RAKT, the operating times of the RDNs did not change over time. Thus, the obvious lack of a typical learning curve illustrates that for LDNs, the learning curve had already been passed and for RDNs, significant prior expertise in robotic surgery made it possible to reach stable results from the start [29].

As with the operating time, WIT was not different between RDNs and LDNs (3 vs. 2.45 min). In the RDNs, most grafts were extracted via a GelPOINT® trocar (Applied Medical, Los Angeles, CA, USA), which is an easy and fast, yet expensive method. Wang et al. illustrated significantly longer WIT for RDNs than LDNs in their meta-analysis, which is an often-stated argument against RDNs [17,30]. However, it is unlikely that differences of 30 or 60 s in WIT will harm the graft function in the long-, mid- or even short-term. It has clearly been shown that a WIT longer than 45 min impairs graft survival in living kidney donation [31]. Fortunately, neither our results nor those from other studies have documented WIT longer than 15 min for RDNs, keeping in mind that the consecutive CIT is again followed by another WIT during transplantation.

Intraoperative complication rates were low in both RDNs (5.7%) and LDNs (2.9%), and did not significantly differ. In line with others, most intraoperative complications were bleedings, whereof one in the LDN group made a conversion to open surgery necessary, but none in the RDN group [17]. In contrast, a patient with massive obesity had multiple trocar dislocations within the first minutes of surgery, so the RDN had to be converted to open surgery. Due to a technical defect of the stapler system for one patient in the RDN group, which made it cut but not staple, locking Hem-o-Lok clips were predominantly used later on, as described elsewhere [32]. During LDNs, Hem-o-Lok and titanium clips are used for the renal artery, a stapler for the right vein, and two Hem-o-Lok clips for the left vein. Not only intraoperative but also postoperative complication rates, according to Clavien–Dindo, were low and did not differ between LDN and RDN. Therefore, both surgical approaches had equivalent complication rates, while LDN has less costs, but RDN appears to be superior in complex situations such as bleedings.

The kidney donors were discharged five days after DN, irrespective of the type of surgery (see Table 2). Consequently, the median length of stay was longer than in most other works, ranging from 2–3 days for LDNs and RDNs [11,17,24]. This can be attributed to differences in national health care systems as (i) the German reimbursement system covers a longer hospital stay and (ii) most donors wanted to stay longer as inpatients for psychological reasons. In fact, only 15 (5.8%) patients were discharged two or three days after DN. Early discharge after RDN and LDN is possible from a surgical point of view, however, it has not been a crucial parameter for our perioperative approach, as long as neither patient satisfaction nor health care costs are affected.

As a secondary outcome, the impact of the surgical approach on postoperative kidney function was assessed. Kidney donors had a worse kidney function at discharge, which was comparable between groups and similar to results found in other studies (RDN 1.1 mg/dL vs. LDN 1.23 mg/dL; see Figure 1) [28,33]. Correspondingly, the preoperative kidney function, but not the type of surgical approach for DN, was predictive for the postoperative kidney function of the donor at discharge (see Table 4). Interestingly, patient gender also had a significant impact on postoperative kidney function. However, this should not be over-interpreted, as male kidney donors had a worse kidney function than women, with higher serum creatinine values preoperatively (0.9 vs. 0.72 mg/dL, $p < 0.001$) and postoperatively (1.42 vs. 1.1 mg/dL, $p < 0.001$) in this analysis. For this reason, (male) patient gender was predictive for (worse) postoperative kidney function; this may not be representative for other cohorts.

Similarly, Benoit et al. created a model to predict 1-year postoperative renal function of kidney donors after LDN, which has been externally validated [34,35]. The authors predicted postoperative eGFR by preoperative eGFR and patient age (postoperative eGFR = 31.71 + (0.5 × preoperative eGFR) − 0.314 × age at donation). In our model, patient age was not predictive for postoperative kidney function, potentially because we evaluated the short-term kidney function at discharge and not one year after DN.

Concerning recipients, the DGF rates of 6.3% (LDN) and 11.5% (RDN) did not significantly differ between groups. In general, there is a large variety of reported DGF rates in living kidney donation, ranging from 4 to 10% [36,37]. This not only results from center-specific differences, but also from inconsistent definitions: DGF can be defined by urine output per day, serum creatinine decline, or the need for dialysis after transplantation [36]. We applied a considerably broad definition for DGF (postoperative dialysis within one week after transplantation for any cause or insufficient creatinine decrease not below 2 mg/dL). DGF rates in the RDN group were 11.5% due to transplantation-related surgical, mainly vascular causes. One (1.9%) patient with a mechanic aortic valve developed a perirenal hematoma, causing prolonged creatinine decline without the need for dialysis. In the LDN group, DGF was mainly caused by acute rejections (3.4%), and also comprised one patient (0.5%) who required dialysis for potassium depletion only. Consequently, DGF did not result from the type of DN, but rather transplantation-specific causes.

Regardless, the kidney function of the recipients significantly improved after transplantation, and did not differ between groups during follow-up (see Figure 1). In the multiple regression analysis, not only the preoperative kidney function of the recipient, but also a history of donor smoking, had a significant impact on graft function one week after transplantation (see Table 4). Smoking is a well-known modifiable risk factor for the development of chronic and end-stage kidney disease [38,39]. A history of donor smoking has a negative impact not only on the survival of the donor, but also of the recipient [40]. In our cohort, a positive history of donor smoking increased serum creatinine one week after transplantation by 0.63 mg/dL. This highlights, again, the importance of informing not only transplant patients, but also potential kidney donors, about the risks of tobacco use, and the importance of helping patients to stop smoking.

This analysis is not devoid of limitations. As a bi-centric study, experienced but different surgeons and different teams conducted the RDNs and LDNs. Patient cohorts did not significantly differ in terms of characteristics, but were not equally balanced in terms of caseload. Although surgical results were not affected by inherent learning curves, at least the results in the RDN group were affected by simultaneous robot-assisted kidney transplantation. This procedural aspect highlights the complexity of comparing minimally-invasive donor nephrectomies: the surgical part itself is in high demand, but the high variability of the technical, procedural, and underlying ethical aspects also have to be taken into account [41].

5. Conclusions

Minimally-invasive surgical techniques have increased the acceptance of living kidney donation, but its high variability renders head-to-head comparisons of surgical approaches a complex task. In this bi-centric study, we compared more than 250 cases of 52 transperitoneal robotic DNs with 205 laparoscopic DNs. Operating time and length of stay were no different between groups, but slightly longer than elsewhere, as DNs and transplantations were conducted simultaneously to reduce CIT, and most other national health systems do not allow longer inpatient stays. Other perioperative results (complication rates, WIT) and mid-term kidney function including DGF rates were comparable with published data, and did not differ between RDN and LDN. This was possible because both centers already had prior expertise in either LDN itself or robotic surgery in general. For this reason, patient-specific factors (preoperative kidney function, history of donor smoking) were the more relevant impacts upon donor and graft function.

Author Contributions: P.Z., F.F., and M.S. (Michael Stöckle) designed the study; P.Z. analyzed the data and wrote the manuscript; L.H., R.P., M.S. (Matthias Saar), J.L., S.S., A.M., J.K., L.L., K.B., T.S., F.F., and M.S. (Michael Stöckle) drafted and revised the paper. All authors approved the final version of the manuscript.

Acknowledgments: We would like to thank the working group for kidney transplantation ("Arbeitskreis Nierentransplantation", https://www.nieren-transplantation.com/) of the German Association of Urology for initiating this bi-centric work.

References

1. Shapiro, R. End-stage renal disease in 2010: Innovative approaches to improve outcomes in transplantation. *Nat. Rev. Nephrol.* **2011**, *7*, 68–70. [CrossRef] [PubMed]
2. Murray, J.E.; Merrill, J.P.; Harrison, J.H. Renal homotransplantation in identical twins. *J. Am. Soc. Nephrol. JASN* **2001**, *12*, 201–204. [PubMed]
3. Schweitzer, E.J.; Wilson, J.; Jacobs, S.; Machan, C.H.; Philosophe, B.; Farney, A.; Colonna, J.; Jarrell, B.E.; Bartlett, S.T. Increased rates of donation with laparoscopic donor nephrectomy. *Ann. Surg.* **2000**, *232*, 392–400. [CrossRef] [PubMed]
4. Ratner, L.E.; Ciseck, L.J.; Moore, R.G.; Cigarroa, F.G.; Kaufman, H.S.; Kavoussi, L.R. Laparoscopic live donor nephrectomy. *Transplantation* **1995**, *60*, 1047–1049.
5. Pfaffl, M.W.; Horgan, G.W.; Dempfle, L. Relative expression software tool (REST) for group-wise comparison and statistical analysis of relative expression results in real-time PCR. *Nucleic Acids Res.* **2002**, *30*, e36. [CrossRef]
6. Wolf, J.S., Jr.; Tchetgen, M.B.; Merion, R.M. Hand-assisted laparoscopic live donor nephrectomy. *Urology* **1998**, *52*, 885–887. [CrossRef]
7. Wadstrom, J.; Lindstrom, P. Hand-assisted retroperitoneoscopic living-donor nephrectomy: Initial 10 cases. *Transplantation* **2002**, *73*, 1839–1840. [CrossRef]
8. Gill, I.S.; Canes, D.; Aron, M.; Haber, G.P.; Goldfarb, D.A.; Flechner, S.; Desai, M.R.; Kaouk, J.H.; Desai, M.M. Single port transumbilical (E-NOTES) donor nephrectomy. *J. Urol.* **2008**, *180*, 637–641, discussion 641. [CrossRef]

9. Janki, S.; Dor, F.J.; JN, I.J. Surgical aspects of live kidney donation: An updated review. *Front. Biosci.* **2015**, *7*, 346–365. [CrossRef]

10. Pietrabissa, A.; Abelli, M.; Spinillo, A.; Alessiani, M.; Zonta, S.; Ticozzelli, E.; Peri, A.; Dal Canton, A.; Dionigi, P. Robotic-assisted laparoscopic donor nephrectomy with transvaginal extraction of the kidney. *Am. J. Transplant.* **2010**, *10*, 2708–2711. [CrossRef]

11. LaMattina, J.C.; Alvarez-Casas, J.; Lu, I.; Powell, J.M.; Sultan, S.; Phelan, M.W.; Barth, R.N. Robotic-assisted single-port donor nephrectomy using the da Vinci single-site platform. *J. Surg. Res.* **2018**, *222*, 34–38. [CrossRef] [PubMed]

12. Tzvetanov, I.; Bejarano-Pineda, L.; Giulianotti, P.C.; Jeon, H.; Garcia-Roca, R.; Bianco, F.; Oberholzer, J.; Benedetti, E. State of the art of robotic surgery in organ transplantation. *World J. Surg.* **2013**, *37*, 2791–2799. [CrossRef] [PubMed]

13. Kortram, K.; Ijzermans, J.N.; Dor, F.J. Perioperative Events and Complications in Minimally Invasive Live Donor Nephrectomy: A Systematic Review and Meta-Analysis. *Transplantation* **2016**, *100*, 2264–2275. [CrossRef] [PubMed]

14. Abramowicz, D.; Cochat, P.; Claas, F.H.; Heemann, U.; Pascual, J.; Dudley, C.; Harden, P.; Hourmant, M.; Maggiore, U.; Salvadori, M.; et al. European Renal Best Practice Guideline on kidney donor and recipient evaluation and perioperative care. *Nephrol. Dial. Transplant.* **2015**, *30*, 1790–1797. [CrossRef]

15. Breda, A.; Budde, K.; Figueiredo, A.; Lledó García, E.; Olsburgh, J.; Regele, H.; Boissier, R.; Taylor, C.F.; Hevia, V.; Faba, O.R.; et al. *EAU Guidelines on Renal Transplantation*; EAU Guidelines Office: Arnhem, The Netherlands, 2020; ISBN 978-94-92671-07-3.

16. Wilson, C.H.; Sanni, A.; Rix, D.A.; Soomro, N.A. Laparoscopic versus open nephrectomy for live kidney donors. *Cochrane Database Syst. Rev.* **2011**, CD006124. [CrossRef] [PubMed]

17. Wang, H.; Chen, R.; Li, T.; Peng, L. Robot-assisted laparoscopic vs laparoscopic donor nephrectomy in renal transplantation: A meta-analysis. *Clin. Transplant.* **2019**, *33*, e13451. [CrossRef] [PubMed]

18. Janssen, M.S.U.; Kopper, B.; Gerber, M.; Ohlmann, C.-H.; Akcetin, Z.; Kamradt, D.; Siemer, S.; Stöckle, M. Lectures: 088 Robotic-assisted donor nephrectomy for living donor kidney transplantation—Results of the first series in Germany. *Transplant. Int.* **2011**, *24*, 3–24. [CrossRef]

19. Territo, A.; Gausa, L.; Alcaraz, A.; Musquera, M.; Doumerc, N.; Decaestecker, K.; Desender, L.; Stockle, M.; Janssen, M.; Fornara, P.; et al. European experience of robot-assisted kidney transplantation: Minimum of 1-year follow-up. *BJU Int.* **2018**, *122*, 255–262. [CrossRef] [PubMed]

20. Zeuschner, P.; Siemer, S.; Stockle, M. Robot-assisted kidney transplantation. *Urol. A* **2020**, *59*, 3–9. [CrossRef] [PubMed]

21. Turk, I.A.; Deger, S.; Davis, J.W.; Giesing, M.; Fabrizio, M.D.; Schonberger, B.; Jordan, G.H.; Loening, S.A. Laparoscopic live donor right nephrectomy: A new technique with preservation of vascular length. *J. Urol.* **2002**, *167*, 630–633. [CrossRef]

22. Giessing, M.; Deger, S.; Schonberger, B.; Turk, I.; Loening, S.A. Laparoscopic living donor nephrectomy: From alternative to standard procedure. *Transplant. Proc.* **2003**, *35*, 2093–2095. [CrossRef]

23. Cohen, A.J.; Williams, D.S.; Bohorquez, H.; Bruce, D.S.; Carmody, I.C.; Reichman, T.; Loss, G.E., Jr. Robotic-assisted laparoscopic donor nephrectomy: Decreasing length of stay. *Ochsner J.* **2015**, *15*, 19–24. [PubMed]

24. Serrano, O.K.; Kirchner, V.; Bangdiwala, A.; Vock, D.M.; Dunn, T.B.; Finger, E.B.; Payne, W.D.; Pruett, T.L.; Sutherland, D.E.; Najarian, J.S.; et al. Evolution of Living Donor Nephrectomy at a Single Center: Long-term Outcomes With 4 Different Techniques in Greater Than 4000 Donors Over 50 Years. *Transplantation* **2016**, *100*, 1299–1305. [CrossRef] [PubMed]

25. Basiri, A.; Simforoosh, N.; Heidari, M.; Moghaddam, S.M.; Otookesh, H. Laparoscopic v open donor nephrectomy for pediatric kidney recipients: Preliminary report of a randomized controlled trial. *J. Endourol.* **2007**, *21*, 1033–1036. [CrossRef] [PubMed]

26. Simforoosh, N.; Basiri, A.; Tabibi, A.; Shakhssalim, N.; Hosseini Moghaddam, S.M. Comparison of laparoscopic and open donor nephrectomy: A randomized controlled trial. *BJU Int.* **2005**, *95*, 851–855. [CrossRef] [PubMed]

27. Horgan, S.; Galvani, C.; Gorodner, M.V.; Jacobsen, G.R.; Moser, F.; Manzelli, A.; Oberholzer, J.; Fisichella, M.P.; Bogetti, D.; Testa, G.; et al. Effect of robotic assistance on the "learning curve" for laparoscopic hand-assisted donor nephrectomy. *Surg. Endosc.* **2007**, *21*, 1512–1517. [CrossRef] [PubMed]

28. Janki, S.; Klop, K.W.J.; Hagen, S.M.; Terkivatan, T.; Betjes, M.G.H.; Tran, T.C.K.; Ijzermans, J.N.M. Robotic surgery rapidly and successfully implemented in a high volume laparoscopic center on living kidney donation. *Int. J. Med. Robot.* **2017**, *13*. [CrossRef]

29. Friedersdorff, F.; Werthemann, P.; Cash, H.; Kempkensteffen, C.; Magheli, A.; Hinz, S.; Waiser, J.; Liefeldt, L.; Miller, K.; Deger, S.; et al. Outcomes after laparoscopic living donor nephrectomy: Comparison of two laparoscopic surgeons with different levels of expertise. *BJU Int.* **2013**, *111*, 95–100. [CrossRef]

30. Kawan, F.; Theil, G.; Fornara, P. Robotic Donor Nephrectomy: Against. *Eur. Urol. Focus* **2018**, *4*, 142–143. [CrossRef]

31. Hellegering, J.; Visser, J.; Kloke, H.J.; D'Ancona, F.C.; Hoitsma, A.J.; van der Vliet, J.A.; Warle, M.C. Deleterious influence of prolonged warm ischemia in living donor kidney transplantation. *Transplant. Proc.* **2012**, *44*, 1222–1226. [CrossRef]

32. Brunotte, M.; Rademacher, S.; Weber, J.; Sucher, E.; Lederer, A.; Hau, H.-M.; Stolzenburg, J.-U.; Seehofer, D.; Sucher, R. Robotic assisted nephrectomy for living kidney donation (RANLD) with use of multiple locking clips or ligatures for renal vascular closure. *Ann. Transl. Med.* **2020**, *8*, 305. [CrossRef] [PubMed]

33. Luke, P.P.; Aquil, S.; Alharbi, B.; Sharma, H.; Sener, A. First Canadian experience with robotic laparoendoscopic single-site vs. standard laparoscopic living-donor nephrectomy: A prospective comparative study. *Can. Urol. Assoc. J.* **2018**, *12*, E440–E446. [CrossRef] [PubMed]

34. Benoit, T.; Game, X.; Roumiguie, M.; Sallusto, F.; Doumerc, N.; Beauval, J.B.; Rischmann, P.; Kamar, N.; Soulie, M.; Malavaud, B. Predictive model of 1-year postoperative renal function after living donor nephrectomy. *Int. Urol. Nephrol.* **2017**, *49*, 793–801. [CrossRef] [PubMed]

35. Kulik, U.; Gwiasda, J.; Oldhafer, F.; Kaltenborn, A.; Arelin, V.; Gueler, F.; Richter, N.; Klempnauer, J.; Schrem, H. External validation of a proposed prognostic model for the prediction of 1-year postoperative eGFR after living donor nephrectomy. *Int. Urol. Nephrol.* **2017**, *49*, 1937–1940. [CrossRef]

36. Perico, N.; Cattaneo, D.; Sayegh, M.H.; Remuzzi, G. Delayed graft function in kidney transplantation. *Lancet* **2004**, *364*, 1814–1827. [CrossRef]

37. Narayanan, R.; Cardella, C.J.; Cattran, D.C.; Cole, E.H.; Tinckam, K.J.; Schiff, J.; Kim, S.J. Delayed graft function and the risk of death with graft function in living donor kidney transplant recipients. *Am. J. Kidney Dis.* **2010**, *56*, 961–970. [CrossRef]

38. Xia, J.; Wang, L.; Ma, Z.; Zhong, L.; Wang, Y.; Gao, Y.; He, L.; Su, X. Cigarette smoking and chronic kidney disease in the general population: A systematic review and meta-analysis of prospective cohort studies. *Nephrol. Dial. Transplant.* **2017**, *32*, 475–487. [CrossRef]

39. Orth, S.R.; Hallan, S.I. Smoking: A risk factor for progression of chronic kidney disease and for cardiovascular morbidity and mortality in renal patients–absence of evidence or evidence of absence? *Clin. J. Am. Soc. Nephrol.* **2008**, *3*, 226–236. [CrossRef]

40. Aref, A.; Sharma, A.; Halawa, A. Smoking in Renal Transplantation; Facts beyond Myth. *World J. Transplant.* **2017**, *7*, 129–133. [CrossRef]

41. Ahlawat, R.K.; Jindal, T. Robotic Donor Nephrectomy: The Right Way Forward. *Eur. Urol. Focus* **2018**, *4*, 140–141. [CrossRef]

7

Urinary Excretion of N^1-Methylnicotinamide, as a Biomarker of Niacin Status, and Mortality in Renal Transplant Recipients

Carolien P.J. Deen [1,2,3,*], Anna van der Veen [2], Martijn van Faassen [2], Isidor Minović [2],
António W. Gomes-Neto [1,4], Johanna M. Geleijnse [5], Karin J. Borgonjen-van den Berg [5],
Ido P. Kema [2] and Stephan J.L. Bakker [1,3,4]

[1] Department of Internal Medicine, University of Groningen, University Medical Center Groningen,
9713 GZ Groningen, The Netherlands; a.w.gomes.neto@umcg.nl (A.W.G.-N.); s.j.l.bakker@umcg.nl (S.J.L.B.)
[2] Department of Laboratory Medicine, University of Groningen, University Medical Center Groningen,
9713 GZ Groningen, The Netherlands; a.van.der.veen03@umcg.nl (A.v.d.V.);
h.j.r.van.faassen@umcg.nl (M.v.F.); i.minovic@umcg.nl (I.M.); i.p.kema@umcg.nl (I.P.K.)
[3] Top Institute Food and Nutrition, 6709 PA Wageningen, The Netherlands
[4] TransplantLines Food and Nutrition Biobank and Cohort Study, University of Groningen,
University Medical Center Groningen, 9713 GZ Groningen, The Netherlands
[5] Division of Human Nutrition and Health, Wageningen University, 6708 PB Wageningen, The Netherlands;
marianne.geleijnse@wur.nl (J.M.G.); karin.borgonjen@wur.nl (K.J.B.-v.d.B.)
* Correspondence: c.p.j.deen@umcg.nl

Abstract: Renal transplant recipients (RTR) commonly suffer from vitamin B_6 deficiency and its functional consequences add to an association with poor long-term outcome. It is unknown whether niacin status is affected in RTR and, if so, whether this affects clinical outcomes, as vitamin B_6 is a cofactor in nicotinamide biosynthesis. We compared 24-h urinary excretion of N^1-methylnicotinamide (N^1-MN) as a biomarker of niacin status in RTR with that in healthy controls, in relation to dietary intake of tryptophan and niacin as well as vitamin B_6 status, and investigated whether niacin status is associated with the risk of premature all-cause mortality in RTR. In a prospective cohort of 660 stable RTR with a median follow-up of 5.4 (4.7–6.1) years and 275 healthy kidney donors, 24-h urinary excretion of N^1-MN was measured with liquid chromatography-tandem mass spectrometry LC-MS/MS. Dietary intake was assessed by food frequency questionnaires. Prospective associations of N^1-MN excretion with mortality were investigated by Cox regression analyses. Median N^1-MN excretion was 22.0 (15.8–31.8) μmol/day in RTR, compared to 41.1 (31.6–57.2) μmol/day in healthy kidney donors ($p < 0.001$). This difference was independent of dietary intake of tryptophan (1059 ± 271 and 1089 ± 308 mg/day; $p = 0.19$), niacin (17.9 ± 5.2 and 19.2 ± 6.2 mg/day; $p < 0.001$), plasma vitamin B_6 (29.0 (17.5–49.5), and 42.0 (29.8–60.3) nmol/L; $p < 0.001$), respectively. N^1-MN excretion was inversely associated with the risk of all-cause mortality in RTR (HR 0.57; 95% CI 0.45–0.71; $p < 0.001$), independent of potential confounders. RTR excrete less N^1-MN in 24-h urine than healthy controls, and our data suggest that this difference cannot be attributed to lower dietary intake of tryptophan and niacin, nor vitamin B_6 status. Importantly, lower 24-h urinary excretion of N^1-MN is independently associated with a higher risk of premature all-cause mortality in RTR.

Keywords: urinary excretion of N^1-methylnicotinamide; kidney transplantation; mortality; niacin status; dietary intake; tryptophan; vitamin B_3

1. Introduction

Kidney transplantation is the preferred treatment for end-stage renal disease in terms of survival, quality of life and costs [1,2]. Advances in transplantation medicine have lifted the 1-year patient survival higher than 90% [3]. While short-term patient outcomes are continuing to improve, the long-term posttransplant survival has remained largely unchanged over the past few decades [4]. Compared with the general population, renal transplant recipients (RTR) are at highly increased risk of premature mortality [5]. Improving perspectives relies on the management of modifiable factors that impact long-term outcome in RTR, of which nutrition is increasingly acknowledged [6,7].

Recently, we found that RTR commonly suffer from vitamin B_6 deficiency and its functional consequences that add to an association with poor long-term outcomes [8]. As vitamin B_6 is an essential cofactor of key enzymes involved in de novo biosynthesis of nicotinamide from tryptophan [9], niacin deficiency might be lurking in these patients as well. Nicotinamide, nicotinic acid, and nicotinamide riboside are collectively referred to as niacin or vitamin B_3, and are precursors of the metabolically active NAD^+. Besides dietary intake of pre-formed niacin, the so-called tryptophan-nicotinamide pathway is critical to maintaining niacin status [10]. Ongoing NAD^+ supply from its metabolic precursors, collectively referred to as "niacin equivalents", is required to provide reducing equivalents for energy metabolism and substrates of NAD^+ consuming enzymes [11]. NAD^+ is catabolized to N^1-methylnicotinamide (N^1-MN) through methylation of nicotinamide in the liver, and the 24-h urinary excretion of N^1-MN is considered the most reliable biomarker of niacin status [12–14].

It is unknown whether niacin status is affected in RTR and, if so, whether this affects clinical outcomes. Hence, this study aims to compare 24-h urinary excretion of N^1-MN in RTR with that in healthy kidney donors, in relation to dietary intake of tryptophan and niacin as well as vitamin B_6 status, and to investigate whether niacin status is associated with the risk of premature all-cause mortality in RTR.

2. Materials and Methods

2.1. Study Population

This prospective study was conducted in a well-characterized, single-center cohort of 707 RTR (aged ≥18 years) with a functioning graft for at least 1 year who visited the outpatient clinic of the University Medical Center Groningen, Groningen, the Netherlands, between 2008 and 2011 [15–17]. As a control group, 367 healthy kidney donors were included who participated in a screening program before kidney donation. Signed informed consent was obtained from all participating subjects and the study protocol was approved by the institutional review board (METc 2008/186) adhering to the Declaration of Helsinki. Exclusion of subjects with missing biomaterial or niacin supplementation use left 660 RTR and 275 kidney donors eligible for statistical analyses (Figure S1).

2.2. Data Collection

All baseline measurements were obtained during a morning visit to the outpatient clinic. Participants were instructed to collect a 24-h urine sample on the day before their visit, and to fast overnight for 8 to 12 h. Urine samples were collected under oil, and chlorhexidine was added as an antiseptic agent. Fasting blood samples were drawn after completion of the urine collection. Blood was collected in a series of evacuated tubes with different additives (Vacutainer®; BD, Franklin Lakes, NJ, USA) for preparation of plasma and serum. Body composition and hemodynamic parameters were measured according to a previously described, strict protocol [15]. Serum parameters, including lipid, inflammation, and glucose homeostasis variables were measured with spectrophotometric-based routine clinical laboratory methods (Roche Diagnostics, Rotkreuz, Switzerland). Diabetes was diagnosed if fasting plasma glucose was ≥7.0 mmol/L or antidiabetic medication was used [15]. Plasma vitamin B_6 was determined as its principal, metabolically active form pyridoxal-5'-phosphate using a

HPLC method (Waters Alliance, Milford, MA, USA) with fluorescence detection (JASCO, Inc., Easton, MD, USA) [8].

Renal function was assessed by estimation of the glomerular filtration rate (eGFR) and detection of proteinuria. The eGFR was calculated using the combined creatinine and cystatin C-based Chronic Kidney Disease Epidemiology Collaboration equation [18], which has been shown to be the most accurate equation in RTR [19]. Proteinuria was diagnosed if total urinary protein excretion was ≥0.5 g/day as measured by a biuret reaction-based assay (MEGA AU510; Merck Diagnostica, Darmstadt, Germany).

Dietary intake including tryptophan and niacin intakes was assessed with a validated semi-quantitative food frequency questionnaire (FFQ) [20–22]. The self-administered questionnaire was filled out at home and inquired about 177 food items during the last month, taking seasonal variations into account. During the visit to the outpatient clinic, the FFQ was checked for completeness by a trained researcher and inconsistent answers were verified with the participant. The FFQ was validated for RTR as previously reported [16]. Dietary data were converted into daily nutrient intake using the Dutch Food Composition Table of 2006 [23]. Alcohol consumption and smoking behavior were assessed with a separate questionnaire [6]. Additional data on medical history and use of medication and vitamin supplements were obtained from medical records [6].

2.3. Assessment of N^1-MN Excretion

Measurement of N^1-MN concentration was performed with a validated liquid chromatography (Luna HILIC column; Phenomenex, Torrance, CA, USA) isotope dilution-tandem mass spectrometry (LC-MS/MS) (Quattro Premier; Waters, Milford, MA, USA) method, as described previously [24]. The 24-h urinary excretion of N^1-MN (μmol/day) was obtained after multiplying N^1-MN concentration (μmol/L) by total urine volume calculated from weight (L/day). The reference range of N^1-MN excretion in healthy individuals was previously established at 17.3–115 μmol/day [24].

2.4. Clinical Endpoints

The primary outcome of this study was all-cause mortality which was recorded until 30 September 2015 with no loss due to follow-up. RTR status was kept up-to-date through the continuous surveillance system of the outpatient program.

2.5. Statistical Analysis

Data are presented as the mean ± SD, median (IQR) and absolute number (percentage) for normally distributed, skewed, and nominal data, respectively. Assumptions for normality were checked by visual judgments of the corresponding frequency distribution and Q-Q plot.

Baseline characteristics of RTR and healthy kidney donors were compared by means of t, Mann-Whitney, and Chi-Square tests. Niacin status in RTR and healthy kidney donors was compared by linear regression analyses of 2-base log-transformed N^1-MN excretion, with subsequent cumulative adjustment for age and sex (model 1), eGFR (model 2) and intake of energy, tryptophan, and niacin and plasma vitamin B_6 (model 3).

RTR characteristics were divided into tertiles of N^1-MN excretion stratified by sex (T1, T2, and T3) and compared by means of ANOVA, Kruskal-Wallis, and Chi-Square tests.

For prospective analyses, a Cox proportional hazards regression model for all-cause mortality outcome was fitted to N^1-MN excretion as a sex-stratified tertile-based categorical variable, as well as a continuous variable adjusted for sex (model 1). Confounding was controlled for by including potential confounders as covariates in the regression model. Crude associations were adjusted cumulatively for age (model 2), smoking and body surface area (model 3) and, to prevent overfitting, additionally for intake of alcohol and energy and plasma vitamin B_6 (model 4), kidney function (model 5), medication use (model 6), and high-sensitivity C-reactive protein (hs-CRP) (model 7). Variables that could lie in the causal pathway of N^1-MN excretion and all-cause mortality were not adjusted for because this might obscure otherwise existing associations unintentionally. Assumptions of proportionality of the hazard functions and the linearity of log-hazards were checked by visual judgements of Kaplan Meier plots of the survival and log-survival function entering the sex-stratified N^1-MN excretion tertile group variable.

In secondary analyses, effect modification was assessed by including the cross product term of each potential confounder and 2-base log-transformed N^1-MN excretion in the Cox regression model adjusted for age and sex (model 2). Subsequent stratified analyses were performed for subgroups of significant effect modifiers on the association of N^1-MN excretion with all-cause mortality.

For all statistical analyses, a two-sided p-value of less than 0.05 was considered to indicate statistical significance and SPSS Statistics version 23.0 (IBM, Armonk, NY, USA) was used as software.

3. Results

3.1. Baseline Characteristics and Comparison of N^1-MN Excretion

This study included 660 stable RTR (57% male; mean age 53.0 ± 12.7 years), at a median time of 5.6 (2.0–12.0) years after transplantation, and 275 healthy kidney donors (41% male; mean age 53.3 ± 10.7 years) (Table 1). Intake of tryptophan was similar in both groups (1059 ± 271 and 1089 ± 308 mg/day, respectively; $p = 0.19$), while intake of niacin was lower in RTR than in kidney donors (17.9 ± 5.2 and 19.2 ± 6.2 mg/day, respectively; $p = 0.01$). Taken together, intake of niacin equivalents was lower in RTR than in kidney donors (35.6 ± 9.2 mg/day and 37.4 ± 10.8, respectively; $p = 0.03$) (Figure 1). All RTR and kidney donors complied with the recommended daily intake that is set at a minimum of 6.6 niacin equivalents per 1000 kcal (≥ 9.6 and ≥ 11.7 mg/1000 kcal, respectively) [12]. As previously reported, RTR had significantly lower plasma vitamin B_6 compared to kidney donors (29.0 (17.5–49.5) and 42.0 (29.8–60.3) nmol/L, respectively; $p < 0.001$). Median N^1-MN excretion was 22.0 (15.8–31.8) μmol/day in RTR, compared to 41.1 (31.6–57.2) μmol/day in kidney donors ($p < 0.001$) (Figure 1). Furthermore, urinary excretion of N^1-MN was below the reference limit of 17.3 μmol/day in 202 (31%) RTR, against 4 (2%) kidney donors. The difference in N^1-MN excretion between RTR and kidney donors was independent of age, sex, eGFR, intake of energy, tryptophan, and niacin and plasma vitamin B_6 (Table 2). Cyclosporine, azathioprine, and anticonvulsants were used by, respectively, 253 (38%), 112 (17%) of 19 (3%) of RTR, and none of the controls received drugs that are known to potentially affect niacin status.

Table 1. Baseline characteristics of stable RTR compared to that in healthy kidney donors [1].

Variable	Donors $n = 275$	RTR $n = 660$	p-Value [2]
Age, years	53.3 ± 10.7	53.0 ± 12.7	0.68
Male, n (%)	112 (41)	379 (57)	0.001
Body surface area, m^2	1.9 ± 0.2	1.9 ± 0.2	0.90
Current smoker, n (%)	39 (14)	78 (12)	<0.001
Alcohol intake, g/day	6.7 (1.1–16.4)	3.1 (0.1–11.9)	<0.001
Energy intake, kcal/day	2295 ± 746	2182 ± 642	0.04
Niacin equivalents intake, mg/day [3]	37.4 ± 10.8	35.6 ± 9.2	0.03
Tryptophan intake, mg/day	1089 ± 308	1059 ± 271	0.19
Niacin intake, mg/day	19.2 ± 6.2	17.9 ± 5.2	0.01
N^1-MN excretion, μmol/day	41.4 (31.6–57.2)	22.0 (15.8–31.8)	<0.001
<17.3 μmol/day, n (%)	4 (2)	202 (31)	0.03
Plasma vitamin B_6 (nmol/L)	42.0 (29.8–60.3)	29.0 (17.5–49.5)	<0.001
Systolic blood pressure, mmHg	125.1 ± 13.9	135.8 ± 17.3	<0.001
Diastolic blood pressure, mmHg	75.6 ± 9.1	82.5 ± 11.0	<0.001
Triglycerides, mmol/L	1.2 (0.9–1.7)	1.7 (1.2–2.3)	<0.001
HbA1c, (%)	5.6 (5.4–5.8)	5.8 (5.5–6.2)	<0.001

Table 1. *Cont.*

Variable	Donors $n = 275$	RTR $n = 660$	p-Value [2]
eGFR, ml/min/1.73 m^2	91.0 ± 14.2	53.0 ± 20.0	<0.001
Acetylsalicylic acid, n (%)	4 (2)	127 (19)	<0.001
Proton pump inhibitor, n (%)	5 (2)	326 (49)	<0.001
Diuretic, n (%)	9 (3)	261 (40)	<0.001

[1] Data are presented as mean ± SD, median (IQR) and absolute number (percentage) for normally distributed, skewed and nominal data, respectively. [2] p-value for difference was tested by t and Mann-Whitney tests for normally and skewed distributed continuous variables, respectively, and Chi-Square tests for nominal variables. [3] Intake of niacin equivalents was calculated by adding up niacin and one-sixtieth of tryptophan intake. Subjects who were using niacin supplementation were excluded. eGFR, estimated glomerular filtration rate; HbA1c, hemoglobin A1c; N^1-MN, N^1-methylnicotinamide; RTR, renal transplant recipients.

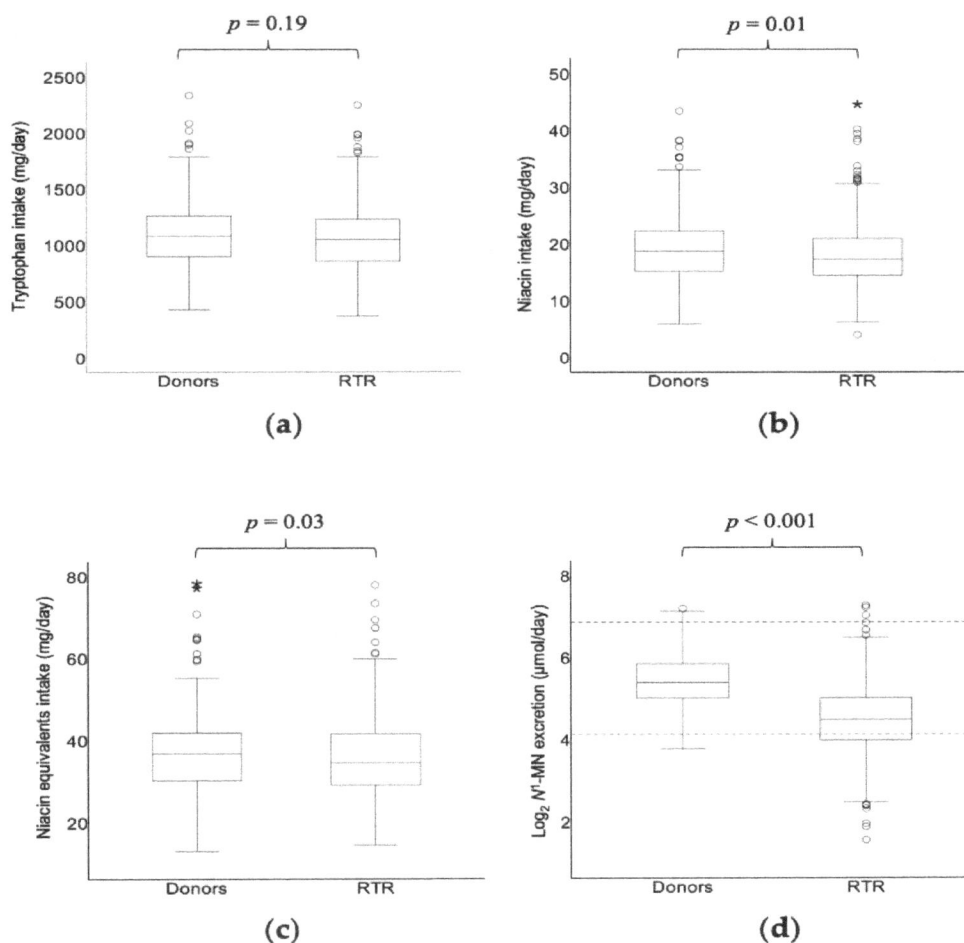

Figure 1. Box plots of dietary intake of (**a**) tryptophan, (**b**) niacin and (**c**) niacin equivalents and (**d**) log$_2$ 24-h urinary excretion of N^1-MN in RTR compared to that in healthy kidney donors. Boxes, bars and whiskers represent IQRs, medians and values <1.5 × IQR, respectively, whereas outliers (1.5–3 × IQR) are indicated by circles and extreme outliers (>3 × IQR) by asterisks. Log$_2$ of the lower and upper bound of the reference range of N^1-MN excretion in healthy individuals (17.3–115.0) μmol/day [24] are indicated with dotted lines (**d**). p-value for difference between RTR and donors was tested by t and Mann-Whitney tests for normally and skewed distributed continuous variables, respectively. Intake of niacin equivalents was calculated by adding up niacin and one-sixtieth of tryptophan intake. N^1-MN, N^1-methylnicotinamide; RTR, renal transplant recipients.

Table 2. Association of RTR and healthy kidney donors grouping with N^1-MN excretion [1].

Variable	Model 1 [2]		Model 2 [3]		Model 3 [4]		Model 4 [5]	
	Std.β	p-Value	Std.β	p-Value	Std.β	p-Value	Std.β	p-Value
Grouping	−0.42	<0.001	−0.44	<0.001	−0.25	<0.001	−0.21	<0.001
Sex	-	-	−0.15	<0.001	−0.14	<0.001	−0.10	0.002
Age, years	-	-	−0.16	<0.001	−0.11	<0.001	−0.07	0.02
eGFR, ml/min/1.73 m^2	-	-	-	-	0.31	<0.001	0.29	<0.001
Energy intake, kcal/day	-	-	-	-	-	-	−0.10	0.08
Tryptophan intake, mg/day	-	-	-	-	-	-	0.007	0.91
Niacin intake, mg/day	-	-	-	-	-	-	0.25	<0.001
Plasma vitamin B$_6$, nmol/L	-	-	-	-	-	-	0.23	<0.001
R^2	0.18		0.23		0.28		0.37	

[1] Linear regression analyses were performed to investigate the association of RTR and healthy kidney donors as grouping variable with N^1-MN excretion, with adjustment for potential confounders. [2] Model 1: crude model. [3] Model 2: adjusted for age and sex. [4] Model 3: adjusted as for model 2 and for eGFR. [5] Model 4: adjusted as for model 3 and for intake of energy, tryptophan and niacin and plasma vitamin B$_6$. eGFR, estimated glomerular filtration rate; N^1-MN, N^1-methylnicotinamide; RTR, renal transplant recipients; std.β, standardized beta coefficient.

RTR characteristics across tertiles of sex-stratified N^1-MN excretion (M: <19.2, 19.2–28.8, >28.8 μmol/day; F: <16.1, 16.1–25.6, >25.6 μmol/day in T1, T2, and T3, respectively) are shown in Table 3. Age and the presence of acetylsalicylic acid, proton pump inhibitors, diuretics and post mortem donors were lower with increasing tertiles of N^1-MN excretion, while intake of alcohol, energy, tryptophan and niacin, plasma vitamin B$_6$, kidney function and the presence of proliferation inhibitors and primary glomerular disease were higher with increasing tertiles of N^1-MN excretion.

Table 3. Baseline characteristics of RTR across tertiles of N^1-MN excretion stratified by sex [1].

Variable	Tertiles of Sex-Stratified N^1-MN Excretion			p-Value [2]
	T1 n = 219	T2 n = 221	T3 n = 220	
Males, μmol/day	<19.2	19.2–28.8	>28.8	
Females, μmol/day	<16.1	16.1–25.6	>25.6	
Male, n (%)	126 (58)	127 (58)	126 (57)	-
Age, years	54.6 ± 12.7	53.7 ± 13.1	50.7 ± 12.1	0.004
BMI, kg/m^2	25.8 (22.7–29.4)	26.1 (23.3–29.0)	26.0 (23.6–29.6)	0.41
Body surface area, m^2	1.9 ± 0.2	1.9 ± 0.2	2.0 ± 0.2	0.13
Lifestyle				
Current smoker, n (%)	21 (10)	25 (11)	32 (15)	0.26
Alcohol consumption, g/day	0.5 (0.0–7.0)	3.2 (0.1–11.3)	6.7 (0.8–20.9)	<0.001
Vegetarian, n (%)	7 (3)	2 (1)	3 (1)	0.16
Dietary intake				
Energy, kcal/day	2065 ± 586	2197 ± 675	2285 ± 647	0.002
Tryptophan, mg/day	1001 ± 253	1063 ± 273	1112 ± 274	<0.001
Niacin, mg/day	16.6 ± 4.9	17.6 ± 4.8	19.5 ± 5.5	<0.001
Plasma vitamin B$_6$, nmol/L	20.3 (14.0–39.0)	29.5 (19.0–47.0)	39.0 (22.0–65.0)	<0.001
Hemodynamic				
Systolic blood pressure, mmHg	139 ± 18	134 ± 18	135 ± 16	0.01
Diastolic blood pressure, mmHg	83 ± 11	82 ± 12	83 ± 11	0.20
Mean arterial pressure, mmHg	109 ± 15	106 ± 15	106 ± 14	0.07
Heart rate, beats per minute	69 ± 11	68 ± 12	68 ± 12	0.52
Antihypertensive use, n (%)	199 (91)	193 (87)	189 (86)	0.26

Table 3. *Cont.*

Variable	Tertiles of Sex-Stratified N^1-MN Excretion			*p*-Value [2]
	T1 *n* = 219	T2 *n* = 221	T3 *n* = 220	
Lipids				
Total cholesterol, mmol/L	5.1 ± 1.2	5.2 ± 1.1	5.0 ± 1.1	0.36
HDL, mmol/L	1.3 (1.0–1.6)	1.3 (1.1–1.6)	1.3 (1.1–1.7)	0.06
LDL, mmol/L	3.0 ± 0.9	3.1 ± 0.9	2.9 ± 0.9	0.31
Triglycerides, mmol/L	1.7 (1.3–2.3)	1.7 (1.3–2.3)	1.6 (1.1–2.2)	0.03
Statin, *n* (%)	122 (56)	115 (52)	112 (51)	0.55
Glucose homeostasis				
Glucose, mmol/L	5.3 (4.8–6.0)	5.3 (4.8–5.9)	5.2 (4.7–6.2)	0.58
HbA1c, (%)	5.8 (5.5–6.3)	5.9 (5.6–6.1)	5.7 (5.4–6.1)	0.05
Diabetes, *n* (%)	58 (27)	44 (20)	50 (23)	0.26
Antidiabetic, *n* (%)	41 (19)	28 (13)	27 (12)	0.10
Other serum parameters				
Hs-CRP, mg/L	1.7 (0.8–5.3)	1.6 (0.6–3.8)	1.4 (0.7–4.6)	0.42
Phosphate, mmol/L	1.0 ± 0.2	1.0 ± 0.2	0.9 ± 0.2	0.01
Immunosuppressant medication				
Prednisolon dose, mg/day	10 (7.5–10)	10 (7.5–10)	10 (7.5–10)	0.18
Calcineurin inhibitor, *n* (%)	136 (62)	125 (57)	112 (51)	0.06
Cyclosporine, *n* (%)	87 (40)	82 (37)	84 (38)	0.85
Azathioprine, *n* (%)	35 (16)	36 (16)	41 (19)	0.72
Proliferation inhibitor, *n* (%)	171 (78)	186 (84)	191 (87)	0.04
Other medication				
Acetylsalicylic acid, *n* (%)	55 (25)	47 (21)	25 (11)	0.001
Anticonvulsant, *n* (%)	7 (3)	5 (2)	7 (3)	0.80
Proton pump inhibitor, *n* (%)	127 (58)	107 (48)	92 (42)	0.003
Diuretic, *n* (%)	104 (48)	79 (36)	78 (36)	0.01
Kidney function				
Serum creatinine, μmol/L	138 (104–189)	122 (101–153)	114 (94–140)	<0.001
Cystatin C, mg/L	2.0 (1.4–2.8)	1.6 (1.3–2.1)	1.4 (1.2–1.9)	<0.001
eGFR, ml/min/1.73 m^2	39.0 ± 18.7	45.8 ± 16.9	52.7 ± 18.0	<0.001
Proteinuria ≥ 0.5 g/day, *n* (%)	55 (25)	39 (18)	38 (17)	0.07
Kidney transplantation				
Time since transplantation, years	5.6 (1.7–12.9)	5.0 (1.5–11.0)	6.5 (2.9–12.3)	0.16
Donor				
Age, years	46 (33–54)	47 (29–57)	43 (29–53)	0.22
Male, *n* (%)	104 (48)	110 (50)	112 (51)	0.60
Post mortem status, *n* (%)	161 (74)	143 (65)	121 (55)	<0.001
Primary kidney disease				
Primary glomerular disease, *n* (%)	48 (22)	67 (30)	71 (32)	0.04
Glomerulonephritis, *n* (%)	12 (6)	17 (8)	21 (10)	0.27
Tubulointerstitial disease, *n* (%)	27 (12)	30 (14)	20 (9)	0.32
Polycystic renal disease, *n* (%)	52 (24)	45 (20)	40 (18)	0.35
Dysplasia and hypoplasia, *n* (%)	9 (4)	10 (5)	9 (4)	0.97
Renovascular disease, *n* (%)	17 (8)	8 (4)	11 (5)	0.15
Diabetic nephropathy, *n* (%)	15 (7)	7 (3)	13 (6)	0.20
Other or unknown cause, *n* (%)	39 (18)	36 (16)	35 (16)	0.85

[1] Data are presented as mean ± SD, median (IQR) and absolute number (percentage) for normally distributed, skewed and nominal data, respectively. [2] *p*-value for difference was tested by ANOVA and Kruskal-Wallis tests for normally and skewed distributed continuous variables, respectively, and Chi-Square tests for nominal variables. eGFR, estimated glomerular filtration rate; HbA1c, hemoglobin A1c; hs-CRP, high-sensitivity C-reactive protein; N^1-MN, N^1-methylnicotinamide; RTR, renal transplant recipients.

3.2. N^1-MN Excretion and Mortality

During a median follow-up time of 5.4 (4.7–6.1) years, 143 (22%) RTR died. The risk of all-cause mortality increased with lower tertiles of N^1-MN excretion, as depicted by Kaplan-Meier curves (Figure 2). Cox regression analyses revealed an inverse association of N^1-MN excretion with all-cause mortality (Model 2: HR 0.57; 95% CI 0.45–0.71; $p < 0.001$), independent of potential confounders (Table 4). The same held for analyses across tertiles of sex-stratified N^1-MN excretion (Table 4). RTR in the lowest and middle tertiles were at higher risk of all-cause mortality compared to those in the highest tertile as reference (Model 2: HR 2.68; 95% CI 1.67–4.33; $p < 0.001$ and HR 2.04; 95% CI 1.25–3.34; $p = 0.004$, respectively), independent of potential confounders (Table 4).

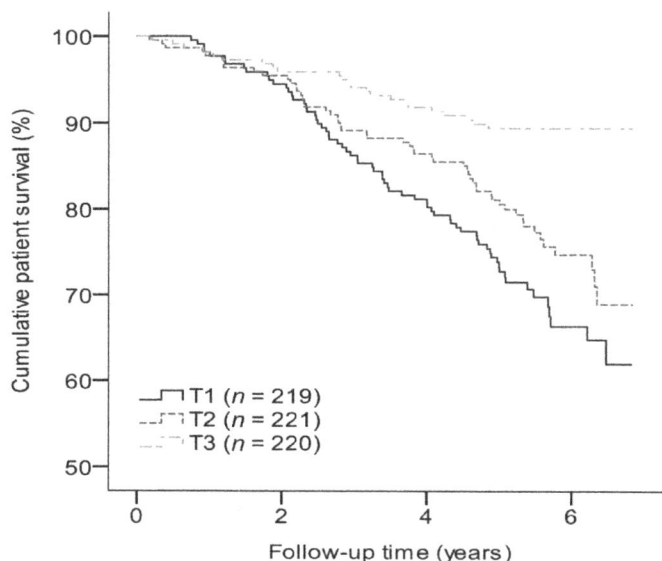

Figure 2. Survival curves for all-cause mortality in RTR according to tertiles of sex-stratified N^1-MN excretion. N^1-MN excretion was <19.2, 19.2–28.8, and >28.8 µmol/day for males, and <16.1, 16.1–25.6 and >25.6 µmol/day for females in T1, T2, and T3, respectively. N^1-MN, N^1-methylnicotinamide; RTR, renal transplant recipients.

Table 4. Association of N^1-MN excretion with risk of all-cause mortality in RTR [1].

Model	N^1-MN Excretion (log$_2$) As Continuous Variable $n = 660$		Tertiles of Sex-Stratified N^1-MN Excretion [2]					
			T1 $n = 219$		T2 $n = 221$		T3 $n = 220$
	HR (95% CI)	p-Value	HR (95% CI)	p-Value	HR (95% CI)	p-Value	Reference HR
1 [3]	0.53 (0.43–0.65)	<0.001	3.28 (2.04–5.26)	<0.001	2.41 (1.48–3.93)	<0.001	1.00
2 [4]	0.57 (0.45–0.71)	<0.001	2.68 (1.67–4.33)	<0.001	2.04 (1.25–3.34)	0.004	1.00
3 [5]	0.59 (0.47–0.74)	<0.001	2.65 (1.60–4.39)	<0.001	2.10 (1.25–3.52)	0.005	1.00
4 [6]	0.69 (0.53–0.90)	0.005	2.10 (1.17–3.78)	0.01	2.04 (1.15–3.63)	0.02	1.00
5 [7]	0.75 (0.58–0.96)	0.02	1.86 (1.07–3.25)	0.02	1.80 (1.04–3.13)	0.04	1.00
6 [8]	0.65 (0.51–0.82)	<0.001	2.25 (1.35–3.75)	0.002	2.06 (1.23–3.46)	0.006	1.00
7 [9]	0.60 (0.48–0.76)	<0.001	2.59 (1.54–4.35)	<0.001	2.13 (1.26–3.61)	0.005	1.00
Events (n)	143		67		53		23

[1] Cox regression analyses were performed to investigate the association of N^1-MN excretion with risk of all-cause mortality in RTR, with adjustment for potential confounders. [2] N^1-MN excretion was <19.2, 19.2–28.8, and >28.8 µmol/day for males, and <16.1, 16.1–25.6, and >25.6 µmol/day for females in T1, T2, and T3, respectively. [3] Model 1: not adjusted in tertiles of sex-stratified N^1-MN excretion, adjusted for sex in continuous analyses. [4] Model 2: adjusted as for model 1 and for age. [5] Model 3: adjusted as for model 2 and for smoking and body surface area. [6] Model 4: adjusted as for model 3 and for intake of alcohol and energy and plasma vitamin B$_6$. [7] Model 5: adjusted as for model 3 and for eGFR, proteinuria, donor status and primary glomerular disease. [8] Model 6: adjusted as for model 3 and for use of proliferation inhibitors, acetylsalicylic acid, proton pump inhibitors and diuretics. [9] Model 7: adjusted as for model 3 and for hs-CRP. eGFR, estimated glomerular filtration rate; hs-CRP, high-sensitivity C-reactive protein; N^1-MN, N^1-methylnicotinamide; RTR, renal transplant recipients.

Secondary analyses exposed significant effect modification of hs-CRP on the association of N^1-MN excretion with all-cause mortality ($p = 0.05$), independent of age and sex. The inverse association of N^1-MN excretion with all-cause mortality was stronger for individuals in the subgroup with serum hs-CRP <2.4 mg/L (HR 0.47; 95% CI 0.35–0.64; $p < 0.001$), than in the subgroup with serum hs-CRP ≥2.4 mg/L (HR 0.70; 95% CI 0.50–0.96; $p = 0.03$) according to subsequent stratified analysis.

4. Discussion

In this large prospective cohort study, we showed that RTR excrete less N^1-MN in 24-h urine than healthy controls and our data suggest that this difference cannot be attributed to lower dietary intake of tryptophan and niacin, nor vitamin B_6 status. Furthermore, lower 24-h urinary excretion of N^1-MN as a biomarker of niacin status was independently associated with a higher risk of premature all-cause mortality in RTR.

To the best of our knowledge, niacin status has not been studied within the context of kidney transplantation and its concomitant long-term implications yet. In fact, prospective data on the urinary excretion of N^1-MN have been limited to one previous study in patients recovering from leukemia treatment [25]. Studies on niacin nutrition in relation to prospective outcomes are likewise scarce, as the prevailing intake of niacin equivalents is suggested to be not sufficiently low to compromise survival. Presumed health benefits of niacin are pharmacological rather than physiological [26–29], although higher survival with higher niacin intake in elderly has been reported previously [30] in congruence with our findings.

Niacin is considered the least critical vitamin to meet the recommendations through dietary intake in western societies [31], as niacin equivalents are found in a wide range of foods [12]. In line with this, dietary intake of niacin equivalents was sufficient according to WHO guidelines in all RTR and healthy kidney donors, while we found that urinary excretion of N^1-MN was commonly below the established reference bound in RTR. The observed disparity of N^1-MN excretion between RTR and healthy kidney donors could moreover not be explained by lower dietary intake of niacin equivalents in RTR in the present study.

The fact that we found a positive association of plasma vitamin B_6 concentration with N^1-MN excretion strengthens our hypothesis that inadequacies of this cofactor might affect niacin status in RTR. Adjustment for plasma vitamin B_6, however, neither did alter the discrepancy of N^1-MN excretion between RTR and healthy kidney donors. Therefore, one should consider other factors that could interfere with N^1-MN excretion as a biomarker of niacin status, and add to poor long-term outcome in RTR.

Whereas secondary dietary inadequacies may interrupt niacin metabolism, this also holds for certain medications including specific antituberculosis, anticonvulsant and antiproliferative drugs, as well as cyclosporine and azathioprine [32–34], which are common immunosuppressant drugs in RTR, although in our population those did not appear to affect N^1-MN excretion.

We can furthermore speculate on the presence of enhanced consumption of tryptophan for protein biosynthesis at the cost of niacin status in RTR. Interestingly, tryptophan is argued to be quantitatively the most important NAD^+ precursor, as it is more effective in elevating liver NAD^+ and urinary excretion of N^1-MN than the salvageable precursors [35–38]. The tryptophan-nicotinamide pathway is, however, mainly regulated by tryptophan intake rather than niacin status, since the generally accepted conversion ratio of 60:1 falls when dietary tryptophan is limiting [39]. Indeed, tryptophan is used primarily for protein biosynthesis and only after nitrogen balance has been achieved for the nicotinamide pathway [40]. This allows us to speculate on protein catabolism and negative protein balance as part of protein-energy wasting in RTR, engendered by metabolic derangement, systemic inflammation, acidemia, and the use of immunosuppressive drugs, to induce tryptophan consumption for protein synthesis in this population [41,42]. However, as our study was not designed to assess protein-energy wasting, we cannot conclusively address such an effect on N^1-MN excretion in RTR.

On the contrary, the tryptophan-nicotinamide pathway is implicated in disease states in which systemic inflammation is present, by the enhanced action of indoleamine 2,3-dioxygenase in response to inflammatory cytokines and mediators. This upregulation of tryptophan degradation towards nicotinamide is known to yield relativity large amounts of quinolinic acid to fuel NAD$^+$-consuming poly (ADP-ribose) polymerase (PARP) reaction in response to immune-related (oxidative) damage [35]. Although we observed lower serum hs-CRP levels as a low-grade inflammation biomarker with higher tertiles of N^1-MN excretion, this difference did not reach significance.

Finally, the renal clearance of N^1-MN itself can also be affected by several factors and not in the least by impaired kidney function. In fact, N^1-MN is eliminated almost exclusively by the kidneys, being partly excreted partly by glomerular filtration and partly by tubular secretion with negligible and saturable tubular reabsorption [43]. Whereas renal clearance of N^1-MN has been investigated as a model of renal secretory function [43] and to predict renal clearance of cationic drugs in renal insufficiency [44], plasma concentrations are suggested to be less sensitive to kidney function because of the contribution of aldehyde oxidase to N^1-MN clearance, yielding N^1-methyl-2-pyridone-5-carboxamide (2Py) [45]. Although our findings appeared independent of kidney function, future studies are warranted to rule out enhanced oxidative metabolism, causing a shift towards urinary excretion of 2Py in this population.

Regarding potential mechanisms for the association of N^1-MN excretion with mortality, NAD$^+$ homeostasis has been linked to increased resistance against a range of pathophysiological processes that are predominant and impact poor long-term outcome in RTR, including cardiovascular, inflammatory, malignant and metabolic disorders [46]. The availability of NAD$^+$ is determined by its production from niacin equivalents, as well as its degradation in NAD$^+$ consuming activities [47]. NAD$^+$ levels remain constant when used as a coenzyme, being recycled back and forth between its oxidized and reduced forms [11], but are depleted by three distinct classes of enzymes that consume NAD$^+$ as a substrate: PARP, cyclic ADP ribose synthases (CD38 and CD157), and sirtuins [48]. Excessive activation of PARP and CD38 is induced by stresses such as inflammation, oxidative stress and DNA damage that are predominant in in RTR [48,49]. As a result, NAD$^+$ availability might become limiting for beneficial sirtuin activities; in particular with lower niacin status. These beneficial effects of sirtuins have been described more specifically for renal diseases, including renoprotective effects by inhibition of renal cell apoptosis, inflammation, and fibrosis and regulation of mitochondrial function and glucose, lipid, and energy metabolism [50–53].

Whereas we did not find an association of N^1-MN excretion with hs-CRP, this low-grade inflammation biomarker appeared to affect the magnitude of the inverse association of N^1-MN excretion with all-cause mortality. Although we can only speculate on the underlying mechanism, earlier mentioned inflammation-related overconsumption of NAD$^+$ limiting its downstream beneficial activities might at least partly explain the lower protective effect of niacin status on mortality in the subgroup with higher serum hs-CRP levels.

The current study should be interpreted within its strengths and limitations. First, its observational nature prohibits causal inferences, but it also did not allow us to draw conclusions on underlying mechanisms of lower N^1-MN excretion in RTR and its contribution to worse survival. Second, the generalizability of our findings might be compromised by overrepresentation of Caucasian individuals from a single center, despite being controlled for by the inclusion of a large, representative control group. Third, the reliability of FFQ data is subject to sources of measurement error, including recall and social desirability biases and limitations in food composition databases [54]. Higher similarity in dietary sources could be achieved by including spouses as a control group. Finally, the present study is confined to the 24-h urinary excretion of N^1-MN as the recommended biomarker of niacin nutritional status by authorities, including the WHO and the European Food Safety Authority [12–14]. Future studies are, however, encouraged to elaborate on plasma concentrations of niacin and its metabolites, or NAD^+ and the ratio of NAD^+ to $NADP^+$ in erythrocytes as additional indices of niacin status. Although observational evidence is inherent to limitations, prospective cohort studies provide a strong design to address nutritional status and health outcome associations over a long period of time. Strengths of our study include its large sample size, with a sufficient number of incident cases and no loss to follow-up, and therefore minimizing the risk of bias in the assessment of outcome. The extensive characterization of participants, moreover, allowed us to control for confounding and effect modification in estimates of the effect.

5. Conclusions

In conclusion, 24-h urinary excretion of N^1-MN as a biomarker of niacin status is lower in RTR than in healthy controls, and other factors than dietary intake of niacin equivalents and vitamin B_6 status appear to reinforce this discrepancy. Importantly, 24-h urinary excretion of N^1-MN is inversely associated with a higher risk of premature all-cause mortality in RTR and niacin status is therefore revealed as a potential target for nutritional strategies to improve long-term outcome after kidney transplantation. However, further research is warranted to unravel underlying mechanisms that potentially interfere with N^1-MN excretion in RTR, and to strengthen causal inferences for health outcomes to support dietary recommendation.

Author Contributions: The authors' responsibilities were as follows—S.J.L.B. and I.P.K.: designed research; M.v.F., A.W.G.-N., J.M.G. and K.J.B.-v.d.B.: provided essential materials; C.P.J.D. and A.v.d.V.: analyzed data; C.P.J.D. and S.J.L.B.: wrote paper and had primary responsibility for final content; A.v.d.V., M.v.F., I.M., A.W.G.-N. and J.M.G.: critically revised the manuscript for important intellectual content; and all authors: read and approved the final manuscript.

Acknowledgments: Supported by FrieslandCampina and Danone Nutricia Research. The cohort on which the study was based is registered at clinicaltrials.gov as "TransplantLines Food and Nutrition Biobank and Cohort Study (TxL-FN)" with number NCT02811835.

References

1. Garcia, G.G.; Harden, P.; Chapman, J.; World Kidney Day Steering Committee 2012. The Global Role of Kidney Transplantation. *Nephrol. Dial. Transplant.* **2013**, *28*, e1–e5. [CrossRef] [PubMed]
2. Nerini, E.; Bruno, F.; Citterio, F.; Schena, F.P. Nonadherence to Immunosuppressive Therapy in Kidney Transplant Recipients: Can Technology Help? *J. Nephrol.* **2016**, *29*, 627–636. [CrossRef] [PubMed]
3. Nankivell, B.J.; Kuypers, D.R. Diagnosis and Prevention of Chronic Kidney Allograft Loss. *Lancet* **2011**, *378*, 1428–1437. [CrossRef]
4. Tong, A.; Budde, K.; Gill, J.; Josephson, M.A.; Marson, L.; Pruett, T.L.; Reese, P.P.; Rosenbloom, D.; Rostaing, L.; Warrens, A.N.; et al. Standardized Outcomes in Nephrology-Transplantation: A Global Initiative to Develop a Core Outcome Set for Trials in Kidney Transplantation. *Transplant. Direct* **2016**, *2*, e79. [CrossRef] [PubMed]
5. Neuberger, J.M.; Bechstein, W.O.; Kuypers, D.R.; Burra, P.; Citterio, F.; De Geest, S.; Duvoux, C.; Jardine, A.G.; Kamar, N.; Kramer, B.K.; et al. Practical Recommendations for Long-Term Management of Modifiable Risks in Kidney and Liver Transplant Recipients: A Guidance Report and Clinical Checklist by the Consensus on Managing Modifiable Risk in Transplantation (COMMIT) Group. *Transplantation* **2017**, *101*, S1–S56. [CrossRef] [PubMed]
6. Eisenga, M.F.; Kieneker, L.M.; Soedamah-Muthu, S.S.; van den Berg, E.; Deetman, P.E.; Navis, G.J.; Gans, R.O.; Gaillard, C.A.; Bakker, S.J.; Joosten, M.M. Urinary Potassium Excretion, Renal Ammoniagenesis, and Risk of Graft Failure and Mortality in Renal Transplant Recipients. *Am. J. Clin. Nutr.* **2016**, *104*, 1703–1711. [CrossRef] [PubMed]

7.   Sotomayor, C.G.; Gomes-Neto, A.W.; Eisenga, M.F.; Nolte, I.M.; Anderson, J.L.C.; de Borst, M.H.; Oste, M.C.J.; Rodrigo, R.; Gans, R.O.B.; Berger, S.P.; et al. Consumption of Fruits and Vegetables and Cardiovascular Mortality in Renal Transplant Recipients: A Prospective Cohort Study. *Nephrol. Dial. Transplant.* **2018**, 1–9. [CrossRef] [PubMed]

8.   Minovic, I.; van der Veen, A.; van Faassen, M.; Riphagen, I.J.; van den Berg, E.; van der Ley, C.; Gomes-Neto, A.W.; Geleijnse, J.M.; Eggersdorfer, M.; Navis, G.J.; et al. Functional Vitamin B-6 Status and Long-Term Mortality in Renal Transplant Recipients. *Am. J. Clin. Nutr.* **2017**, *106*, 1366–1374. [CrossRef] [PubMed]

9.   Combs, G.F.; McClungh, J.P. Vitamin B6. In *The Vitamins*, 5th ed.; Academic Press: Cambridge, MA, USA, 2017; pp. 350–371.

10.   Fukuwatari, T.; Shibata, K. Nutritional Aspect of Tryptophan Metabolism. *Int. J. Tryptophan Res.* **2013**, *6*, 3–8. [CrossRef] [PubMed]

11.   Bogan, K.L.; Brenner, C. Nicotinic Acid, Nicotinamide, and Nicotinamide Riboside: A Molecular Evaluation of NAD+ Precursor Vitamins in Human Nutrition. *Annu. Rev. Nutr.* **2008**, *28*, 115–130. [CrossRef] [PubMed]

12.   World Health Organization and United Nations High Commissions for Refugees. *Pellagra and Its Prevention and Control in Major Emergencies*; WHO/NHD/00.10.2000; Available online: https://www.who.int/nutrition/publications/emergencies/WHO_NHD_00.10/en/ (accessed on 26 March 2018).

13.   Menon, R.M.; Gonzalez, M.A.; Adams, M.H.; Tolbert, D.S.; Leu, J.H.; Cefali, E.A. Effect of the Rate of Niacin Administration on the Plasma and Urine Pharmacokinetics of Niacin and its Metabolites. *J. Clin. Pharmacol.* **2007**, *47*, 681–688. [CrossRef] [PubMed]

14.   EFSA NDA Panel. Scientific Opinion on Dietary Reference Values for Niacin. *EFSA J.* **2014**, *12*, 3759. [CrossRef]

15.   Van den Berg, E.; Engberink, M.F.; Brink, E.J.; van Baak, M.A.; Joosten, M.M.; Gans, R.O.; Navis, G.; Bakker, S.J. Dietary Acid Load and Metabolic Acidosis in Renal Transplant Recipients. *Clin. J. Am. Soc. Nephrol.* **2012**, *7*, 1811–1818. [CrossRef] [PubMed]

16.   Van den Berg, E.; Engberink, M.F.; Brink, E.J.; van Baak, M.A.; Gans, R.O.; Navis, G.; Bakker, S.J. Dietary Protein, Blood Pressure and Renal Function in Renal Transplant Recipients. *Br. J. Nutr.* **2013**, *109*, 1463–1470. [CrossRef] [PubMed]

17.   Van den Berg, E.; Pasch, A.; Westendorp, W.H.; Navis, G.; Brink, E.J.; Gans, R.O.; van Goor, H.; Bakker, S.J. Urinary Sulfur Metabolites Associate with a Favorable Cardiovascular Risk Profile and Survival Benefit in Renal Transplant Recipients. *J. Am. Soc. Nephrol.* **2014**, *25*, 1303–1312. [CrossRef] [PubMed]

18.   Inker, L.A.; Schmid, C.H.; Tighiouart, H.; Eckfeldt, J.H.; Feldman, H.I.; Greene, T.; Kusek, J.W.; Manzi, J.; Van Lente, F.; Zhang, Y.L.; et al. Estimating Glomerular Filtration Rate from Serum Creatinine and Cystatin C. *N. Engl. J. Med.* **2012**, *367*, 20–29. [CrossRef] [PubMed]

19.   Salvador, C.L.; Hartmann, A.; Asberg, A.; Bergan, S.; Rowe, A.D.; Morkrid, L. Estimating Glomerular Filtration Rate in Kidney Transplant Recipients: Comparing a Novel Equation with Commonly used Equations in this Population. *Transplant. Direct* **2017**, *3*, e332. [CrossRef] [PubMed]

20.   Feunekes, G.I.; Van Staveren, W.A.; De Vries, J.H.; Burema, J.; Hautvast, J.G. Relative and Biomarker-Based Validity of a Food-Frequency Questionnaire Estimating Intake of Fats and Cholesterol. *Am. J. Clin. Nutr.* **1993**, *58*, 489–496. [CrossRef] [PubMed]

21.   Feunekes, I.J.; Van Staveren, W.A.; Graveland, F.; De Vos, J.; Burema, J. Reproducibility of a Semiquantitative Food Frequency Questionnaire to Assess the Intake of Fats and Cholesterol in the Netherlands. *Int. J. Food Sci. Nutr.* **1995**, *46*, 117–123. [CrossRef] [PubMed]

22.   Verkleij-Hagoort, A.C.; de Vries, J.H.; Ursem, N.T.; de Jonge, R.; Hop, W.C.; Steegers-Theunissen, R.P. Dietary Intake of B-Vitamins in Mothers Born a Child with a Congenital Heart Defect. *Eur. J. Nutr.* **2006**, *45*, 478–486. [CrossRef] [PubMed]

23.   Dutch Nutrient Databank. *NEVO Table 2006*; Voorlichtingsbureau Voor de Voeding: The Hague, The Netherlands, 2006.

24.   Bouma, G.; van Faassen, M.; Kats-Ugurlu, G.; de Vries, E.G.; Kema, I.P.; Walenkamp, A.M. Niacin (Vitamin B3) Supplementation in Patients with Serotonin-Producing Neuroendocrine Tumor. *Neuroendocrinology* **2016**, *103*, 489–494. [CrossRef] [PubMed]

25. Tamulevicius, P.; Streffer, C. N-Methylnicotinamide as a Possible Prognostic Indicator of Recovery from Leukaemia in Patients Treated with Total-Body Irradiation and Bone Marrow Transplants. *Strahlentherapie* **1984**, *160*, 249–254. [PubMed]

26. Canner, P.L.; Berge, K.G.; Wenger, N.K.; Stamler, J.; Friedman, L.; Prineas, R.J.; Friedewald, W. Fifteen Year Mortality in Coronary Drug Project Patients: Long-Term Benefit with Niacin. *J. Am. Coll. Cardiol.* **1986**, *8*, 1245–1255. [CrossRef]

27. Qiao, Y.L.; Dawsey, S.M.; Kamangar, F.; Fan, J.H.; Abnet, C.C.; Sun, X.D.; Johnson, L.L.; Gail, M.H.; Dong, Z.W.; Yu, B.; et al. Total and Cancer Mortality After Supplementation with Vitamins and Minerals: Follow-Up of the Linxian General Population Nutrition Intervention Trial. *J. Natl. Cancer Inst.* **2009**, *101*, 507–518. [CrossRef] [PubMed]

28. Duggal, J.K.; Singh, M.; Attri, N.; Singh, P.P.; Ahmed, N.; Pahwa, S.; Molnar, J.; Singh, S.; Khosla, S.; Arora, R. Effect of Niacin Therapy on Cardiovascular Outcomes in Patients with Coronary Artery Disease. *J. Cardiovasc. Pharmacol. Ther.* **2010**, *15*, 158–166. [CrossRef] [PubMed]

29. Schandelmaier, S.; Briel, M.; Saccilotto, R.; Olu, K.K.; Arpagaus, A.; Hemkens, L.G.; Nordmann, A.J. Niacin for Primary and Secondary Prevention of Cardiovascular Events. *Cochrane Database Syst. Rev.* **2017**, *6*, CD009744. [CrossRef] [PubMed]

30. Huang, Y.C.; Lee, M.S.; Wahlqvist, M.L. Prediction of all-Cause Mortality by B Group Vitamin Status in the Elderly. *Clin. Nutr.* **2012**, *31*, 191–198. [CrossRef] [PubMed]

31. Troesch, B.; Hoeft, B.; McBurney, M.; Eggersdorfer, M.; Weber, P. Dietary Surveys Indicate Vitamin Intakes below Recommendations are Common in Representative Western Countries. *Br. J. Nutr.* **2012**, *108*, 692–698. [CrossRef] [PubMed]

32. Hegyi, J.; Schwartz, R.A.; Hegyi, V. Pellagra: Dermatitis, Dementia, and Diarrhea. *Int. J. Dermatol.* **2004**, *43*, 1–5. [CrossRef] [PubMed]

33. Li, R.; Yu, K.; Wang, Q.; Wang, L.; Mao, J.; Qian, J. Pellagra Secondary to Medication and Alcoholism: A Case Report and Review of the Literature. *Nutr. Clin. Pract.* **2016**, *31*, 785–789. [CrossRef] [PubMed]

34. Muller, F.; Sharma, A.; Konig, J.; Fromm, M.F. Biomarkers for in Vivo Assessment of Transporter Function. *Pharmacol. Rev.* **2018**, *70*, 246–277. [CrossRef] [PubMed]

35. Badawy, A.A. Kynurenine Pathway of Tryptophan Metabolism: Regulatory and Functional Aspects. *Int. J. Tryptophan Res.* **2017**, *10*, 1178646917691938. [CrossRef] [PubMed]

36. Bender, D.A.; Magboul, B.I.; Wynick, D. Probable Mechanisms of Regulation of the Utilization of Dietary Tryptophan, Nicotinamide and Nicotinic Acid as Precursors of Nicotinamide Nucleotides in the Rat. *Br. J. Nutr.* **1982**, *48*, 119–127. [CrossRef] [PubMed]

37. McCreanor, G.M.; Bender, D.A. The Metabolism of High Intakes of Tryptophan, Nicotinamide and Nicotinic Acid in the Rat. *Br. J. Nutr.* **1986**, *56*, 577–586. [CrossRef] [PubMed]

38. Williams, J.N., Jr.; Feigelson, P.; Elvehjem, C.A. Relation of Tryptophan and Niacin to Pyridine Nucleotides of Tissue. *J. Biol. Chem.* **1950**, *187*, 597–604. [PubMed]

39. Kirkland, J.B. Niacin Status, NAD Distribution and ADP-Ribose Metabolism. *Curr. Pharm. Des.* **2009**, *15*, 3–11. [CrossRef] [PubMed]

40. Shibata, K.; Matsuo, H. Effect of Dietary Tryptophan Levels on the Urinary Excretion of Nicotinamide and its Metabolites in Rats Fed a Niacin-Free Diet Or a Constant Total Protein Level. *J. Nutr.* **1990**, *120*, 1191–1197. [CrossRef] [PubMed]

41. Teplan, V.; Valkovsky, I.; Teplan, V., Jr.; Stollova, M.; Vyhnanek, F.; Andel, M. Nutritional Consequences of Renal Transplantation. *J. Ren. Nutr.* **2009**, *19*, 95–100. [CrossRef] [PubMed]

42. Ter Wee, P.M. Protein Energy Wasting and Transplantation. *J. Ren. Nutr.* **2013**, *23*, 246–249. [CrossRef] [PubMed]

43. Nasseri, K.; Daley-Yates, P.T. A Comparison of N-1-Methylnicotinamide Clearance with 5 Other Markers of Renal Function in Models of Acute and Chronic Renal Failure. *Toxicol. Lett.* **1990**, *53*, 243–245. [CrossRef]

44. Maiza, A.; Daley-Yates, P.T. Estimation of the Renal Clearance of Drugs using Endogenous N-1-Methylnicotinamide. *Toxicol. Lett.* **1990**, *53*, 231–235. [CrossRef]

45. Maiza, A.; Waldek, S.; Ballardie, F.W.; Daley-Yates, P.T. Estimation of Renal Tubular Secretion in Man, in Health and Disease, using Endogenous N-1-Methylnicotinamide. *Nephron* **1992**, *60*, 12–16. [CrossRef] [PubMed]

46.   Yang, Y.; Sauve, A.A. NAD (+) Metabolism: Bioenergetics, Signaling and Manipulation for Therapy. *Biochim. Biophys. Acta* **2016**, *1864*, 1787–1800. [CrossRef] [PubMed]
47.   Stein, L.R.; Imai, S. The Dynamic Regulation of NAD Metabolism in Mitochondria. *Trends Endocrinol. Metab.* **2012**, *23*, 420–428. [CrossRef] [PubMed]
48.   Chini, C.C.S.; Tarrago, M.G.; Chini, E.N. NAD and the Aging Process: Role in Life, Death and Everything in Between. *Mol. Cell. Endocrinol.* **2017**, *455*, 62–74. [CrossRef] [PubMed]
49.   Canto, C.; Menzies, K.J.; Auwerx, J. NAD (+) Metabolism and the Control of Energy Homeostasis: A Balancing Act between Mitochondria and the Nucleus. *Cell. Metab.* **2015**, *22*, 31–53. [CrossRef] [PubMed]
50.   Hao, C.M.; Haase, V.H. Sirtuins and their Relevance to the Kidney. *J. Am. Soc. Nephrol.* **2010**, *21*, 1620–1627. [CrossRef] [PubMed]
51.   Kitada, M.; Kume, S.; Takeda-Watanabe, A.; Kanasaki, K.; Koya, D. Sirtuins and Renal Diseases: Relationship with Aging and Diabetic Nephropathy. *Clin. Sci.* **2013**, *124*, 153–164. [CrossRef] [PubMed]
52.   Wakino, S.; Hasegawa, K.; Itoh, H. Sirtuin and Metabolic Kidney Disease. *Kidney Int.* **2015**, *88*, 691–698. [CrossRef] [PubMed]
53.   Dong, Y.J.; Liu, N.; Xiao, Z.; Sun, T.; Wu, S.H.; Sun, W.X.; Xu, Z.G.; Yuan, H. Renal Protective Effect of Sirtuin 1. *J. Diabetes Res.* **2014**, *2014*, 843786. [CrossRef] [PubMed]
54.   Naska, A.; Lagiou, A.; Lagiou, P. Dietary Assessment Methods in Epidemiological Research: Current State of the Art and Future Prospects. *F1000Research* **2017**, *6*, 926. [CrossRef] [PubMed]

8

Biopsy-Controlled Non-Invasive Quantification of Collagen Type VI in Kidney Transplant Recipients: A Post-Hoc Analysis of the MECANO Trial

Manuela Yepes-Calderón [1,†], Camilo G. Sotomayor [1,*,†], Daniel Guldager Kring Rasmussen [2],
Ryanne S. Hijmans [1], Charlotte A. te Velde-Keyzer [1], Marco van Londen [1], Marja van Dijk [1],
Arjan Diepstra [3], Stefan P. Berger [1], Morten Asser Karsdal [2], Frederike J. Bemelman [4],
Johan W. de Fijter [5], Jesper Kers [6,7,8,9], Sandrine Florquin [6,7,8], Federica Genovese [2],
Stephan J. L. Bakker [1], Jan-Stephan Sanders [1] and Jacob Van Den Born [1]

[1] Division of Nephrology, Department of Internal Medicine, University Medical Center Groningen, University of Groningen, 9713 AV Groningen, The Netherlands; manueyepes@gmail.com (M.Y.-C.); r.s.hijmans@umcg.nl (R.S.H.); c.a.keyzer@umcg.nl (C.A.t.V.-K.); m.van.londen@umcg.nl (M.v.L.); m.van.dijk02@umcg.nl (M.v.D.); s.p.berger@umcg.nl (S.P.B.); s.j.l.bakker@umcg.nl (S.J.L.B.); j.sanders@umcg.nl (J.-S.S.); j.van.den.born@umcg.nl (J.V.D.B.)
[2] Nordic Bioscience A/S, 2730 Herlev, Denmark; dgr@nordicbio.com (D.G.K.R.); MK@nordicbioscience.com (M.A.K.); fge@nordicbio.com (F.G.)
[3] Department of Pathology and Medical Biology, University Medical Center Groningen, University of Groningen, 9713 AV Groningen, The Netherlands; a.diepstra@umcg.nl
[4] Department of Nephrology, Amsterdam University Medical Center, University of Amsterdam, 1105 AZ Amsterdam, The Netherlands; f.j.bemelman@amsterdamumc.nl
[5] Department of Nephrology, Leiden University Medical Center, University of Leiden, 2300 RC Leiden, The Netherlands; J.W.de_Fijter@lumc.nl
[6] Amsterdam Institute for Infection and Immunity (AII), Amsterdam UMC, University of Amsterdam, 1098 XH Amsterdam, The Netherlands; j.kers@amsterdamumc.nl (J.K.); s.florquin@amsterdamumc.nl (S.F.)
[7] Amsterdam Cardiovascular Sciences (ACS), Amsterdam UMC, University of Amsterdam, 1098 XH Amsterdam, The Netherlands
[8] Leiden Transplant Center, Department of Pathology, Leiden University Medical Center, 2300 RC Leiden, The Netherlands
[9] Van 't Hoff Institute for Molecular Sciences (HIMS), University of Amsterdam, 1098 XH Amsterdam, The Netherlands
* Correspondence: c.g.sotomayor.campos@umcg.nl
† These authors contributed equally to this work.

Abstract: The PRO-C6 assay, a reflection of collagen type VI synthesis, has been proposed as a non-invasive early biomarker of kidney fibrosis. We aimed to investigate cross-sectional and longitudinal associations between plasma and urine PRO-C6 and proven histological changes after kidney transplantation. The current study is a post-hoc analysis of 94 participants of the MECANO trial, a 24-month prospective, multicenter, open-label, randomized, controlled trial aimed at comparing everolimus-based vs. cyclosporine-based immunosuppression. PRO-C6 was measured in plasma and urine samples collected 6 and 24 months post-transplantation. Fibrosis was evaluated in biopsies collected at the same time points by Banff interstitial fibrosis/tubular atrophy (IF/TA) scoring and collagen staining (Picro Sirius Red; PSR); inflammation was evaluated by the tubulo-interstitial inflammation score (ti-score). Linear regression analyses were performed. Six-month plasma PRO-C6 was cross-sectionally associated with IF/TA score (Std. β = 0.34), and prospectively with 24-month IF/TA score and ti-score (Std. β = 0.24 and 0.23, respectively) ($p < 0.05$ for all). No significant associations were found between urine PRO-C6 and any of the biopsy findings. Fibrotic changes and urine PRO-C6 behaved differently over time according to immunosuppressive therapy. These results are a first step towards non-invasive fibrosis detection after kidney transplantation by means of collagen VI synthesis measurement, and further research is required.

Keywords: kidney transplantation; fibrosis; inflammation; extracellular matrix; collagen type VI

---

1. Introduction

Kidney transplantation is the best available treatment for patients with end-stage kidney disease [1,2]. In recent times, short-term graft survival has seen great improvement, which unfortunately has not been paralleled by equivalent improvement in long-term graft survival [3]. An important threat to long-term graft survival is progressive loss of kidney allograft function related to progressive fibrosis [4]. Despite its clinical importance, early identification of fibrosis appearance remains a challenge [5]. Currently, biopsy samples are the gold standard for the detection of established kidney fibrosis, but this has the evident drawback as a follow-up measurement of requiring an invasive procedure, which generates discomfort for the patients and can be complicated by bleeding. Other drawbacks are sampling variability and sampling errors [5,6]. Therefore, great interest exists in finding non-invasive biomarkers that can detect fibrosis formation, ideally at early stages [4].

Kidney allograft fibrosis reflects a pathological response to injury where the equilibrium between extracellular matrix formation and degradation is deregulated and progressive deposition of collagens, among other matrix constituents, takes place [7,8]. Assessment of active collagen formation may identify kidney transplant recipients (KTRs) at high risk of fibrosis progression and therefore development of chronic graft failure [9,10]. Among the different collagens, collagen type VI (COL VI) is found in the kidney and is constantly produced by fibroblasts at relative low levels in the interstitium, the intima and adventitia layers of the kidney vasculature, as well as in the glomeruli [11–13]. Under normal conditions, COL VI has an important physiological role in maintaining extracellular matrix (ECM) structure and function, controlling matrix and cell orientation [14]. However, under pathological conditions (e.g., chronic kidney disease), its active deposition in the kidneys is massively increased [9,12]. During production of COL VI, the C5 domain at the C-terminal of the α3 chain is released from the immediate pericellular matrix [15]. The PRO-C6 assay detects the C-terminal end of this domain and is proposed as a surrogate biomarker for COL VI active formation [9]. Moreover, the cleavage of part of this domain gives rise to a bioactive molecule, named endotrophin, which is also detected by the PRO-C6 assay [15,16]. Endotrophin has important biological effects, such as attracting macrophages, increasing transforming growth factor-β (TGFβ) signaling, promoting epithelial–mesenchymal transition, adipose tissue fibrosis, and metabolic dysfunction [17]. Increased plasma levels of PRO-C6 have previously been associated with the progression of chronic kidney disease and, specifically in the post-transplantation setting, with reduced graft function in KTR [4,9,18,19]. Whether associations between PRO-C6 and decreased graft function indeed correspond to increased fibrotic or inflammatory changes in the kidneys and whether it could be used as a non-invasive biomarker for fibrosis development in KTR remain unknown.

In the current study, we aimed to investigate the cross-sectional and longitudinal associations between PRO-C6 in plasma and urine, and proven histological changes in KTR of the minimization of maintenance immunosuppression early after kidney transplantation (MECANO) trial, which is a randomized, controlled, open-label, multicenter trial testing early cyclosporine A (CsA) elimination. Furthermore, since it is known that CsA nephrotoxicity includes pathological increased production and decreased degradation of extracellular matrix proteins, including collagen, and TGF-β up-regulation [20–22], we explored a potential differential role of PRO-C6 as a biomarker of fibrosis among patients under different immunosuppressive regimens.

2. Materials and Methods

2.1. Study Design and Population

Between November 2005 and June 2009, 361 de novo KTRs were recruited in three Dutch transplantation centers to participate in the MECANO trial (trial registration: NTR1615). The study was conducted according to the Good Clinical Practice guidelines, in accordance with the ethical principles of the Declaration of Helsinki, and was approved by the Dutch Medical Ethical Board for medical research (METC 04/154, 1 October 2004) [23,24]. All patients signed written informed consent forms. This study was a 24-month, prospective, multi-center, open-label, randomized, controlled trial, aiming at optimizing maintenance immunosuppression and reducing side effects. During the first six months after enrollment, all patients had a similar quadruple immunosuppressive regimen: induction with basiliximab, followed by CsA, mycophenolate sodium (MPS), and prednisolone [24]. At month six, a protocol biopsy was performed. When no histological signs of rejection were seen, patients were randomized to receive dual immunosuppressive therapy with CsA ($n = 89$), MPS, or everolimus (EVL) ($n = 96$), all in combination with prednisolone. In case of (borderline) rejection patients, were not randomized. The primary endpoint of the MECANO study was the development of interstitial fibrosis at the 24-months protocol biopsy.

After enrollment of 39 patients, the MPS-group was prematurely stopped by the Data Safety Monitoring Board because of an unacceptably high rejection percentage (21%). The trial continued as a two-group trial, comparing CsA and EVL. The results of the primary outcome of the study were published in 2016 [23].

2.2. Protocol Kidney Biopsies and Histological Analyses

Protocol biopsies were scheduled at 6 and 24 months after transplantation. At six months, biopsies were obtained in 99% and 98% of patients in the CsA group and the EVL group, respectively. Of the available biopsies, 78% and 81% in the CsA group and the EVL group were considered adequate, respectively. At 24 months, biopsies were obtained in 84% and 79% of patients in the CsA group and the EVL group, respectively. The prevalence of adequate samples was 81% and 73% in the CsA group and the EVL group, respectively ($p = 0.4$, two-tailed). The current study reports the results of the 94 patients (51 in the CsA group and 43 in the EVL group) whose 6-month biopsies met the minimal adequacy threshold of seven glomeruli and one artery.

Tissues were formalin-fixed and paraffin-embedded and stained with periodic-acid Schiff diastase, hematoxylin/eosin, and Jones' methenamine silver. Two independent kidney pathologists (Amsterdam University Medical Center (UMC) and Leiden UMC, The Netherlands), unaware of any clinical data, classified the biopsies according to the 2015 update of the Banff classification [25] and assigned a Banff interstitial fibrosis/tubular atrophy (IF/TA) score. Morphometric analysis of cortical interstitial fibrosis was centralized at the Amsterdam UMC. Adequate protocol biopsy sections were stained with Picro Sirius Red (PSR, Aldrich, Munich, Germany), which is used for the detection of collagen fibers. PSR-stained slides were digitalized using a slide virtual microscope system (Olympus, Tokyo, Japan) with a 20× magnification objective and saved in Tagged Image File Format (TIFF format). Image analyses were performed with the ImageJ software package (National Institutes of Health, Bethesda, MD, USA) where the PSR-stained area was aut omatically assessed by means of a macro. All input was verified manually. Inflammation was evaluated by the total percentage of inflamed cortical area (ti-score) as a continuous score [26].

2.3. PRO-C6 Detection

Plasma and urine PRO-C6 concentrations were measured using a competitive enzyme-linked immunosorbent assay (Nordic Bioscience, Herlev, Denmark) that specifically detects the last 10 amino acids of the alpha-3 chain of COL VI (3168'KPGVISVMGT3177') and is validated for both sample matrices [27]. The assay has a detection limit of 0.15 ng/mL and a 95% confidence interval for inter-

and intra-assay variability in plasma samples reported as 3.4%–12.4% and 1.1%–5.3%, respectively [19]. For urine samples, the detection limit was the same as plasma, and inter- and intra-assay variability are reported as 7.9% and 3.2%, respectively [9]. To account for variations in urine concentration, urinary PRO-C6 was divided by urinary creatinine, measured by the QuantiChrom™ Creatinine Assay Kit (BioAssay Systems, Hayward, CA, USA), and the PRO-C6/creatinine ratio was used in all analyses.

2.4. Statistical Analyses

Data analyses, computations, and graphs were performed with SPSS 25.0 software (IBM Corporation, Chicago, IL, USA). To test whether variables were normally distributed, a histogram was generated for each variable. For descriptive statistics data were presented as mean (standard deviation (SD)) for normally distributed data, and as median (interquartile range (IQR)) for variables with a non-normal distribution. Categorical data were expressed as number (percentage).

Differences in plasma and urine PRO-C6 and biopsy changes (IF/TA score, PSR, and ti-score) among subgroups of KTRs according to their treatment regimen and to their primary kidney disease were tested by one-way ANOVA for continuous variables with normal distribution, Mann–Whitney U test for continuous variables with skewed distribution, and X^2 test for categorical variables. Linear regression analyses were performed to study the association of plasma and urine PRO-C6 with biopsy changes at 6 and 24 months and the delta between the two visits. Furthermore, subgroup analyses were performed by dividing patients by the immunosuppressive regimen used. We also performed sensitivity analyses, in which patients who were grouped under "unknown cause" as primary kidney disease were recoded as if they have been suffering from glomerulonephritis as primary kidney disease. For all statistical analyses, a 2-sided $p < 0.05$ was considered significant.

3. Results

3.1. Baseline Characteristics

The characteristics at enrollment and at randomization of a total of 94 patients, 51 in the CsA group and 43 in the EVL group, are displayed in Tables 1 and 2. At enrollment, in the overall population, the mean (SD) age was 52 (13) years-old, and most patients were male and Caucasian. The main cause of end-stage kidney disease in this trial was polycystic kidney disease (24%), followed by glomerulonephritis (17%) and hypertension (16%). The mean donor age was 50 (13) years old, and the most frequent type of donors was living unrelated (31%), followed closely by deceased after brain death (30%). The median antigen mismatch was 3, and the median (IQR) of total time on kidney replacement therapy was 24 (5–46) months.

At randomization, 6 months after the beginning of the trial, patients had a mean graft function, as assessed by the estimated glomerular filtration rate (eGFR), of 49 (42–62) mL/min/1.73 m². Patients had a mean weight of 79 (14) kg and a mean systolic blood pressure of 144 (20) mmHg. Mean low-density lipoprotein (LDL) was 3.19 (2.39–3.75) mmol/L, and 59% of patients were statin users. Mean glycated hemoglobin was 6.08% (1.10), and only two patients had the diagnosis of diabetes mellitus. Fifteen patients (16%) were active smokers. Concerning subgroup differences, patients in the CsA group had an apparent higher weight (81 vs. 78 kg), a more frequent use of statins (63% vs. 54%), and a higher percentage were active smokers (20% vs. 12%) when compared to the EVL group. Also, the two diabetic patients were both in the EVL group. None of these differences was of statistical significance.

Table 1. Characteristics at enrollment of study population, overall kidney transplant recipients (KTRs), and randomization groups.

Characteristics at Enrollment	Overall	Randomized Group		p Value
		CsA	EVL	
Number of patients, n	94	51	43	
Age, years (SD)	52 (13)	51 (13)	54 (12)	0.30
Sex (male), n (%)	64 (68)	33 (65)	31 (72)	0.44
Race (Caucasian), n (%)	83 (88)	47 (92)	36 (84)	0.21
Primary kidney disease, n (%)				0.81
Polycystic kidney disease	24 (26)	13 (26)	11 (26)	
Glomerulonephritis	16 (17)	9 (18)	7 (16)	
Hypertension	15 (16)	7 (14)	8 (19)	
Urologic	8 (9)	3 (6)	5 (12)	
Vascular	5 (5)	2 (4)	3 (7)	
Focal segmental glomerulosclerosis	3 (3)	1 (2)	2 (5)	
Diabetes mellitus	3 (3)	2 (4)	1 (2)	
Unknown cause	16 (17)	11 (22)	5 (12)	
Donor type, n (%)				0.81
Living unrelated	29 (31)	15 (29)	14 (33)	
Deceased after brain death	28 (30)	15 (29)	13 (30)	
Living related	22 (23)	14 (28)	8 (19)	
Deceased after cardiac death	14 (15)	7 (14)	7 (16)	
Donor age, years (SD) [a]	50 (13)	51 (13)	49 (12)	0.55
Antigen mismatch, n (IQR)	3 (2–4)	3 (2–3)	3 (2–4)	0.52
TTKRT, months (IQR)	24 (5–46)	18 (6–46)	24 (5–48)	0.53

[a] Data available in 87 patients.   CsA: cyclosporine A; EVL: everolimus; TTKRT: total time on kidney replacement therapy.

Table 2. Characteristics at randomization of study population, overall KTRs, and randomization groups.

Characteristics at Randomization	Overall	Randomized Group		p Value
		CsA	EVL	
eGFR, mL/min/1.73 m^2	49 (42–62)	49 (43–57)	49 (40–67)	0.89
Weight, kg (SD) [a]	79 (14)	81 (15)	78 (13)	0.24
BMI, kg/m^2 (SD) [a]	26.7 (3.5)	26.0 (3.9)	25.4 (3.1)	0.44
SBP, mmHg (SD) [b]	144 (20)	144 (20)	145 (21)	0.82
DBP, mmHg (SD) [b]	84 (12)	84 (11)	83 (12)	0.68
LDL, mmol/L (SD) [b]	3.19 (2.39–3.75)	3.19 (2.37–3.95)	3.15 (2.40–3.70)	0.84
HDL, mmol/L (SD) [b]	1.39 (1.20–1.73)	1.30 (1.17–1.71)	1.49 (1.20–1.76)	0.49
Cholesterol, mmol/L (SD) [b]	5.13 (4.34–6.10)	5.16 (4.26–6.23)	5.08 (4.40–6.07)	0.92
Statins use, n (%)	55 (59)	32 (63)	23 (54)	0.36
Glucose, mmol/L [c]	5.10 (4.50–5.80)	5.10 (4.70–5.80)	4.90 (4.50–5.90)	0.35
HbA1c, % (SD) [c]	6.08 (1.10)	6.14 (1.25)	6.01 (0.88)	0.60
Diabetes mellitus, n (%)	2 (2)	0 (0)	2 (5)	0.12
Smoking current, n (%)	15 (16)	10 (20)	5 (12)	0.29

Data available in [a] 90, [b] 92, and [c] 88 patients. eGFR: estimated glomerular filtration rate; BMI: body mass index; SPB: systolic blood pressure; DBP: diastolic blood pressure; LDL: low-density lipoprotein; HDL: high-density lipoprotein; HbA1c: glycated hemoglobin.

3.2. PRO-C6 and Biopsy-Proven Histological Changes over Follow-Up

Mean (SD) plasma PRO-C6 at 6 and 24 months was 9.5 (3.4) and 9.4 (4.3) ng/mL, respectively, without significant differences between the two groups. As for urine, median (IQR) PRO-C6 at 6 and 24 months after correction by creatinine was 6.7 (4.8–12.4) and 5.9 (3.4–21.5) ng/mg, respectively. Plasma and urine PRO-C6 did not correlate at either 6 or 24 months (Spearman's ρ 0.226, $p = 0.09$; Spearman's ρ 0.311, $p = 0.11$; respectively). No difference in urine PRO-C6 between the two study groups was present at 6 months, but at 24 months mean urine PRO-C6 was significantly higher in the EVL group compared to the CsA group (7.5 vs. 4.5 ng/mg; $p = 0.02$). Delta plasma PRO-C6 was positive in both subgroups and was not significantly different. As for delta urine PRO-C6, it was positive in the EVL group and negative in the CsA group; this difference was statistically significant (0.9 vs. -1.4 ng/mg; $p = 0.01$). (Table 3).

Table 3. Biomarkers and histological characteristics during follow-up of overall KTRs and randomization groups.

Biomarkers and Histological Characteristics	Overall	Randomized Group		p
		CsA	EVL	
Biomarkers				
6 Months				
Plasma				
PRO-C6 (ng/mL) [a]	9.5 (3.4)	9.5 (3.1)	9.4 (3.9)	0.93
Creatinine, μmol/L (SD)	130 (33)	130 (31)	130 (35)	0.96
Urine				
PRO-C6 (ng/mg creat) [b]	6.7 (4.8–12.4)	6.6 (4.9–12.9)	6.8 (3.8–12.8)	0.70
24 Months				
Plasma				
PRO-C6 (ng/mL) [c]	9.4 (4.3)	9.6 (4.5)	9.1 (4.3)	0.72
Creatinine, μmol/L (SD)	143 (49)	149 (46)	136 (53)	0.22
Urine				
PRO-C6 (ng/mg creat) [b]	5.9 (3.4–21.5)	4.5 (3.2–10.2)	7.5 (4.6–40.7)	0.02
Delta$_{24-6}$				
Plasma				
PRO-C6 (ng/mL) [c]	0.3 (3.9)	0.6 (3.1)	0.01 (4.6)	0.67
Urine				
PRO-C6 (ng/mg creat) [b]	-0.5 (-2.6–4.8)	-1.4 (-3.6–0.27)	0.9 (-2.2–23.9)	0.01
Histological analyses				
6 Months				
IF/TA-score	1 (0–1)	1 (0–1)	1 (1–2)	0.56
PSR, %	13.3 (6.0)	13.0 (6.1)	13.6 (6.0)	0.65
ti-score, %	10.0 (5.0–15.8)	10.0 (5.0–10.0)	10.0 (5.0–20.0)	0.38
24 Months				
IF/TA-score	1 (1–2)	1 (0–1)	1 (1–2)	0.36
PSR, %	17.3 (10.6)	19.7 (11.7)	14.5 (8.5)	0.02
ti-score, %	20.0 (10.0–41.3)	20.0 (10.0–50.0)	15.0 (10.0–30.0)	0.16
Delta$_{24-6}$				
IF/TA-score	0.5 (0–1)	1 (0–1)	0 (0–1)	0.23
PSR, %	4.0 (11.4)	6.7 (13.1)	0.9 (7.9)	0.01
ti-score, %	10 (0–30)	10 (0–45)	5 (0–20)	0.09

Data available in [a] 73, [b] 62, [c] 36 patients. CsA: cyclosporine group; EVL: everolimus group; PRO-C6: released pro-peptide of collagen type VI (endotrophin); IF/TA: interstitial fibrosis/tubular atrophy; PSR: Picro Sirius Red; ti-score: total inflammation score.

Histological analyses at 6 months showed a median IF/TA score of 1 (0–1) points and a mean PSR staining percentage of 13.3% (6.0), with no significant differences between patients in the CsA and EVL groups. Inflammation, as evaluated by the ti-score, was also not significantly different between the two groups. At 24 months, the overall population showed a higher IF/TA score, PSR percentage, and ti-score when compared to the previous biopsy. At this time point, the PSR staining percentage was higher in the CsA group compared to the EVL group (19.7% vs. 14.5%; $p = 0.02$); no significant difference was present in the other histological parameters (Table 3).

When patients were stratified by their primary kidney disease, no significant differences were found in the plasma and urine concentrations of PRO-C6 at any time point during follow-up. No significant difference was found either in fibrosis (IF/TA and PRO-C6) or inflammation (ti-score) at 6 and 24 months (Table S1). Also, no significant differences were found in sensitivity analyses in which all KTRs with unknown cause of primary kidney disease were considered as patients with glomerulonephritis as primary kidney disease (Table S2).

3.3. Association between PRO-C6 and Biopsy Changes

Plasma PRO-C6 at 6 months post transplantation was significantly associated with 6-month and 24-month IF/TA scores (Std. $\beta = 0.34$ and 0.24, respectively; both $p < 0.05$). A prospective association was also present for 6-month plasma PRO-C6 with 24-month biopsy proven inflammation (ti-score) and the delta inflammation between the two biopsies (Std. $\beta = 0.23$ and 0.22, respectively; both $p < 0.05$). No association was found between 6-month plasma PRO-C6 and 6- or 24-month PSR. Also, no cross-sectional association was found between 24-month plasma PRO-C6 and histological evidence of fibrosis or inflammation. Urine PRO-C6 at 6 months only showed a prospective and inverse association with 24-month PSR (Std. $\beta = -0.30$; $p < 0.05$), and there were no cross-sectional associations at 24 months. Delta plasma and urine PRO-C6 did not correlate with either histological evidence of fibrosis or inflammation (Table 4).

Table 4. Association of histological analyses with plasma and urine PRO-C6.

Histological Analyses	6-Months PRO-C6		24-Months PRO-C6		Delta$_{24-6}$ PRO-C6	
	Plasma, ng/mL	Urine, ng/mg	Plasma, ng/mL	Urine, ng/mg	Plasma, ng/mL	Urine, ng/mg
	Std. β	Std. β	Std. β	Std. β	Std. β	Std. β
6 Months						
IF/TA	0.34 **	0.20				
PSR	0.11	−0.18				
ti-score	0.04	0.08				
24 Months						
IF/TA	0.24 *	0.06	0.08	0.13	−0.04	0.02
PSR	0.01	−0.30 *	0.06	−0.24	−0.01	0.04
ti-score	0.23 *	0.23	0.16	0.09	0.05	−0.03
Delta$_{24-6}$						
IF/TA	−0.03	−0.08	−0.20	−0.07	−0.16	0.01
PSR	−0.06	−0.17	−0.009	−0.19	0.04	−0.04
ti-score	0.22 *	0.20	0.11	−0.02	0.01	−0.02

* p value < 0.05; ** p value < 0.01. Linear regression analyses were performed. Std. β coefficients represent the difference (in standard deviations) in each biomarker per 1 standard deviation increment in each individual biopsy score. PRO-C6: pro-peptide of collagen VI (endotrophin); Std. β: standardized beta coefficient; IF/TA: interstitial fibrosis/tubular atrophy; PSR: Picro Sirius Red; ti-score: total inflammation score.

When patients were divided by randomization group, no significant associations were found between 24-month plasma PRO-C6 and histological changes. Urine PRO-C6 was significantly and inversely associated with the delta of IF/TA score in patients among the CsA group, and no other significant association was found. Delta plasma and urine PRO-C6 were not significantly associated with any histological changes (Table 5).

Table 5. Association of histological analyses with plasma and urine PRO-C6 among CsA and EVL groups.

Histological Analyses	24 Months				$Delta_{24-6}$			
	Plasma PRO-C6, ng/mL		Urine PRO-C6, ng/mg		Plasma PRO-C6, ng/mL		Urine PRO-C6, ng/mg	
	CsA	EVL	CsA	EVL	CsA	EVL	CsA	EVL
	Std. β	Std. β	Std. β	Std. β	Std. β	Std. β	Std. β	Std. β
24 Months								
IF/TA	−0.11	0.32	−0.25	0.30	−0.31	0.16	0.13	−0.11
PSR	−0.07	0.18	−0.09	−0.31	−0.47	0.25	0.12	−0.11
ti-score	−0.07	0.40	0.18	0.14	−0.37	0.32	0.08	−0.07
$Delta_{24-6}$								
IF/TA	−0.30	−0.07	−0.43 *	0.07	−0.40	−0.01	0.12	−0.003
PSR	0.001	−0.06	−0.10	−0.27	−0.28	0.25	0.03	−0.18
ti-score	−0.08	0.33	0.07	0.05	−0.35	0.25	0.09	0.04

* p value < 0.05. Linear regression analyses were performed. Std. β coefficients represent the difference (in standard deviations) in each biomarker per 1 standard deviation increment in each individual biopsy score. PRO-C6: pro-peptide of collagen type VI (endotrophin); CsA: cyclosporine group; EVL: everolimus group; Std. β: standardized beta coefficient; IF/TA: interstitial fibrosis/tubular atrophy; PSR: Picro Sirius Red; ti-score: total inflammation score.

4. Discussion

This study shows, in a homogeneous well-characterized cohort of KTRs who were participants of the MECANO clinical trial, that 6-month post-transplant plasma concentration of PRO-C6 associates with graft biopsy-proven fibrotic and inflammatory changes, both cross-sectionally (IF/TA score) and longitudinally (IF/TA score and ti-score). Further, we show that these same associations are not found with 6-month urine PRO-C6, and that at 24 months, no cross-sectional association was present between fibrotic changes and either urine or plasma PRO-C6. Subgroup analyses comparing patients under CsA vs. EVL immunosuppressive therapy showed higher urinary concentration of PRO-C6 in the EVL group compared to the CsA groups during follow-up, despite lower fibrosis scorings.

The progression of kidney diseases is characterized by the appearance of progressive fibrosis, which reflects a pathological disequilibrium between the synthesis and degradation of ECM constituents, including collagens, within scarred kidneys [8,28]. COL VI is an ECM molecule distributed in the kidney interstitium, vasculature, and in the glomeruli, which is constantly produced by fibroblasts at relative low levels [12,13]. Under healthy conditions, it has an important physiological role in maintaining structure and function of the ECM by controlling organization and cell orientation [14]. However, its markedly increased synthesis and deposition has been reported under a wide spectrum of kidney pathologies [29,30].

COL VI biosynthesis and assembly involves a complex multi-step pathway [14,31]. During active deposition in the ECM, a pro-peptide in the α3 chain of COL VI is released; in turn, this gives rise to the bioactive molecule endotrophin [15,27], which is known to have a role in shaping a pro-inflammatory and pro-fibrotic microenvironment by, amongst other processes, triggering an increase in cytokines such as TGFβ [16]. The PRO-C6 assay measures both the release of endotrophin and of the pro-peptide, reflecting newly formed molecules of mature COL VI [9,27]. In the post-transplantation setting, the assessment of active collagen formation has been proposed as a way of early identifying KTRs that are at high risk of fibrosis progression [9,10], and since allograft function loss is closely related to the appearance and progression of interstitial fibrosis and tubular atrophy [10,32,33], it could identify also KTRs at future risk of developing chronic graft failure [9,10].

Clinically, increased deposition of COL VI has been reported in multiple scenarios of chronic kidney disease [28,31], and specifically in the post-transplantation setting, a strong association was found between increased plasma concentration of PRO-C6 and a decrease in graft function over time [4]. In agreement with this evidence, we found a positive prospective association between 6-month

PRO-C6 concentration and biopsy evidence of increased graft fibrosis (IF/TA). However, no associations were found with PSR staining. Following the evidence that patients receiving CsA are at risk of developing nephrotoxicity, which is also a condition with unregulated ECM deposition and TGF-β upregulation [20–22,34], we performed exploratory analysis by subgroups of immunosuppressive therapy. When dividing the population into subgroups, we found that patients in the CsA group had higher PSR% at 24 months, but urine PRO-C6 was higher in the EVL group.

This analysis shows that PRO-C6 measurement, as reflection of collagen VI synthesis, is associated with, but not identical to, quantification of fibrosis in transplanted kidneys, especially not under different treatment conditions. The next considerations should be taken into account: first, by measuring plasma or urine PRO-C6, the cells/tissues where the existing collagen VI synthesis takes place cannot be identified and might be (partially) different from the transplanted kidney. Second, PRO-C6, by definition, only measures a collagen split product of the alpha3 chain of collagen VI [15,27], whereas PSR staining is the resultant of all collagen deposits. As we know, there are >20 different types of collagens, all of which can be stained by PSR [35]. So, changes in PSR staining do not necessarily correspond with changes in COL VI synthesis. Third, the PRO-C6 assay measures a split product of collagen VI that is cleaved off after cellular synthesis and thus reflects synthesis of collagen VI. Collagen deposition in a tissue, however, is the resultant of collagen synthesis and collagen degradation (mainly by metalloproteinases). So, the PRO-C6 assay shows one side of the coin (synthesis), whereas the other side of the coin (degradation) is not measured. We anticipate that various treatment regimens might not only influence collagen VI synthesis but collagen VI degradation as well. Next, since we did not perform immunofluorescent studies, we cannot assure that there was recurrence or enhanced interstitial inflammation; however, when stratified analyses by primary kidney disease were performed, there was no significant difference in biomarkers or histological evidence of inflammation. Also, the possibility that incidence of glomerulonephritis was underestimated due to low use of immunofluorescence in the evaluation of biopsy materials in the regular clinical setting in which the current study was performed, and the possibility that such potential underestimation may have biased our results, is a limitation of our study. Although we performed sensitivity analyses in which we found no indication of the presence of such bias, it can, of course, not be excluded. Future studies are warranted to confirm our findings, and it would be relevant to apply immunofluorescence in such studies in order to maximize the accuracy of estimation of glomerulonephritis recurrence. It would also be interesting if future studies would compare the pre- and post-transplantation behavior of PRO-C6. Furthermore, patients receiving CsA had a more marked decline in eGFR compared to the EVL group, as was shown in the main outcomes of the MECANO publication [23]. This might have influenced both plasma and urine PRO-C6 values and differences between both treatment arms. Finally, we do not have information on eGFR at inclusion, therefore the eGFR changes before randomization could not be evaluated, and this prevents us from exploring the causes underlying early fibrotic lesions.

The present study has several strengths. Being a randomized clinical trial, we have a very homogenous population regarding time since transplantation and initial immunosuppressive regimen. Also, we studied PRO-C6 against the current gold standard for fibrosis detection, which is kidney biopsy [5,6], taken at the same time point as the biomarkers, allowing both cross-sectional and longitudinal analyses. Several limitations must also be considered. Most of our patients are from a European background, and care should be taken when extrapolating our findings to other ethnic groups. Also, especially at 24 months, we had a reduced number of available samples and a longer follow-up would have allowed us to further explore the prospective behavior of PRO-C6.

In conclusion, 6-month post-transplantation plasma concentration PRO-C6 has a good longitudinal association with graft biopsy-proven IFTA scores, which could make it potentially useful as a follow-up tool. On the other hand, urine PRO-C6 did not associate with fibrotic parameters measured at time of biopsy or in future protocol biopsies. Additionally, we showed a differential evolution of PRO-C6 during follow-up dependent on immunosuppressive regimen. For the first time, this study provides biopsy-controlled data of PRO-C6 as a potential non-invasive biomarker of graft fibrosis in KTRs.

This is a first step towards non-invasive detection by plasma PRO-C6 of pro-fibrotic ECM turnover early after transplantation. The potential utility of the implementation of PRO-C6 in clinical follow-up of KTRs requires further clinical studies.t The detection of causes underlying early kidney fibrosis was not the scope of the current study, yet we hold a plea for future studies aiming at evaluating whether primary kidney disease may influence he performance of PRO-C6 as a biomarker in KTRs. Furthermore, it would be interesting if future studies would also compare the pre- and post-transplantation behavior of PRO-C6.

Author Contributions: Conceptualization: C.G.S., D.G.K.R., and J.V.D.B.; Data curation: D.G.K.R., R.S.H., C.A.t.V.-K., M.v.L., M.v.D., and A.D.; Formal analysis: M.Y.-C., C.G.S., S.J.L.B., and J.V.D.B.; Investigation: D.G.K.R., R.S.H., C.A.t.V.-K., M.v.L., M.v.D., A.D., M.A.K., F.J.B., J.W.d.F., S.F., J.K., F.G., and S.J.L.B.; Methodology: S.P.B., M.A.K., F.J.B., J.W.d.F., S.F., J.K., and F.G.; Project administration: S.P.B., S.J.L.B., J.-S.S., and J.V.D.B.; Resources: D.G.K.R., M.A.K., and F.G.; Supervision: S.P.B., S.J.L.B, J.-S.S., and J.V.D.B.; Writing—original draft: M.Y.-C. and C.G.S.; Writing—review and editing: M.Y.-C., C.G.S., D.G.K.R., R.S.H, C.A.t.V.-K., M.v.L., M.v.D., A.D., S.P.B., M.A.K., F.J.B., J.W.d.F., S.F., J.K., F.G., S.J.L.B., J.-S.S., and J.V.D.B. All authors have read and agreed to the published version of the manuscript.

References

1. Laupacis, A.; Keown, P.; Pus, N.; Krueger, H.; Ferguson, B.; Wong, C.; Muirhead, N. A study of the quality of life and cost-utility of renal transplantation. *Kidney Int.* **1996**, *50*, 235–242. [CrossRef] [PubMed]
2. Wolfe, R.A.; Ashby, V.B.; Milford, E.L.; Ojo, A.O.; Ettenger, R.E.; Agodoa, L.Y.C.; Held, P.J.; Port, F.K. Comparison of Mortality in All Patients on Dialysis, Patients on Dialysis Awaiting Transplantation, and Recipients of a First Cadaveric Transplant. *N. Engl. J. Med.* **1999**, *341*, 1725–1730. [CrossRef] [PubMed]
3. Meier-Kriesche, H.-U.; Schold, J.D.; Srinivas, T.R.; Kaplan, B. Lack of Improvement in Renal Allograft Survival Despite a Marked Decrease in Acute Rejection Rates Over the Most Recent Era. *Am. J. Transplant.* **2004**, *4*, 378–383. [CrossRef] [PubMed]
4. Stribos, E.G.D.; Nielsen, S.H.; Brix, S.; Karsdal, M.A.; Seelen, M.A.; van Goor, H.; Bakker, S.J.L.; Olinga, P.; Mutsaers, H.A.M.; Genovese, F. Non-invasive quantification of collagen turnover in renal transplant recipients. *PLoS ONE* **2017**, *12*, e0175898. [CrossRef]
5. Hijmans, R.S.; Rasmussen, D.G.K.; Yazdani, S.; Navis, G.; van Goor, H.; Karsdal, M.A.; Genovese, F.; van den Born, J. Urinary collagen degradation products as early markers of progressive renal fibrosis. *J. Transl. Med.* **2017**, *15*, 63. [CrossRef]
6. Farris, A.B.; Colvin, R.B. Renal interstitial fibrosis: Mechanisms and evaluation. *Curr. Opin. Nephrol. Hypertens.* **2012**, *21*, 289–300. [CrossRef]
7. Karsdal, M.A.; Nielsen, M.J.; Sand, J.M.; Henriksen, K.; Genovese, F.; Bay-Jensen, A.-C.; Smith, V.; Adamkewicz, J.I.; Christiansen, C.; Leeming, D.J. Extracellular matrix remodeling: The common denominator in connective tissue diseases. Possibilities for evaluation and current understanding of the matrix as more than a passive architecture, but a key player in tissue failure. *Assay Drug Dev. Technol.* **2013**, *11*, 70–92. [CrossRef]
8. Soylemezoglu, O.; Wild, G.; Dalley, A.J.; MacNeil, S.; Milford-Ward, A.; Brown, C.B.; el Nahas, A.M. Urinary and serum type III collagen: Markers of renal fibrosis. *Nephrol. Dial. Transplant.* **1997**, *12*, 1883–1889. [CrossRef]
9. Rasmussen, D.G.K.; Fenton, A.; Jesky, M.; Ferro, C.; Boor, P.; Tepel, M.; Karsdal, M.A.; Genovese, F.; Cockwell, P. Urinary endotrophin predicts disease progression in patients with chronic kidney disease. *Sci. Rep.* **2017**, *7*, 17328. [CrossRef]
10. Serón, D.; Moreso, F.; Ramón, J.M.; Hueso, M.; Condom, E.; Fulladosa, X.; Bover, J.; Gil-Vernet, S.; Castelao, A.M.; Alsina, J.; et al. Protocol renal allograft biopsies and the design of clinical trials aimed to prevent or treat chronic allograft nephropathy. *Transplantation* **2000**, *69*, 1849–1855. [CrossRef]
11. Magro, G.; Grasso, S.; Colombatti, A.; Lopes, M. Immunohistochemical distribution of type VI collagen in developing human kidney. *Histochem. J.* **1996**, *28*, 385–390. [CrossRef] [PubMed]
12. Groma, V. Demonstration of collagen type VI and alpha-smooth muscle actin in renal fibrotic injury in man. *Nephrol. Dial. Transplant.* **1998**, *13*, 305–312. [CrossRef] [PubMed]

13. Lennon, R.; Byron, A.; Humphries, J.D.; Randles, M.J.; Carisey, A.; Murphy, S.; Knight, D.; Brenchley, P.E.; Zent, R.; Humphries, M.J. Global analysis reveals the complexity of the human glomerular extracellular matrix. *J. Am. Soc. Nephrol.* **2014**, *25*, 939–951. [CrossRef]

14. Cescon, M.; Gattazzo, F.; Chen, P.; Bonaldo, P. Collagen VI at a glance. *J. Cell Sci.* **2015**, *128*, 3525–3531. [CrossRef] [PubMed]

15. Aigner, T.; Hambach, L.; Söder, S.; Schlötzer-Schrehardt, U.; Pöschl, E. The C5 domain of Col6A3 is cleaved off from the Col6 fibrils immediately after secretion. *Biochem. Biophys. Res. Commun.* **2002**, *290*, 743–748. [CrossRef] [PubMed]

16. Fenton, A.; Jesky, M.D.; Ferro, C.J.; Sørensen, J.; Karsdal, M.A.; Cockwell, P.; Genovese, F. Serum endotrophin, a type VI collagen cleavage product, is associated with increased mortality in chronic kidney disease. *PLoS ONE* **2017**, *12*, e0175200. [CrossRef]

17. Sun, K.; Park, J.; Gupta, O.T.; Holland, W.L.; Auerbach, P.; Zhang, N.; Goncalves Marangoni, R.; Nicoloro, S.M.; Czech, M.P.; Varga, J.; et al. Endotrophin triggers adipose tissue fibrosis and metabolic dysfunction. *Nat. Commun.* **2014**, *5*, 3485. [CrossRef]

18. Rasmussen, D.G.K.; Hansen, T.W.; von Scholten, B.J.; Nielsen, S.H.; Reinhard, H.; Parving, H.-H.; Tepel, M.; Karsdal, M.A.; Jacobsen, P.K.; Genovese, F.; et al. Higher Collagen VI Formation Is Associated with All-Cause Mortality in Patients with Type 2 Diabetes and Microalbuminuria. *Diabetes Care* **2018**, *41*, 1493–1500. [CrossRef]

19. Pilemann-Lyberg, S.; Rasmussen, D.G.K.; Hansen, T.W.; Tofte, N.; Winther, S.A.; Holm Nielsen, S.; Theilade, S.; Karsdal, M.A.; Genovese, F.; Rossing, P. Markers of Collagen Formation and Degradation Reflect Renal Function and Predict Adverse Outcomes in Patients with Type 1 Diabetes. *Diabetes Care* **2019**, *42*, 1760–1768. [CrossRef]

20. Gooch, J.L.; King, C.; Francis, C.E.; Garcia, P.S.; Bai, Y. Cyclosporine A alters expression of renal microRNAs: New insights into calcineurin inhibitor nephrotoxicity. *PLoS ONE* **2017**, *12*, e0175242. [CrossRef]

21. Sanchez-Pozos, K.; Lee-Montiel, F.; Perez-Villalva, R.; Uribe, N.; Gamba, G.; Bazan-Perkins, B.; Bobadilla, N.A. Polymerized type I collagen reduces chronic cyclosporine nephrotoxicity. *Nephrol. Dial. Transplant.* **2010**, *25*, 2150–2158. [CrossRef] [PubMed]

22. Slattery, C.; Campbell, E.; McMorrow, T.; Ryan, M.P. Cyclosporine A-Induced Renal Fibrosis. *Am. J. Pathol.* **2005**, *167*, 395–407. [CrossRef]

23. Bemelman, F.J.; de Fijter, J.W.; Kers, J.; Meyer, C.; Peters-Sengers, H.; de Maar, E.F.; van der Pant, K.A.M.I.; de Vries, A.P.J.; Sanders, J.-S.; Zwinderman, A.; et al. Early Conversion to Prednisolone/Everolimus as an Alternative Weaning Regimen Associates With Beneficial Renal Transplant Histology and Function: The Randomized-Controlled MECANO Trial. *Am. J. Transplant.* **2017**, *17*, 1020–1030. [CrossRef]

24. Bemelman, F.J.; de Maar, E.F.; Press, R.R.; van Kan, H.J.; ten Berge, I.J.; Homan van der Heide, J.J.; de Fijter, H.W. Minimization of Maintenance Immunosuppression Early After Renal Transplantation: An Interim Analysis. *Transplantation* **2009**, *88*, 421–428. [CrossRef]

25. Loupy, A.; Haas, M.; Solez, K.; Racusen, L.; Glotz, D.; Seron, D.; Nankivell, B.J.; Colvin, R.B.; Afrouzian, M.; Akalin, E.; et al. The Banff 2015 Kidney Meeting Report: Current Challenges in Rejection Classification and Prospects for Adopting Molecular Pathology. *Am. J. Transplant.* **2017**, *17*, 28–41. [CrossRef] [PubMed]

26. Mengel, M.; Reeve, J.; Bunnag, S.; Einecke, G.; Jhangri, G.S.; Sis, B.; Famulski, K.; Guembes-Hidalgo, L.; Halloran, P.F. Scoring Total Inflammation Is Superior to the Current Banff Inflammation Score in Predicting Outcome and the Degree of Molecular Disturbance in Renal Allografts. *Am. J. Transplant.* **2009**, *9*, 1859–1867. [CrossRef]

27. Sun, S.; Henriksen, K.; Karsdal, M.A.; Byrjalsen, I.; Rittweger, J.; Armbrecht, G.; Belavy, D.L.; Felsenberg, D.; Nedergaard, A.F. Collagen Type III and VI Turnover in Response to Long-Term Immobilization. *PLoS ONE* **2015**, *10*, e0144525. [CrossRef]

28. Bülow, R.D.; Boor, P. Extracellular Matrix in Kidney Fibrosis: More Than Just a Scaffold. *J. Histochem. Cytochem.* **2019**, *67*, 643–661. [CrossRef]

29. Nerlich, A.G.; Schleicher, E.D.; Wiest, I.; Specks, U.; Timpl, R. Immunohistochemical localization of collagen VI in diabetic glomeruli. *Kidney Int.* **1994**, *45*, 1648–1656. [CrossRef]

30. Wu, Q.; Jinde, K.; Nishina, M.; Tanabe, R.; Endoh, M.; Okada, Y.; Sakai, H.; Kurokawa, K. Analysis of prognostic predictors in idiopathic membranous nephropathy. *Am. J. Kidney Dis.* **2001**, *37*, 380–387. [CrossRef]

31. Knupp, C.; Pinali, C.; Munro, P.M.; Gruber, H.E.; Sherratt, M.J.; Baldock, C.; Squire, J.M. Structural correlation between collagen VI microfibrils and collagen VI banded aggregates. *J. Struct. Biol.* **2006**, *154*, 312–326. [CrossRef] [PubMed]

32. Boor, P.; Floege, J. Renal allograft fibrosis: Biology and therapeutic targets. *Am. J. Transplant.* **2015**, *15*, 863–886. [CrossRef] [PubMed]

33. Scian, M.J.; Maluf, D.G.; Archer, K.J.; Suh, J.L.; Massey, D.; Fassnacht, R.C.; Whitehill, B.; Sharma, A.; King, A.; Gehr, T.; et al. Gene expression changes are associated with loss of kidney graft function and interstitial fibrosis and tubular atrophy: Diagnosis versus prediction. *Transplantation* **2011**, *91*, 657–665. [CrossRef] [PubMed]

34. Busauschina, A.; Schnuelle, P.; van der Woude, F. Cyclosporine nephrotoxicity. *Transplant. Proc.* **2004**, *36*, S229–S233. [CrossRef] [PubMed]

35. Fitzgerald, J.; Holden, P.; Hansen, U. The expanded collagen VI family: New chains and new questions. *Connect. Tissue Res.* **2013**, *54*, 345–350. [CrossRef] [PubMed]

9

Plasma Vitamin C and Cancer Mortality in Kidney Transplant Recipients

Tomás A. Gacitúa [1], Camilo G. Sotomayor [1,*], Dion Groothof [1], Michele F. Eisenga [1], Robert A. Pol [2], Martin H. de Borst [1], Rijk O.B. Gans [1], Stefan P. Berger [1], Ramón Rodrigo [3], Gerjan J. Navis [1] and Stephan J.L. Bakker [1]

[1] Department of Internal Medicine, University Medical Center Groningen, University of Groningen, 9713 GZ Groningen, The Netherlands; t.a.gacitua.guzman@umcg.nl (T.A.G.); d.groothof@umcg.nl (D.G.); m.f.eisenga@umcg.nl (M.F.E.); m.h.de.borst@umcg.nl (M.H.d.B.); r.o.b.gans@umcg.nl (R.O.B.G.); s.p.berger@umcg.nl (S.P.B.); g.j.navis@umcg.nl (G.J.N.); s.j.l.bakker@umcg.nl (S.J.L.B.)
[2] Department of Surgery, University Medical Center Groningen, University of Groningen, 9713 GZ Groningen, The Netherlands; r.pol@umcg.nl
[3] Molecular and Clinical Pharmacology Program, Institute of Biomedical Sciences, Faculty of Medicine, University of Chile, CP 8380453 Santiago, Chile; rrodrigo@med.uchile.cl
* Correspondence: c.g.sotomayor.campos@umcg.nl

Abstract: There is a changing trend in mortality causes in kidney transplant recipients (KTR), with a decline in deaths due to cardiovascular causes along with a relative increase in cancer mortality rates. Vitamin C, a well-known antioxidant with anti-inflammatory and immune system enhancement properties, could offer protection against cancer. We aimed to investigate the association of plasma vitamin C with long-term cancer mortality in a cohort of stable outpatient KTR without history of malignancies other than cured skin cancer. Primary and secondary endpoints were cancer and cardiovascular mortality, respectively. We included 598 KTR (mean age 51 ± 12 years old, 55% male). Mean (SD) plasma vitamin C was 44 ± 20 µmol/L. At a median follow-up of 7.0 (IQR, 6.2–7.5) years, 131 patients died, of which 24% deaths were due to cancer. In Cox proportional hazards regression analyses, vitamin C was inversely associated with cancer mortality (HR 0.50; 95%CI 0.34–0.74; $p < 0.001$), independent of potential confounders, including age, smoking status and immunosuppressive therapy. In secondary analyses, vitamin C was not associated with cardiovascular mortality (HR 1.16; 95%CI 0.83–1.62; $p = 0.40$). In conclusion, plasma vitamin C is inversely associated with cancer mortality risk in KTR. These findings underscore that relatively low circulating plasma vitamin C may be a meaningful as yet overlooked modifiable risk factor of cancer mortality in KTR.

Keywords: Kidney transplant; vitamin C; cancer mortality; oxidative stress.

1. Introduction

Although kidney transplantation improves the prognosis of patients with end-stage renal disease (ESRD), kidney transplant recipients (KTR) remain at higher mortality risk compared to healthy individuals [1]. Since the beginning of kidney transplantation, the main cause of death has been cardiovascular [2–4]. In recent years, however, there has been a changing trend in mortality causes in KTR, with a decline in death due to cardiovascular causes along with a relative increase in cancer mortality [2,5–7]. Among non-cardiovascular deaths, malignancies lead the individual causes of death [8,9]. Noteworthy is that overall risk of death associated with cancer in KTR is ten-fold higher than in the general population [9]. Given this relative increase in cancer mortality in KTR, further studies to explore potential risk factors and underlying mechanisms are needed.

Post-transplantation immunosuppression as well as chronic uremic state have been recently proposed as risk factors, with oxidative stress as a potential underlying mechanism [2,10,11]. Vitamin C is a well-known radical scavenger and reducing agent [12], and due to its antioxidant, anti-inflammatory and immune system enhancement properties, it could offer protection against cancer incidence in KTR [13]. There is evidence supporting that low plasma vitamin C may lead to an increased risk of dying from cancer in the general male population [13], and is also inversely associated with gastric cancer risk in the general population [14].

Increased oxidative stress occurs when there is an imbalance between antioxidant and pro-oxidant species, leading to oxidative damage. Malondialdehyde (MDA), a decomposition product of peroxidized polyunsaturated fatty acids, is a widely used and sensitive biomarker of oxidative damage [15]. Gamma-glutamyl transpeptidase (GGT) is also currently used as an indicator of whole body oxidative stress [16,17]. Uric acid in plasma acts as antioxidant in presence of vitamin C [18]. Higher levels of free thiol groups have been proposed to be protective against oxidative damage, similarly to vitamin C [19]. Under the hypothesis that anti-carcinogenic properties of vitamin C are mainly driven by its antioxidant properties, the potential protective effect of vitamin C against cancer mortality would be expected to vary upon changes in oxidative stress biomarkers.

This evidence suggests that vitamin C could be a simple and widely available modifiable risk factor for cancer mortality in KTR. Nevertheless, studies focusing on the prospective association of vitamin C and long-term cancer mortality in this clinical setting are lacking. In this study, in primary analyses we aimed to investigate the association of circulating plasma vitamin C concentrations with long-term cancer mortality in a large cohort of KTR. As oxidative stress is considered a potential underlying mechanism, we aimed to assess whether the potential association of plasma vitamin C with cancer mortality would vary upon changes in oxidative stress biomarkers, i.e., uric acid, free thiol groups, MDA and GGT. In secondary analyses, we aimed to investigate the association of circulating plasma vitamin C concentrations with cardiovascular mortality.

2. Materials and Methods

2.1. Study Design and Patients

We performed a post hoc analysis in the TransplantLines Insulin Resistance and Inflammation Biobank and Cohort Study, number NCT03272854. Outpatient KTR (≥18 years old) with a functioning graft for at least 1 year were invited to participate between August 2001 and July 2003. Patients with overt congestive heart failure and patients diagnosed with cancer other than cured skin cancer (squamous cell or basal cell carcinoma successfully treated by a dermatologist) were not considered eligible for the study. The outpatient follow-up constitutes a continuous surveillance system in which patients visit the outpatient clinic with declining frequency, in accordance with the American Transplantation Society guidelines [20]. A total of 847 KTR were invited to be enrolled, of which 606 (72%) patients provided written informed consent to participate. Data were extensively collected at baseline. Patients with missing plasma vitamin C concentration ($n = 8$) were excluded for the statistical analysis, resulting in 598 KTR, of whom data are presented in the current study (Figure S1). The present study was approved by the Institutional Review Board (METc 2001/039), and was conducted in accordance with declarations of Helsinki and Istanbul.

2.2. Kidney Transplant Recipients Characteristics

Relevant characteristics including recipient age, gender, and transplant date were extracted from the Groningen Renal Transplant Database. This database contains detailed information on all kidney transplantations that have been performed at the University Medical Center Groningen since 1968. Details of the standard immunosuppressive treatment were described previously [21]. Smoking status was obtained using a self-report questionnaire at inclusion. Details about collection of dietary history have been described before [22]. In brief, a semi-quantitative food-frequency questionnaire was used to assess fruit and vegetable intake. Fruit intake was assessed by asking participants 'How many servings of fruit do you eat per day on average?' Vegetable intake was assessed by asking participants 'How many tablespoons of vegetable do you eat per day on average?' Respondents were asked to choose among five possible frequency categories: 0, 1, 2, 3, ≥4 per day. Collection of data on use of vitamin C or multivitamin supplements containing vitamin C was systematically performed, by means of self-report, at baseline.

2.3. Laboratory Measurements

All measurements were performed during a morning visit to the outpatient clinic. Diabetes mellitus was defined according to the guidelines of the American Diabetes Association [23]. Proteinuria was defined as urinary protein excretion ≥0.5 g/24 h. Kidney function was assessed by estimated Glomerular Filtration Rate (eGFR) applying the Chronic Kidney Disease Epidemiology Collaboration equation [24].

Blood was drawn after a fasting period of 8–12 h, which included no medication intake. According to a strict protocol, patients were instructed to collect a 24-hour urine sample the day before their visit to the outpatient clinic. Total cholesterol, low-density lipoprotein cholesterol (LDL), plasma triglycerides, plasma glucose levels, plasma insulin concentration, and glycated hemoglobin (HbA$_{1C}$) were determined as described previously [25]. Plasma high sensitivity C-reactive protein (hs-CRP) was measured by enzyme-linked immunosorbent assay, as described previously [26]. MDA was measured fluorescently after binding to thiobarbituric acid as described before [27]. Ellman's reagent was used for the determination of free thiol groups in cell culture and a cell-free solution of L-cysteine as described previously [28]. Plasma creatinine concentration was determined using a modified version of the Jaffé method (MEGA AU510; Merck Diagnostica). Total urinary protein concentration was analyzed using the Biuret reaction (MEGA AU510; Merck Diagnostica).

2.4. Plasma Vitamin C Measurement

After phlebotomy, blood was directly transferred to the laboratory on ice, deproteinized and stored in the dark at −20°C until analysis. For quantitative measurement ascorbic acid is enzymatically transformed to dehydroascorbic acid, which in turn is derivatized to 3-(1,2-dihydroxyethyl) furo-[3,4-b] quinoxaline-1-one. Then, reversed phase liquid chromatography with fluorescence detection is applied (excitation 355 nm, emission 425 nm).

2.5. Cause-Specific Mortality and Graft Failure

The primary endpoint for analyses was mortality from cancer, defined according to a previously specified list of International Classification of Diseases, Ninth Revision (ICD-9) codes 140–239 [29]. Secondary endpoint was mortality from cardiovascular causes, defined as death due to cerebrovascular disease, ischemic heart disease, heart failure, or sudden cardiac death according to ICD-9 codes 410–447. Information on the cause of death was derived from the patients' medical records and was assessed by an adjudication committee. Information about death-related type of cancer was ascertained by contacting the general practitioners who were in charge of deceased cancer patients. Graft failure was defined as return to dialysis or need for a re-transplantation. The continuous surveillance system of the outpatient program ensures up-to-date information on patient status and cause of death. There was no loss to follow-up.

2.6. Statistical Analyses

Data analysis was performed using SPSS version 23.0 software (SPSS Inc., Chicago, IL, USA), STATA 14.1 (STATA Corp., College Station, TX, USA), and R version 3.2.3 (R Foundation for Statistical Computing, Vienna, Austria). In all analyses, a two-sided $p < 0.05$ was considered significant. Continuous variables were summarized using mean (standard deviation; SD) for normally distributed data, whereas skewed distributed variables are given as median (interquartile range; IQR). Categorical variables were summarized as numbers (percentage). Multiple imputation was performed to account for missingness of data among variables other than data on plasma vitamin C [30]. The percentages of missing data were 0.2, 0.2, 0.2, 0.2, 0.3, 0.3, 0.3, 0.3, 0.5, 0.7, and 0.7% for waist circumference, HbA_{1C}, albumin, alkaline phosphatase, proteinuria, leukocyte concentration, MDA, cumulative dose of prednisolone, uric acid, GGT, and prior history of cardiovascular disease, respectively. The percentages of missing data were maximally 11, 21, and 33% for free thiol groups, free fatty acids, and fruit and vegetable intake, respectively.

Age- and sex-adjusted linear regression analyses were performed to evaluate the association of plasma vitamin C concentrations with baseline characteristics. Residuals were checked for normality and variables were natural log-transformed when appropriate. In order to study in an integrated manner which patient- and transplant-related variables of interest were independently associated with and were determinants of plasma vitamin C concentrations, we performed forward selection of baseline characteristics by including all the variables that were associated with plasma vitamin C with a $p < 0.1$ in the preceding age- and sex-adjusted linear regression analyses. Selected variables were then used to perform stepwise backwards multivariable linear regression analyses ($P_{out} > 0.05$). Standardized beta coefficients represent the difference (in standard deviations) in plasma vitamin C per 1 standard deviation increment in continuous baseline characteristics, or for categorical characteristics the difference (in standard deviations) in plasma vitamin C compared to the implied reference group.

To analyze whether plasma vitamin C was prospectively and independently associated with cancer mortality, we performed multivariable-adjusted Cox proportional hazards regression analyses. For these analyses plasma vitamin C concentrations were used as log-transformed values with a log2 base, in order to obtain the best fitting model. We tested proportionality assumptions of Cox proportional hazards regression analyses, and they were satisfied, indicating that the association of baseline vitamin C with outcome is constant over follow-up time of the current study. The selection of covariates was made a priori, considering their potential confounding effect based on previously described risk factors for all-cause mortality in KTR and generally accepted risk factors for cancer mortality in the general population and in KTR [9,10,13,31]. We adjusted for age, sex, and smoking status (Model 1); eGFR, dialysis vintage, time since transplantation and proteinuria (Model 2); and, fruit and vegetable intake (Model 3). To avoid overfitting and inclusion of too many variables for the number of events, further models were performed with additive adjustments to Model 3 [32]. We performed additional adjustments for diabetes mellitus, hs-CRP and prior history of cardiovascular disease (Model 4); immunosuppressive therapy (use of calcineurin inhibitors (CNI), use of antimetabolites, use of mammalian target of rapamycin (m-TOR) inhibitors, and cumulative dose of prednisolone, calculated as the sum of maintenance dose of prednisolone since kidney transplantation until inclusion in the study and the dose of prednisolone or methylprednisolone required for treatment of acute rejection (a conversion factor of 1.25 was used to convert methylprednisolone to prednisolone dose). For acute rejection, different amounts of prednisolone or methylprednisolone were administered, which was taken into account in the calculations. Rejection episodes after inclusion were not included [33]; Model 5); and transplantation era (Model 6). Transplantation eras, with corresponding immunosuppressing medications, have been previously well described [34]. In secondary analyses, the aforementioned Cox proportional hazards regression analyses were performed for cardiovascular mortality. The analyses for both cancer death and cardiovascular death were performed by fitting multivariable-adjusted proportional cause-specific hazard models. In each of these models, the competing events were treated as censored observations, causing the regression parameters to directly quantify the hazard ratio among those individuals who are actually at risk of developing the event of interest, i.e., cancer mortality or cardiovascular mortality [35]. Hazard ratios (HR) are reported with 95% confidence interval (CI). The HR of each model is given per doubling of vitamin C concentration.

To adhere to existing recommendations for good reporting on survival analyses [36,37], we tested for potential interaction of all potential confounders and the oxidative stress biomarkers with vitamin C, namely, uric acid, free thiol groups (corrected by total serum protein) [19], MDA, and GGT by fitting models containing both main effects and their cross product terms. For these analyses, $P_{\text{interaction}} < 0.05$

was considered to indicate significant interaction. We also performed subgroup analyses according to the aforementioned oxidative stress biomarkers, with adjustment for age, sex, smoking status, eGFR, dialysis vintage, time since transplantation, proteinuria, and fruit and vegetable intake. Cut-off points of originally continuous variables used in the stratified analyses were determined so they would allow for an as much as possible similar number of events in each subgroup, and thus allow for similar statistical power for the assessment of the primary association under study (plasma vitamin C and cancer mortality) in each subgroup after stratification of the overall population. Whenever and as much as possible, these criteria were matched with clinical cut-off points.

In sensitivity analyses, we performed graft failure-censored Cox proportional hazards regression analyses of the association of plasma vitamin C with cancer mortality and cardiovascular mortality. In addition, we performed Cox proportional hazards regression analyses of the association of plasma vitamin C with cancer mortality with adjustment for HbA1c instead of diabetes mellitus.

3. Results

3.1. Baseline Characteristics

A total of 598 patients (51 ± 12 years old, 55% male) were included at a median of 5.9 (IQR, 2.6–11.4) years after kidney transplantation. None of the patients used vitamin C supplements or multivitamin supplements containing vitamin C. Mean plasma vitamin C concentration was 44 ± 20 µmol/L, mean eGFR was 47 ± 16 mL/min/1.73 m^2. Patient-related variables of interest, including transplant-related characteristics and immunosuppressive therapy are summarized in Table 1. The results of the age- and sex-adjusted linear regression analyses are shown in Table 2. In stepwise backward multivariable linear regression analysis, fruit intake (std. $\beta = 0.22$; $p < 0.01$), dialysis vintage (std. $\beta = -0.09$; $p < 0.05$), proteinuria ≥ 0.5 g/24 h (std. $\beta = -0.11$; $p < 0.05$), HbA$_{1C}$ (std. $\beta = -0.14$; $p < 0.01$), diastolic blood pressure (std. $\beta = -0.16$; $p < 0.01$), alkaline phosphatase (std. $\beta = -0.15$; $p < 0.01$), hs-CRP (std. $\beta = -0.17$; $p < 0.01$) and male sex (std. $\beta = -0.18$; $p < 0.01$) were identified as independent determinants of plasma vitamin C (Table 2). The overall R^2 of the final model was 0.21.

Table 1. Baseline characteristics of 598 kidney transplant recipients.

Baseline Characteristics	All Patients
Study subjects, n (%)	598 (100)
Plasma vitamin C, µmol/L, mean (SD)	44 (20)
Demographics	
Age, years, mean (SD)	51 (12)
Sex, male, n (%)	328 (55)
Caucasian ethnicity, n (%)	577 (97)
Body composition	
Body mass index, kg/m^2, mean (SD)	26.0 (4.3)
Body surface area, m^2, mean (SD)	1.9 (0.2)
Waist circumference, cm, mean (SD) [a]	97 (14)
Kidney allograft function	
estimated Glomerular Filtration Rate, mL/min/1.73 m^2, mean (SD)	47 (16)
Proteinuria ≥ 0.5 g/24 h, n (%) [b]	166 (28)
Tobacco use	
Never smoker, n (%)	214 (36)
Ex-smoker, n (%)	251 (42)
Current smoker, n (%)	131 (22)
Blood pressure	
Systolic blood pressure, mmHg, mean (SD)	153 (23)
Diastolic blood pressure, mmHg, mean (SD)	90 (10)
Prior history of cardiovascular disease	
History of myocardial infarction, n (%) [c]	48 (8)
History of cerebrovascular accident or transient ischemic attack, n (%) [c]	32 (5)

Table 1. *Cont.*

Baseline Characteristics	All Patients
Diet	
Fruit intake, servings/day, mean (SD) [d]	1.5 (1.0)
Vegetable intake, tablespoons/day, mean (SD) [d]	2.5 (0.8)
Diabetes and glucose homeostasis	
Diabetes, n (%)	105 (18)
HbA$_{1C}$, %, mean (SD) [a]	6.5 (1.1)
Insulin, μU/mL, median (IQR)	11.2 (8.0–16.3)
Glucose, mmol/L, median (IQR)	4.5 (4.1–5.0)
Laboratory measurements	
Leukocyte concentration, $\times 10^9$/L, mean (SD) [b]	8.6 (2.4)
hs-CRP, mg/L, median (IQR)	2.0 (0.8–4.8)
Albumin, g/L, mean (SD) [a]	41 (3)
Lipids	
Total cholesterol, mmol/L, mean (SD)	5.6 (1.1)
HDL cholesterol, mmol/L, mean (SD)	1.1 (0.3)
LDL cholesterol, mmol/L, mean (SD)	3.5 (1.0)
Free fatty acids, μmol/L, mean (SD) [e]	403 (180)
Triglycerides, mmol/L, median (IQR)	1.9 (1.4–2.6)
Oxidative stress	
Uric acid, mmol/L, mean (SD) [f]	0.45 (0.13)
Malondialdehyde, μmol/L, mean (SD) [b]	5.6 (1.8)
Gamma-glutamyl transpeptidase, U/L, median (IQR) [c]	24 (18–39)
Alkaline phosphatase, U/L, median (IQR) [a]	72 (57–94)
Kidney transplant and immunosuppressive therapy	
Dialysis vintage, months, median (IQR)	27 (13–48)
Time since transplantation, years, median (IQR)	6 (3–11)
Donor type (living), n (%)	83 (14)
Use of calcineurin inhibitor, n (%)	470 (79)
Cyclosporine, n (%)	386 (65)
Tacrolimus, n (%)	84 (14)
Use of antimetabolites, n (%)	441 (74)
Azathioprine, n (%)	194 (32)
Mycophenolate acid, n (%)	247 (41)
Use of mammalian target of rapamycin inhibitors, n (%)	10 (1.7)
Cumulative dose of prednisolone, g, median (IQR) [b]	21 (11–38)

Data available in: [a] 597, [b] 596, [c] 594, [d] 400, [e] 471, [f] 595. Abbreviations: hs-CRP, high-sensitive C reactive protein; HDL, high-density lipoprotein; IQR, interquartile range; LDL, low-density lipoprotein; HbA$_{1C}$, glycated hemoglobin; SD, standard deviation.

Table 2. Association of baseline characteristics with plasma vitamin C in 598 kidney transplant recipients.

Baseline Characteristics	Plasma Vitamin C (Log$_2$), μmol/L	
	Linear Regression [†]	Backwards Linear Regression [§]
	Std. β	Std. β
Study subjects, n (%)	—	—
Plasma vitamin C, μmol/L, mean (SD)	—	—
Demographics		
Age, years	−0.56	
Sex, male	−0.19 ***	−0.18 ***
Caucasian ethnicity	−0.21	
Body composition		
Body mass index, kg/m^2	−0.08 *	~
Body surface area, m^2	−0.06	
Waist circumference, cm	−0.15 ***	~

Table 2. *Cont.*

Baseline Characteristics	Plasma Vitamin C (Log_2), μmol/L	
	Linear Regression [†] Std. β	Backwards Linear Regression [§] Std. β
Kidney allograft function		
estimated Glomerular Filtration Rate, mL/min/1.73 m^2	0.11 ***	~
Proteinuria ≥0.5 g/24 h	−0.11 ***	−0.11 **
Tobacco use		
Never smoker	0.03	
Ex-smoker	0.08 *	~
Current smoker	−0.11 ***	~
Blood pressure		
Systolic blood pressure, mmHg	−0.12 ***	~
Diastolic blood pressure, mm Hg	−0.1 **	−0.16 ***
Prior history of cardiovascular disease		
History of myocardial infarction	−0.01	
History of cerebrovascular accident or transient ischemic attack	−0.04	
Diet		
Fruit intake, servings/day	0.22 ***	0.22 ***
Vegetable intake, tablespoons/day	0.09*	~
Diabetes and glucose homeostasis		
Diabetes	−0.11 ***	~
HbA$_{1C}$, %	−0.13 ***	−0.14 ***
Insulin, μU/mL	−0.09 **	~
Glucose, mmol/L	−0.07 *	~
Laboratory measurements		
Leukocyte concentration, x × 10^9/L	−0.03	
hs-CRP, mg/L	−0.14 ***	−0.17 ***
Albumin, g/L	0.14 ***	~
Lipids		
Total cholesterol, mmol/L	0.05	
HDL cholesterol, mmol/L	0.12 ***	~
LDL cholesterol, mmol/L	0.07 *	~
Free fatty acids, μmol/L	−0.07	
Triglycerides, mmol/L	−0.09 **	~
Oxidative stress		
Uric acid, mmol/L	−0.14 ***	~
Malondialdehyde, μmol/L	0.01	
Gamma-glutamyl transpeptidase, U/L	−0.05	
Alkaline phosphatase, U/L	−0.18 ***	−0.15 ***
Kidney transplant and immunosuppressive therapy		
Dialysis vintage, months	−0.09 **	−0.09 **
Time since transplantation, years	0.18 ***	~
Donor type (living)	0.02	
Use of calcineurin inhibitor	−0.08 **	~
Cyclosporine	−0.03	
Tacrolimus	−0.06	
Use of antimetabolites	0.01	
Azathioprine	0.10 **	~
Mycophenolate acid	−0.09 **	~
Use of mammalian target of rapamycin inhibitors	−0.09 **	~
Cumulative dose of prednisolone, g	0.17 ***	~

* p Value < 0.1; ** p Value < 0.05; *** p Value < 0.01. [†] Linear regression analysis; adjusted for age and sex. [§] Stepwise backwards linear regression analysis; for inclusion and exclusion in this analysis, p Values were set at 0.1 and 0.05, respectively. ~ Excluded from the final model. Abbreviations: Std. β, standardized beta coefficient; hs-CRP, high-sensitive C reactive protein; HDL, high-density lipoprotein; LDL, low-density lipoprotein; HbA$_{1C}$, glycated hemoglobin.

3.2. Primary Prospective Analyses

At a median follow-up of 7.0 (IQR, 6.2–7.5) years, 131 (22%) patients died, of which 32 (24%) deaths were due to cancer (summary of types of cancer can be found in Table S1). Median time from kidney transplantation to cancer death was 12.0 (IQR, 6.2–20.0). In multivariable-adjusted Cox proportional hazards regression analyses, plasma vitamin C concentration was inversely associated with cancer mortality risk (HR 0.50; 95%CI 0.34–0.74; $p < 0.001$), independent of potential confounders including age, sex, smoking status, eGFR, dialysis vintage, time since transplantation, proteinuria, fruit and vegetable intake, diabetes mellitus, hs-CRP, prior history of cardiovascular disease, immunosuppressive therapy and transplantation era (Table 3, Models 1–6) (Figure 1). Full report of coefficient estimates for both the variable of interest plasma vitamin C as well as for potential confounders included in every multivariable model (Models 1–6) are shown in Table S2. Neither significant interaction of the association of vitamin C with cancer mortality was found for potential confounders (Table S3) nor for oxidative stress biomarkers. Results of interaction and subgroup analyses of oxidative stress biomarkers are presented in Figure 2.

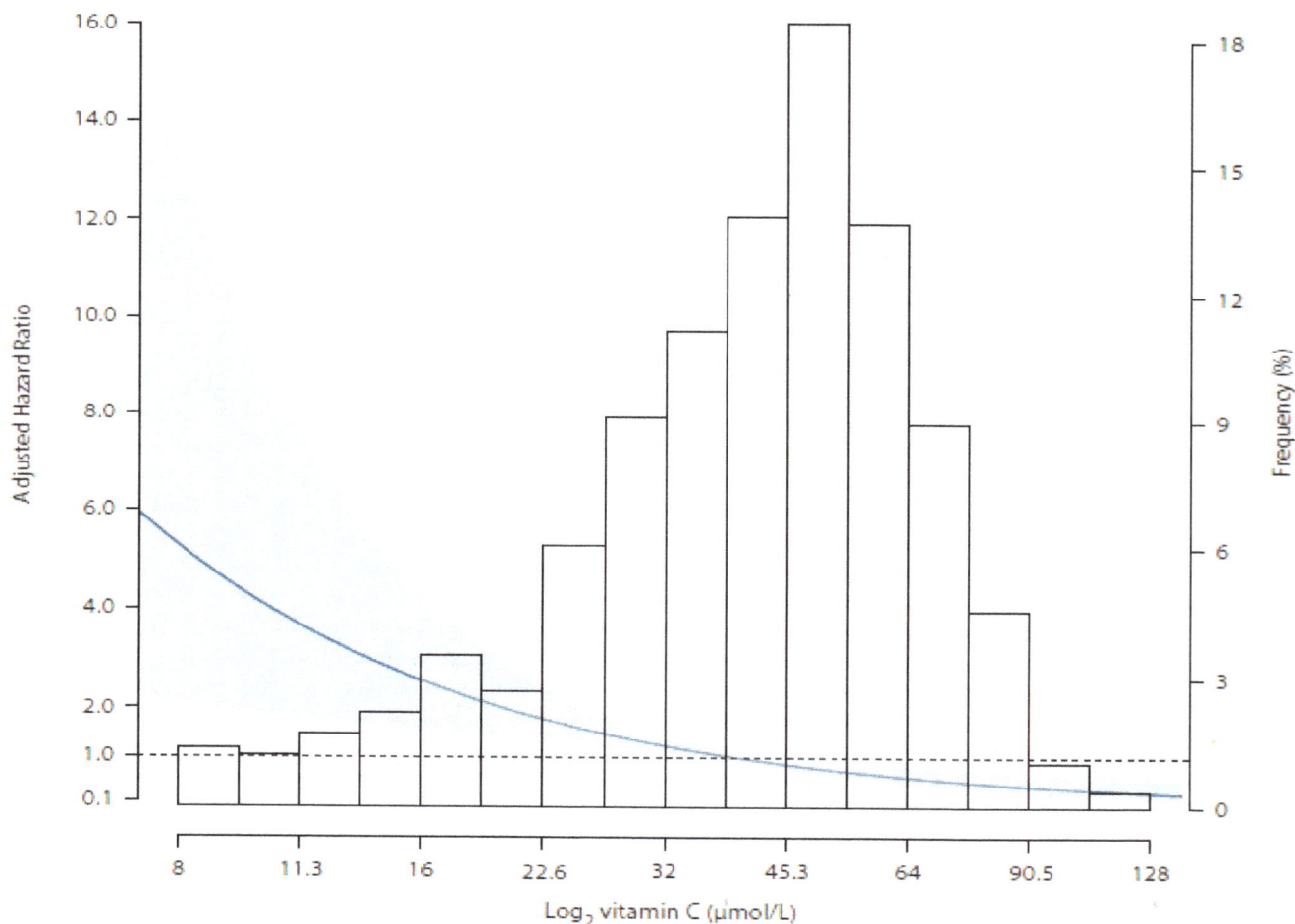

Figure 1. Association of plasma vitamin C with cancer mortality risk in 598 KTR. Data were fitted by a Cox proportional hazards regression model adjusted for age, sex, smoking status, estimated Glomerular Filtration Rate, dialysis vintage, time since transplantation, proteinuria, fruit and vegetable intake, diabetes mellitus, high-sensitivity C-reactive protein, and prior history of cardiovascular disease (Model 4). The gray areas indicate the 95% CIs. The line in the graph represents the hazard ratio.

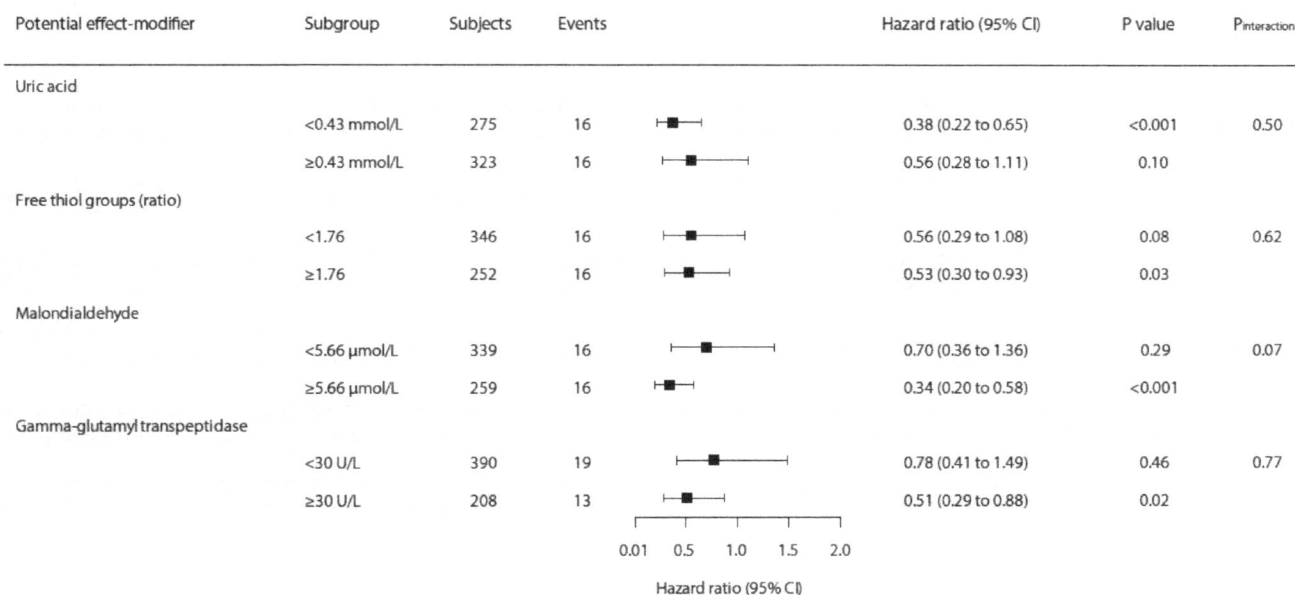

Figure 2. Interaction and subgroup analyses of the association of plasma vitamin C with cancer mortality. $P_{\text{interaction}}$ was calculated by fitting models which contain both main effects as continuous variables and their cross-product term. Hazard ratios were calculated with adjustment for age, sex, smoking status, estimated Glomerular Filtration Rate, dialysis vintage, time since transplantation, proteinuria, and fruit and vegetable intake, analogous to Model 3 of the overall prospective analyses. Abbreviations: CI, confidence interval; MDA, malondialdehyde; GGT, gamma-glutamyl transpeptidase.

Table 3. Association of plasma vitamin C with cancer mortality in 598 kidney transplant recipients.

Models	Vitamin C (Log$_2$), Continuous (μmol/L)		
	HR [a]	95% CI	p Value
Crude	0.63	0.43–0.92	0.016
Model 1	0.61	0.43–0.87	0.006
Model 2	0.52	0.35–0.75	0.001
Model 3	0.50	0.34–0.74	<0.001
Model 4	0.49	0.33–0.72	<0.001
Model 5	0.55	0.38–0.80	0.002
Model 6	0.47	0.32–0.70	<0.001

Cox proportional hazards regression analyses were performed to assess the association of plasma vitamin C with cancer mortality. Model 1: adjustment for age, sex and smoking status. Model 2: Model 1 + adjustment for estimated Glomerular Filtration Rate, dialysis vintage, time since transplantation and proteinuria. Model 3: Model 2 + adjustment for fruit and vegetable intake. Model 4: Model 3 + adjustment for diabetes mellitus, high-sensitivity C-reactive protein and prior history of cardiovascular disease. Model 5: Model 3 + adjustment for immunosuppressive therapy. Model 6: Model 3 + adjustment for transplantation era. Abbreviations: HR, hazard ratio; CI, confidence interval. [a] Each model hazard ratio is given per doubling of vitamin C concentration.

3.3. Secondary Prospective Analyses

In secondary analyses, at a median follow-up of 7.0 (IQR, 6.2–7.5) years, 131 (22%) patients died, of which 67 (49%) deaths were due to cardiovascular causes. Median time from kidney transplantation to cardiovascular death was 11.0 (IQR, 7.6–14.8). There was no significant association of plasma vitamin C with cardiovascular mortality (HR 1.16; 95%CI 0.83–1.62; $p = 0.40$) (Table 4). This finding remained unaltered after adjustment for potential confounders, analogous to Models 1 to 6 of the primary analyses.

Table 4. Association of plasma vitamin C with cardiovascular mortality in 598 kidney transplant recipients.

Models	Vitamin C (Log$_2$), Continuous (μmol/L)		
	HR	95% CI	*p* Value
Crude	0.97	0.70–1.33	0.83
Model 1	0.97	0.71–1.33	0.86
Model 2	1.04	0.75–1.44	0.83
Model 3	1.16	0.83–1.62	0.40
Model 4	1.31	0.92–1.86	0.13
Model 5	1.21	0.86–1.70	0.27
Model 6	1.15	0.82–1.61	0.41

Cox proportional hazards regression analyses were performed to assess the association of plasma vitamin C with cardiovascular mortality. Model 1: adjustment for age, sex, and smoking status. Model 2: Model 1 + adjustment for estimated Glomerular Filtration Rate, dialysis vintage, time since transplantation and proteinuria. Model 3: Model 2 + adjustment for fruit and vegetable intake. Model 4: Model 3 + adjustment for diabetes mellitus, high-sensitivity C-reactive protein and prior history of cardiovascular disease. Model 5: Model 3 + adjustment for immunosuppressive therapy. Model 6: Model 3 + adjustment for transplantation era. Abbreviations: HR, hazard ratio; CI, confidence interval.

3.4. Sensitivity Analyses

After performing graft failure-censored Cox proportional hazards regression analyses, our primary findings of the association of plasma vitamin C with both cancer mortality and cardiovascular mortality remained materially unchanged (Tables S4 and S5, respectively). After performing Cox proportional hazards regression analyses of the association of plasma vitamin C with cancer mortality with adjustment for HbA1c instead of diabetes mellitus the association remained materially unchanged (Table S6).

4. Discussion

In the current study, we show that cancer is a substantially prevalent individual cause of death after kidney transplantation, and that plasma vitamin C concentrations are inversely and independently associated with long-term cancer mortality risk in stable KTR. Secondary analyses did not reveal significant associations with cardiovascular mortality. To the best of our knowledge, this is the first study that provides prospective data supporting vitamin C as a potential risk factor for cancer mortality in KTR.

Our results are in line with previously reported cancer mortality risk data in KTR. Au et al. reported that 16.7% of deaths in a large cohort of KTR were due to cancer after a median follow-up of 6.3 (IQR, 2.3–12.0) years. Although cancer mortality has been previously described as an increasing and imperative problem in KTR [2,5,6,10], there is a paucity of studies exploring potential risk factors and underlying mechanisms leading to this increased cancer mortality in KTR. Immunosuppression following kidney transplant is the most accepted risk factor, specifically CNI [4,6,38,39]. In fact, there is extensive research focused on finding the best combination of immunosuppressants in order to reduce de novo malignancy incidence without increasing rejection rates, where m-TOR inhibitors could have a role in reducing cancer risk [6,40–42]. Noteworthy is that according to our findings, the association of plasma vitamin C concentrations with cancer mortality is independent of immunosuppressive therapies after a kidney transplant.

Low plasma vitamin C has been previously associated with gastric cancer risk in the general population. In this patient setting, mean plasma vitamin C concentration was 39.9 ± 25.2 μmol/L for cases and 41.5 ± 19.4 μmol/L for controls, both comparable to those from our study [14]. Likewise, in the general male population, low plasma vitamin C was linked to an increased risk of mortality with cancer playing a key role. In this study, median plasma vitamin C was 49.4 (IQR, 47.7–51.7) μmol/L [13], also comparable to our study. Furthermore, the anti-cancer properties from vitamin C and other antioxidants have drawn much attention in the oncology research field [43–46]. According to the results of cross-sectional analyses of our study, daily fruit intake was independently associated with plasma vitamin C levels, congruent with evidence suggesting a diet high in fruits to be associated with decreased cancer risk in various patient settings, with antioxidants playing a key-role [47–53]. Surprisingly, our results show that the association of lower plasma vitamin C with cancer mortality risk is independent of fruit and vegetable intake, introducing vitamin C as a specific therapeutic target in this setting of patients.

A possible explanation for the association we found could be the important role that vitamin C plays as epigenetic modulator in health and disease [43–46], and specifically in cancer cell lines [54]. On the other hand, it is well known that oxidative stress can cause cancer [55,56], due to oxidative damage to deoxyribonucleic acid (DNA) [57]. This oxidative damage is usually counteracted by DNA repair enzymes, but in a pro-oxidant environment, e.g., chronic inflammation and uremic state [58,59], this defense-mechanism is held back [56,60,61]. It has been suggested that antioxidant treatment cannot prevent occurrence of gastrointestinal cancer and that it may even increase overall risk of mortality [55]. However, it has been described that kidney transplant recipients (KTR) have increased oxidative stress [19], which in turn can lead to increased oxidative damage to DNA [57]. Together with decreased immunological surveillance secondary to post-transplant immunosuppression, these phenomena can play a role in increased cancer mortality in KTR and an increased contribution of oxidative stress therein. It can therefore not be excluded that other than subjects of the general population, KTR could benefit from anti-oxidant treatment. High dosages of vitamin C supplementation have been linked to higher risk of development of oxalate kidney stones in male subjects of the general population [62,63]. Vitamin C supplementation may also enhance immunity, which could result in increased risk of rejection. Such effects could limit the utility of vitamin C supplementation in clinical practice and should be taken into account when considering vitamin C supplementation strategies in KTR. Of note, no significant interaction of the association of vitamin C with cancer mortality was found by oxidative stress biomarkers. In light of these results, it could be hypothesized that the inverse association of vitamin C with cancer mortality hereby reported may be explained by its potential role as epigenetic modulator rather than through its antioxidant properties. The latter may be further supported by the finding that plasma vitamin C was inversely associated with cancer mortality independently of fruit and vegetable intake, which suggests that the beneficial effect of vitamin C would not be fully related to the classic theory of dietary intake of natural antioxidants as anticarcinogens [53,57].

Our study has important strengths, including its large sample size of stable KTR, which were closely monitored during a considerable follow-up period by regular check-up in the outpatient clinic, without loss of participants to follow-up. Furthermore, data were extensively collected, allowing to adjust our findings for several potential confounders and predictors of the main results, including current or former smoking status. We acknowledge the study's limitations as the following. First, vitamin C was measured at baseline. Like the current study, most epidemiological studies use a single baseline measurement to predict outcomes, which adversely affects predictive properties of variables associated with outcomes [64–67]. If intra-individual variability of predictive biomarkers using repeated measurements is taken into account, this results in strengthening of predictive properties, particularly in case of markers with high intra-individual variation [64,67]. The lower the intra-individual variation from one measurement to the next would be, the more accurate the single measurement represents the usual level of the marker [64–67]. Noteworthy, evidence available for intra-individual variability of plasma vitamin C suggests that its concentrations relatively stable over time, with a single plasma vitamin C measurement being representative of an individual's status for long periods of time [65]. Moreover, previous epidemiological studies have used a baseline measurement of plasma vitamin C to predict clinical outcomes over a period of several years [68–70]. Second, we measured plasma vitamin C rather than leukocyte vitamin C, which could have provided assessment of tissue vitamin C, and therefore additional information on the role of vitamin C in disease prevention [71]. Third, initiation of vitamin C supplementation during follow-up was not recorded, which could have introduced bias that cannot be accounted for in our analyses. Fourth, incidence and types of non-fatal cancer were not documented, while this information would have been of added value to the reported findings. With the presented data, we had no power to discriminate the association with cancer mortality by types of cancer, which does not necessarily imply that associations are similar for all types of cancer. Nevertheless, our results show, for the first time, a prospective association of plasma vitamin C with long-term risk of cancer mortality in stable kidney transplant recipients, which holds a plea for future studies in which data on incidence and types of non-fatal cancer are collected. To allow for such studies we have started a new large, long-lasting prospective cohort study in kidney transplant recipients in which collection of such data is included [72]. Another limitation is that history of cured skin cancer was not documented, it could therefore not be included in multivariable analyses. Finally, due to its observational design, conclusions on causality cannot be drawn from our results.

In conclusion, we show that cancer is a substantially prevalent individual cause of death after kidney transplantation, and that plasma vitamin C concentrations are inversely and independently associated with cancer mortality risk. Remarkably, our findings link for the first time plasma vitamin C concentrations with cancer mortality risk in KTR, which underscores that vitamin C may be a meaningful as yet overlooked modifiable risk factor of cancer mortality in KTR. Considering the relative increase in cancer mortality rates in kidney transplant recipients along with the decline in deaths due to cardiovascular causes, it is expected that novel risk management strategies are to emerge. Whether a novel vitamin C-targeted strategy may represent an opportunity to decrease the burden of cancer mortality in KTR requires further studies.

Author Contributions: Formal analysis, T.A.G., C.G.S. and D.G.; investigation, T.A.G., C.G.S., D.G., M.F.E., R.A.P., M.H.d.B., R.O.B.G., S.P.B., R.R., G.J.N. and S.J.L.B.; data curation, T.A.G., C.G.S. and D.G.; writing—original draft preparation, T.A.G. and C.G.S.; writing—review and editing, T.A.G., C.G.S., D.G., M.F.E., R.A.P., M.H.d.B., R.O.B.G., S.P.B., R.R., G.J.N. and S.J.L.B.; supervision, R.R., G.J.N. and S.J.L.B.; project administration, R.O.B.G., S.P.B., G.J.N. and S.J.L.B.; funding acquisition, T.A.G., C.G.S. and S.J.L.B.

References

1.	Briggs, J.D. Causes of death after renal transplantation. *Nephrol. Dial. Transpl.* **2001**, *16*, 1545–1549. [CrossRef]
2.	Pippias, M.; Jager, K.J.; Kramer, A.; Leivestad, T.; Sánchez, M.B.; Caskey, F.J.; Collart, F.; Couchoud, C.; Dekker, F.W.; Finne, P.; et al. The changing trends and outcomes in renal replacement therapy: Data from the ERA-EDTA Registry. *Nephrol. Dial. Transpl.* **2016**, *31*, 831–841. [CrossRef] [PubMed]
3.	Ojo, A.O.; Hanson, J.A.; Wolfe, R.A.; Leichtman, A.B.; Agodoa, L.Y.; Port, F.K. Long-term survival in renal transplant recipients with graft function. *Kidney Int.* **2000**, *57*, 307–313. [CrossRef] [PubMed]
4.	Lim, W.H.; Russ, G.R.; Wong, G.; Pilmore, H.; Kanellis, J.; Chadban, S.J. The risk of cancer in kidney transplant recipients may be reduced in those maintained on everolimus and reduced cyclosporine. *Kidney Int.* **2017**, *91*, 954–963. [CrossRef] [PubMed]
5.	Pilmore, H.; Dent, H.; Chang, S.; McDonald, S.P.; Chadban, S.J. Reduction in cardiovascular death after kidney transplantation. *Transplantation* **2010**, *89*, 851–857. [CrossRef]
6.	Buell, J.F.; Gross, T.G.; Woodle, E.S. Malignancy after Transplantation. *Transplantation* **2005**, *80*, S254–S264. [CrossRef]
7.	Berthoux, F.; Mariat, C. Cardiovascular Death After Renal Transplantation Remains the First Cause Despite Significant Quantitative and Qualitative Changes. *Transplantation* **2010**, *89*, 806. [CrossRef]
8.	Farrugia, D.; Mahboob, S.; Cheshire, J.; Begaj, I.; Khosla, S.; Ray, D.; Sharif, A. Malignancy-related mortality following kidney transplantation is common. *Kidney Int.* **2014**, *85*, 1395–1403. [CrossRef]
9.	Wong, G.; Chapman, J.R.; Craig, J.C. Death from cancer: A sobering truth for patients with kidney transplants. *Kidney Int.* **2014**, *85*, 1262–1264. [CrossRef]
10.	Au, E.H.; Chapman, J.R.; Craig, J.C.; Lim, W.H.; Teixeira-Pinto, A.; Ullah, S.; McDonald, S.; Wong, G. Overall and Site-Specific Cancer Mortality in Patients on Dialysis and after Kidney Transplant. *J. Am. Soc. Nephrol.* **2019**, *30*, 471–480. [CrossRef]

11. Stoyanova, E.; Sandoval, S.B.; Zúñiga, L.A.; El-Yamani, N.; Coll, E.; Pastor, S.; Reyes, J.; Andrés, E.; Ballarin, J.; Xamena, N.; et al. Oxidative DNA damage in chronic renal failure patients. *Nephrol. Dial. Transpl.* **2010**, *25*, 879–885. [CrossRef] [PubMed]

12. Rodrigo, R.; Guichard, C.; Charles, R. Clinical pharmacology and therapeutic use of antioxidant vitamins. *Fundam. Clin. Pharm.* **2007**, *21*, 111–127. [CrossRef] [PubMed]

13. Loria, C.M.; Klag, M.J.; Caulfield, L.E.; Whelton, P.K. Vitamin C status and mortality in US adults. *Am. J. Clin. Nutr.* **2000**, *72*, 139–145. [CrossRef] [PubMed]

14. Jenab, M.; Riboli, E.; Ferrari, P.; Sabate, J.; Slimani, N.; Norat, T.; Friesen, M.; Tjønneland, A.; Olsen, A.; Overvad, K.; et al. Plasma and dietary vitamin C levels and risk of gastric cancer in the European Prospective Investigation into Cancer and Nutrition (EPIC-EURGAST). *Carcinogenesis* **2006**, *27*, 2250–2257. [CrossRef] [PubMed]

15. Block, G.; Dietrich, M.; Norkus, E.P.; Morrow, J.D.; Hudes, M.; Caan, B.; Packer, L. Factors associated with oxidative stress in human populations. *Am. J. Epidemiol.* **2002**, *156*, 274–285. [CrossRef] [PubMed]

16. Koenig, G.; Seneff, S. Gamma-Glutamyltransferase: A Predictive Biomarker of Cellular Antioxidant Inadequacy and Disease Risk. *Dis. Markers* **2015**, *2015*, 818570. [CrossRef]

17. Lee, D.H.; Blomhoff, R.; Jacobs, D.R. Is serum gamma glutamyltransferase a marker of oxidative stress? *Free Radic. Res.* **2004**, *38*, 535–539. [CrossRef]

18. Frei, B.; Stocker, R.; Amest, B.N. Antioxidant defenses and lipid peroxidation in human blood plasma (oxidants/polymorphonuclear leukocytes/ascorbate/plasma peroxidase). *Proc. Natl. Acad. Sci. USA* **1988**, *85*, 9748–9752. [CrossRef]

19. Frenay, A.S.; de Borst, M.H.; Bachtler, M.; Tschopp, N.; Keyzer, C.A.; van den Berg, E.; Bakker, S.J.L.; Feelisch, M.; Pasch, A.; van Goor, H. Serum free sulfhydryl status is associated with patient and graft survival in renal transplant recipients. *Free Radic. Biol. Med.* **2016**, *99*, 345–351. [CrossRef]

20. Kasiske, B.L.; Vazquez, M.A.; Harmon, W.E.; Brown, R.S.; Danovitch, G.M.; Gaston, R.S.; Roth, D.; Scandling, J.D.; Singer, G.G. Recommendations for the outpatient surveillance of renal transplant recipients. American Society of Transplantation. *J. Am. Soc. Nephrol.* **2000**, *11* (Suppl. 1), S1–S86.

21. Sinkeler, S.J.; Zelle, D.M.; Homan van der Heide, J.J.; Gans, R.O.B.; Navis, G.; Bakker, S.J.L. Endogenous Plasma Erythropoietin, Cardiovascular Mortality and All-Cause Mortality in Renal Transplant Recipients. *Am. J. Transpl.* **2012**, *12*, 485–491. [CrossRef] [PubMed]

22. Sotomayor, C.G.; Gomes-Neto, A.W.; Eisenga, M.F.; Nolte, I.M.; Anderson, J.L.C.; de Borst, M.H.; Osté, M.C.J.; Rodrigo, R.; Gans, R.O.B.; Berger, S.P.; et al. Consumption of fruits and vegetables and cardiovascular mortality in renal transplant recipients: A prospective cohort study. *Nephrol. Dial. Transpl.* **2018**. [CrossRef] [PubMed]

23. Report of the Expert Committee on the Diagnosis and Classification of Diabetes Mellitus. *Diabetes Care* **2003**, *26*, S5–S20. [CrossRef] [PubMed]

24. Levey, A.S.; Stevens, L.A.; Schmid, C.H.; Zhang, Y.; Castro, A.F.; Feldman, H.I.; Kusek, J.W.; Eggers, P.; Van Lente, F.; Greene, T.; et al. A New Equation to Estimate Glomerular Filtration Rate. *Ann. Intern. Med.* **2009**, *150*, 604. [CrossRef]

25. Annema, W.; Dikkers, A.; Freark de Boer, J.; Dullaart, R.P.F.; Sanders, J.-S.F.; Bakker, S.J.L.; Tietge, U.J.F. HDL Cholesterol Efflux Predicts Graft Failure in Renal Transplant Recipients. *J. Am. Soc. Nephrol.* **2016**, *27*, 595–603. [CrossRef]

26. De Leeuw, K.; Sanders, J.S.; Stegeman, C.; Smit, A.; Kallenberg, C.G.; Bijl, M. Accelerated atherosclerosis in patients with Wegener's granulomatosis. *Ann. Rheum. Dis.* **2005**, *64*, 753–759. [CrossRef]

27. Hoeksma, D.; Rebolledo, R.A.; Hottenrott, M.; Bodar, Y.S.; Wiersema-Buist, J.J.; Van Goor, H.; Leuvenink, H.G.D. Inadequate Antioxidative Responses in Kidneys of Brain-Dead Rats. *Transplantation* **2017**, *101*, 746–753. [CrossRef]

28. Van der Toorn, M.; Rezayat, D.; Kauffman, H.F.; Bakker, S.J.L.; Gans, R.O.B.; Koëter, G.H.; Choi, A.M.K.; van Oosterhout, A.J.M.; Slebos, D.-J. Lipid-soluble components in cigarette smoke induce mitochondrial production of reactive oxygen species in lung epithelial cells. *Am. J. Physiol. Cell. Mol. Physiol.* **2009**, *297*, L109–L114. [CrossRef]

29. Weiner, M.G.; Livshits, A.; Carozzoni, C.; McMenamin, E.; Gibson, G.; Loren, A.W.; Hennessy, S. Derivation of malignancy status from ICD-9 codes. In *AMIA Annual Symposium Proceedings*; American Medical Informatics Association: Bethesda, MD, USA, 2003; p. 1050.

30. Tan, F.E.S.; Jolani, S.; Verbeek, H. Guidelines for multiple imputations in repeated measurements with time-dependent covariates: A case study. *J. Clin. Epidemiol.* **2018**, *102*, 107–114. [CrossRef]
31. Sotomayor, C.G.; Eisenga, M.F.; Gomes Neto, A.W.; Ozyilmaz, A.; Gans, R.O.B.; De Jong, W.H.A.; Zelle, D.M.; Berger, S.P.; Gaillard, C.A.J.M.; Navis, G.J.; et al. Vitamin C depletion and all-cause mortality in renal transplant recipients. *Nutrients* **2017**, *9*, 568. [CrossRef]
32. Harrell, F.E.J.; Lee, K.L.; Mark, D.B. Multivariable prognostic models: Issues in developing models, evaluating assumptions and adequacy, and measuring and reducing errors. *Stat. Med.* **1996**, *15*, 361–387. [CrossRef]
33. Oterdoom, L.H.; van Ree, R.M.; de Vries, A.P.J.; Gansevoort, R.T.; Schouten, J.P.; van Son, W.J.; Homan van der Heide, J.J.; Navis, G.; de Jong, P.E.; Gans, R.O.B.; et al. Urinary Creatinine Excretion Reflecting Muscle Mass is a Predictor of Mortality and Graft Loss in Renal Transplant Recipients. *Transplantation* **2008**, *86*, 391–398. [CrossRef] [PubMed]
34. Gomes-Neto, A.W.; Osté, M.C.J.; Sotomayor, C.G.; Berg, E.V.D.; Geleijnse, J.M.; Gans, R.O.B.; Bakker, S.J.L.; Navis, G.J. Fruit and Vegetable Intake and Risk of Post Transplantation Diabetes Mellitus in Renal Transplant Recipients. *Diabetes Care* **2019**, *42*, 1645–1652. [CrossRef] [PubMed]
35. Noordzij, M.; Leffondré, K.; Van Stralen, K.J.; Zoccali, C.; Dekker, F.W.; Jager, K.J. When do we need competing risks methods for survival analysis in nephrology? *Nephrol. Dial. Transpl.* **2013**, *28*, 2670–2677. [CrossRef] [PubMed]
36. Von Elm, E.; Altman, D.G.; Egger, M.; Pocock, S.J.; Gøtzsche, P.C.; Vandenbroucke, J.P. The Strengthening the Reporting of Observational Studies in Epidemiology (STROBE) statement: Guidelines for reporting observational studies. *Lancet* **2007**, *370*, 1453–1457. [CrossRef]
37. Zhu, X.; Zhou, X.; Zhang, Y.; Sun, X.; Liu, H.; Zhang, Y. Reporting and methodological quality of survival analysis in articles published in Chinese oncology journals. *Medicine* **2017**, *96*, e9204. [CrossRef]
38. Dantal, J.; Hourmant, M.; Cantarovich, D.; Giral, M.; Blancho, G.; Dreno, B.; Soulillou, J.P. Effect of long-term immunosuppression in kidney-graft recipients on cancer incidence: Randomised comparison of two cyclosporin regimens. *Lancet* **1998**, *351*, 623–628. [CrossRef]
39. Gutierrez-Dalmau, A.; Campistol, J.M. Immunosuppressive therapy and malignancy in organ transplant recipients: A systematic review. *Drugs* **2007**, *67*, 1167–1198. [CrossRef]
40. Karpe, K.M.; Talaulikar, G.S.; Walters, G.D. Calcineurin inhibitor withdrawal or tapering for kidney transplant recipients. *Cochrane Database Syst. Rev.* **2017**. [CrossRef]
41. Kao, C.C.; Liu, J.S.; Lin, M.H.; Hsu, C.Y.; Chang, F.C.; Lin, Y.C.; Chen, H.H.; Chen, T.W.; Hsu, C.C.; Wu, M.S. Impact of mTOR Inhibitors on Cancer Development in Kidney Transplantation Recipients: A Population-Based Study. *Transpl. Proc.* **2016**, *48*, 900–904. [CrossRef]
42. Piselli, P.; Serraino, D.; Segoloni, G.P.; Sandrini, S.; Piredda, G.B.; Scolari, M.P.; Rigotti, P.; Busnach, G.; Messa, P.; Donati, D.; et al. Risk of de novo cancers after transplantation: Results from a cohort of 7217 kidney transplant recipients, Italy 1997–2009. *Eur. J. Cancer* **2013**, *49*, 336–344. [CrossRef] [PubMed]
43. Mastrangelo, D.; Pelosi, E.; Castelli, G.; Lo-Coco, F.; Testa, U. Mechanisms of anti-cancer effects of ascorbate: Cytotoxic activity and epigenetic modulation. *Blood Cells. Mol. Dis.* **2018**, *69*, 57–64. [CrossRef] [PubMed]
44. Du, J.; Cullen, J.J.; Buettner, G.R. Ascorbic acid: Chemistry, biology and the treatment of cancer. *Biochim. Biophys. Acta* **2012**, *1826*, 443–457. [CrossRef] [PubMed]
45. Cimmino, L.; Neel, B.G.; Aifantis, I. Vitamin C in Stem Cell Reprogramming and Cancer. *Trends Cell Biol.* **2018**, *28*, 698–708. [CrossRef]
46. Shenoy, N.; Creagan, E.; Witzig, T.; Levine, M. Ascorbic Acid in Cancer Treatment: Let the Phoenix Fly. *Cancer Cell* **2018**, *34*, 700–706. [CrossRef]
47. Saglimbene, V.M.; Wong, G.; Ruospo, M.; Palmer, S.C.; Garcia-Larsen, V.; Natale, P.; Teixeira-Pinto, A.; Campbell, K.L.; Carrero, J.-J.; Stenvinkel, P.; et al. Fruit and Vegetable Intake and Mortality in Adults undergoing Maintenance Hemodialysis. *Clin. J. Am. Soc. Nephrol.* **2019**, *14*, 250–260. [CrossRef] [PubMed]
48. Lin, J.; Cook, N.R.; Albert, C.; Zaharris, E.; Gaziano, J.M.; Van Denburgh, M.; Buring, J.E.; Manson, J.E. Vitamins C and E and Beta Carotene Supplementation and Cancer Risk: A Randomized Controlled Trial. *J. Natl. Cancer Inst.* **2009**, *101*, 14–23. [CrossRef]
49. Genkinger, J.M.; Platz, E.A.; Hoffman, S.C.; Comstock, G.W.; Helzlsouer, K.J. Fruit, Vegetable, and Antioxidant Intake and All-Cause, Cancer, and Cardiovascular Disease Mortality in a Community-dwelling Population in Washington County, Maryland. *Am. J. Epidemiol.* **2004**, *160*, 1223–1233. [CrossRef]

50. Lunet, N.; Valbuena, C.; Vieira, A.L.; Lopes, C.; Lopes, C.; David, L.; Carneiro, F.; Barros, H. Fruit and vegetable consumption and gastric cancer by location and histological type: Case–control and meta-analysis. *Eur. J. Cancer Prev.* **2007**, *16*, 312–327. [CrossRef]
51. Gandini, S.; Merzenich, H.; Robertson, C.; Boyle, P. Meta-analysis of studies on breast cancer risk and diet. *Eur. J. Cancer* **2000**, *36*, 636–646. [CrossRef]
52. Pavia, M.; Pileggi, C.; Nobile, C.G.; Angelillo, I.F. Association between fruit and vegetable consumption and oral cancer: A meta-analysis of observational studies. *Am. J. Clin. Nutr.* **2006**, *83*, 1126–1134. [CrossRef] [PubMed]
53. Ames, B.N. Dietary carcinogens and anticarcinogens. Oxygen radicals and degenerative diseases. *Science* **1983**, *221*, 1256–1264. [CrossRef] [PubMed]
54. Mustafi, S.; Sant, D.W.; Liu, Z.J.; Wang, G. Ascorbate induces apoptosis in melanoma cells by suppressing Clusterin expression. *Sci. Rep.* **2017**, *7*, 3671. [CrossRef] [PubMed]
55. Bjelakovic, G.; Nikolova, D.; Simonetti, R.G.; Gluud, C. Antioxidant supplements for prevention of gastrointestinal cancers: A systematic review and meta-analysis. *Lancet* **2004**, *364*, 1219–1228. [CrossRef]
56. Vamvakas, S.; Bahner, U.; Heidland, A. Cancer in End-Stage Renal Disease: Potential Factors Involved. *Am. J. Nephrol.* **1998**, *18*, 89–95. [CrossRef] [PubMed]
57. Ames, B.N.; Gold, L.S.; Willett, W.C. The causes and prevention of cancer. *Proc. Natl. Acad. Sci. USA* **1995**, *92*, 5258–5265. [CrossRef]
58. Maisonneuve, P.; Agodoa, L.; Gellert, R.; Stewart, J.H.; Buccianti, G.; Lowenfels, A.B.; Wolfe, R.A.; Jones, E.; Disney, A.P.S.; Briggs, D.; et al. Cancer in patients on dialysis for end-stage renal disease: An international collaborative study. *Lancet* **1999**, *354*, 93–99. [CrossRef]
59. Malachi, T.; Zevin, D.; Gafter, U.; Chagnac, A.; Slor, H.; Levi, J. DNA repair and recovery of RNA synthesis in uremic patients. *Kidney Int.* **1993**, *44*, 385–389. [CrossRef]
60. Roselaar, S.E.; Nazhat, N.B.; Winyard, P.G.; Jones, P.; Cunningham, J.; Blake, D.R. Detection of oxidants in uremic plasma by electron spin resonance spectroscopy. *Kidney Int.* **1995**, *48*, 199–206. [CrossRef]
61. Xu, H.; Matsushita, K.; Su, G.; Trevisan, M.; Ärnlöv, J.; Barany, P.; Lindholm, B.; Elinder, C.-G.; Lambe, M.; Carrero, J.-J. Estimated Glomerular Filtration Rate and the Risk of Cancer. *Clin. J. Am. Soc. Nephrol.* **2019**, *14*, 530–539. [CrossRef]
62. Thomas, L.D.K.; Elinder, C.-G.; Tiselius, H.-G.; Wolk, A.; Åkesson, A. Ascorbic Acid Supplements and Kidney Stone Incidence Among Men: A Prospective Study. *JAMA Intern. Med.* **2013**, *173*, 386. [CrossRef] [PubMed]
63. Ferraro, P.M.; Curhan, G.C.; Gambaro, G.; Taylor, E.N. Total, Dietary, and Supplemental Vitamin C Intake and Risk of Incident Kidney Stones. *Am. J. Kidney Dis.* **2016**, *67*, 400–407. [CrossRef] [PubMed]
64. Koenig, W.; Sund, M.; Fröhlich, M.; Löwel, H.; Hutchinson, W.L.; Pepys, M.B. Refinement of the association of serum C-reactive protein concentration and coronary heart disease risk by correction for within-subject variation over time: The MONICA Augsburg studies, 1984 and 1987. *Am. J. Epidemiol.* **2003**, *158*, 357–364. [CrossRef] [PubMed]
65. Block, G.; Dietrich, M.; Norkus, E.; Jensen, C.; Benowitz, N.L.; Morrow, J.D.; Hudes, M.; Packer, L. Intraindividual variability of plasma antioxidants, markers of oxidative stress, C-reactive protein, cotinine, and other biomarkers. *Epidemiology* **2006**, *17*, 404–412. [CrossRef] [PubMed]
66. Van Ree, R.M.; De Vries, A.P.J.; Oterdoom, L.H.; Seelen, M.A.; Gansevoort, R.T.; Schouten, J.P.; Struck, J.; Navis, G.; Gans, R.O.B.; Van Der Heide, J.J.H.; et al. Plasma procalcitonin is an independent predictor of graft failure late after renal transplantation. *Transplantation* **2009**, *88*, 279–287. [CrossRef] [PubMed]
67. Danesh, J.; Wheeler, J.G.; Hirschfield, G.M.; Eda, S.; Eiriksdottir, G.; Rumley, A.; Lowe, G.D.O.; Pepys, M.B.; Gudnason, V. C-Reactive Protein and Other Circulating Markers of Inflammation in the Prediction of Coronary Heart Disease. *N. Engl. J. Med.* **2004**, *350*, 1387–1397. [CrossRef] [PubMed]
68. Yokoyama, T.; Date, C.; Kokubo, Y.; Yoshiike, N.; Matsumura, Y.; Tanaka, H. Serum Vitamin C Concentration Was Inversely Associated with Subsequent 20-Year Incidence of Stroke in a Japanese Rural Community. *Stroke* **2000**, *31*, 2287–2294. [CrossRef]
69. Deicher, R.; Ziai, F.; Bieglmayer, C.; Schillinger, M.; Hörl, W.H. Low total vitamin C plasma level is a risk factor for cardiovascular morbidity and mortality in hemodialysis patients. *J. Am. Soc. Nephrol.* **2005**, *16*, 1811–1818. [CrossRef]
70. Czernichow, S.; Vergnaud, A.C.; Galan, P.; Arnaud, J.; Favier, A.; Faure, H.; Huxley, R.; Hercberg, S.; Ahluwalia, N. Effects of long-term antioxidant supplementation and association of serum antioxidant concentrations with risk of metabolic syndrome in adults. *Am. J. Clin. Nutr.* **2009**, *90*, 329–335. [CrossRef]

71. Moyad, M.A.; Combs, M.A.; Vrablic, A.S.; Velasquez, J.; Turner, B.; Bernal, S. Vitamin C metabolites, independent of smoking status, significantly enhance leukocyte, but not plasma ascorbate concentrations. *Adv. Ther.* **2008**, *25*, 995–1009. [CrossRef]

72. Eisenga, M.F.; Gomes-Neto, A.W.; van Londen, M.; Ziengs, A.L.; Douwes, R.M.; Stam, S.P.; Osté, M.C.J.; Knobbe, T.J.; Hessels, N.R.; Buunk, A.M.; et al. Rationale and design of TransplantLines: A prospective cohort study and biobank of solid organ transplant recipients. *BMJ Open* **2018**, *8*, e024502. [CrossRef] [PubMed]

10

Investigating Ethnic Disparity in Living-Donor Kidney Transplantation in the UK: Patient-Identified Reasons for Non-Donation among Family Members

Katie Wong [1,2,*], Amanda Owen-Smith [1], Fergus Caskey [1,2], Stephanie MacNeill [1], Charles R.V. Tomson [3], Frank J.M.F. Dor [4], Yoav Ben-Shlomo [1], Soumeya Bouacida [5], Dela Idowu [6] and Pippa Bailey [1,2]

[1]   Bristol Medical School: Population Health Sciences, University of Bristol, Bristol BS8 2PS, UK;
       a.owen-smith@bristol.ac.uk (A.O.-S.); fergus.caskey@bristol.ac.uk (F.C.);
       stephanie.macneill@bristol.ac.uk (S.M.); y.ben-shlomo@bristol.ac.uk (Y.B.-S.);
       pippa.bailey@bristol.ac.uk (P.B.)
[2]   Southmead Hospital, North Bristol NHS Trust, Bristol BS10 5NB, UK
[3]   The Newcastle upon Tyne Hospitals NHS Foundation Trust, Newcastle upon Tyne NE7 7DN, UK;
       ctomson@doctors.org.uk
[4]   Imperial College Healthcare NHS Trust, London W12 0HS, UK; frank.dor@nhs.net
[5]   Bristol Health Partners' Chronic Kidney Disease Health Integration Team, Bristol BS1 2NT, UK
[6]   Gift of Living Donation (GOLD), London NW10 0NS, UK
*   Correspondence: katie.wong@bristol.ac.uk

Abstract: There is ethnic inequity in access to living-donor kidney transplants in the UK. This study asked kidney patients from Black, Asian and minority ethnic groups why members of their family were not able to be living kidney donors. Responses were compared with responses from White individuals. This questionnaire-based mixed-methods study included adults transplanted between 1/4/13–31/3/17 at 14 UK hospitals. Participants were asked to indicate why relatives could not donate, selecting all options applicable from: Age; Health; Weight; Location; Financial/Cost; Job; Blood group; No-one to care for them after donation. A box entitled 'Other—please give details' was provided for free-text entries. Multivariable logistic regression was used to analyse the association between the likelihood of selecting each reason for non-donation and the participant's self-reported ethnicity. Qualitative responses were analysed using inductive thematic analysis. In total, 1240 questionnaires were returned (40% response). There was strong evidence that Black, Asian and minority ethnic group individuals were more likely than White people to indicate that family members lived too far away to donate (adjusted odds ratio (aOR) = 3.25, 95% Confidence Interval (CI) 2.30–4.58), were prevented from donating by financial concerns (aOR = 2.95, 95% CI 2.02–4.29), were unable to take time off work (aOR = 1.88, 95% CI 1.18–3.02), were "not the right blood group" (aOR = 1.65, 95% CI 1.35–2.01), or had no-one to care for them post-donation (aOR = 3.73, 95% CI 2.60–5.35). Four qualitative themes were identified from responses from Black, Asian and minority ethnic group participants: 'Burden of disease within the family'; 'Differing religious interpretations'; 'Geographical concerns'; and 'A culture of silence'. Patients perceive barriers to living kidney donation in the UK Black, Asian and minority ethnic population. If confirmed, these could be targeted by interventions to redress the observed ethnic inequity.

Keywords: living kidney donation; living-donor kidney transplantation; ethnic disparity

1. Introduction

Living-donor kidney transplantation is the optimal treatment for most people with kidney failure in terms of patient survival, graft survival and quality of life [1–6]. The healthcare costs associated with living-donor kidney transplants (LDKTs) are less than for dialysis and deceased-donor kidney transplants (DDKTs) [7,8]. The medium-term risks of donating a kidney are small [9–12], and the quality of life of donors usually returns to pre-donation levels after donation [13,14].

Only 28% of all kidney transplants performed in the UK each year are from a living donor [6], a proportion below that of the USA and the Netherlands [15]. Individuals from Black, Asian and minority ethnic populations in the UK appear to be particularly disadvantaged as they are less likely to receive a LDKT compared to White people with kidney disease [16,17]; only 18% of living donor kidney transplant recipients in the UK between April 2019–March 2020 were from Black, Asian and minority ethnic group backgrounds, despite individuals from these groups constituting 36% of the kidney transplant waiting list [6]. Improving equity in living-donor kidney transplantation has been highlighted as a UK and international research priority by patients and clinicians [18,19].

Specific religious and cultural beliefs, as well as a lack of specific knowledge about donation, have been identified as reasons for ethnic disparity in deceased organ donation [20,21]. The barriers specifically encountered by Black, Asian and minority ethnic group patients in accessing LDKTs in the UK are not well described.

We have previously investigated reasons why individuals who start assessment for kidney donation do not go on to donate in the UK. In this multicentre study, individuals from Black, Asian and minority ethnic groups were more likely to withdraw from donor evaluation [22]. However, transplant candidates and their families often make decisions regarding the suitability of potential donors before they make contact with hospital services. The perceptions of transplant candidates, regarding the suitability of family members for donation, function as an initial stage of donor screening. Transplant candidates are often uncomfortable broaching the subject of organ donation and make assumptions as to why individuals may or may not be able to donate. Transplant candidates may perceive barriers to donation that prevent potential donors from starting donor assessment. It is important to understand these perceptions in order to fully understand barriers to living-donor kidney transplantation. In this multi-centre questionnaire-based study, we investigated the reasons why family members were perceived by kidney patients as unsuitable as living kidney donors, comparing responses between individuals from White and Black, Asian and minority ethnic groups. Ultimately we aimed to identify potentially modifiable barriers to LDKTs specific to the UK Black, Asian and minority ethnic populations that could be targeted to redress the observed disparity.

2. Experimental Section

2.1. Study Design

We designed this multi-centre questionnaire-based study to investigate the patient-identified and reported reasons potential donors did not donate. We collected both quantitative (checklist item selection) and qualitative (free-text) questionnaire data to gain a greater understanding than that provided by one data type [23]. We collected data on whether participants asked potential donors to donate, whether any offered, and whether any started donor assessment. We collected data from both LDKT and DDKT recipients—LDKT recipients may have had other potential donors who volunteered but did not donate, and we wanted to ensure we captured the reasons for non-donation for all. We compared the responses of Black, Asian and minority ethnic individuals with White individuals to identify barriers that might be specific to Black, Asian and minority ethnic populations and therefore might explain the observed ethnic inequity.

2.2. Participants

The study was based at 14 hospitals in England and Northern Ireland (Supplementary Study Sites). We obtained from each hospital an anonymised list of all individuals who received kidney transplants between 1/4/13 and 31/3/17, stratified by LDKT/DDKT status. Individuals < 18 years at time of transplantation, or who lacked mental capacity according to the Mental Capacity Act 2005 were excluded. We calculated the study sample size using a variable not analysed here: the patient activation variable [24]. The study was designed to detect a 7-point difference in a continuous measure of patient activation (analysis of this variable not presented here) between LDKT cases and DDKT controls with 90% power, assuming a 5% significance level. The calculation indicated that 170 patients would be needed, and that, therefore, a total of 944 would be needed to allow analyses stratified by Index of Multiple Deprivation rank quintile and allow for 10% missing data. This sample size allows for the detection of a far smaller difference (0.16 Standard Deviation) for a dichotomous exposure or between 6–8% for a categorical outcome [24]. We performed stratified random sampling to select, on average, 110 LDKTs and 110 DDKTs from each site, weighted by the number of transplants performed at each study site. Sex and 5-year age group strata matched sampling was used to try to ensure a similar sample distribution by age and sex.

Between October 2017-November 2018, collaborators at study sites mailed paper questionnaires to participants. Questionnaires were accompanied by an invitation letter, a return postage-paid envelope, and a patient information sheet. A website-address was provided for participants who preferred to complete the questionnaire online. Non-responders were sent a second questionnaire after 4–6 weeks. We extracted anonymised data from returned paper questionnaires at the University of Bristol, and uploaded these onto a secure REDCap database [25].

2.3. Questionnaire Content

We have previously reported the development of the questionnaire alongside the findings of a single centre pilot study [24]. Participants were asked to indicate the number of living relatives ≥18 years from a list (spouse/partner, parents, sisters/brothers, children, aunts/uncles, first cousins) as a proxy for their potential living-donor pool. Friends and colleagues were not included, as they contribute very small numbers to the donor pool: between 2006–2017 only 8% of UK living donors were in this category (unpublished data provided by NHS Blood and Transplant to co-author P.B). We asked participants how many relatives had (i) offered to donate, (ii) been asked to donate by the respondent, and (iii) started donor assessment. Participants were asked for the reasons why any of the listed relatives could not donate; individuals were asked to tick all options that applied and were allowed to select multiple reasons from the following list, derived from previous qualitative research into barriers to donation [26]: Age—too old or too young to donate; Health—not healthy enough to donate; Weight—too over or underweight to donate; Location—they live too far away to be able to donate; Financial/Cost—the financial impact of donation would be too much; Job—not able to take the time off work to donate; Blood group—not the right blood group to donate; No-one to care for them after donation. A box entitled "Other—please give details" was provided for free-text entries. Individuals who the respondent considered suitable for donation but who did not donate because another person did were not considered as "not able" to donate. The responses indicated the patient-reported, and therefore the patient-identified, reasons for non-donation.

2.4. Main Exposure and Other Demographics

We collected data on self-reported ethnicity, religion, age, sex, and marital status. Participants could select "Would rather not answer" for all demographic questions. Participants indicated their ethnicity according to the UK's Office for National Statistics (ONS) 2011 census categories [27]: White; Asian/Asian British (Indian, Pakistani, Bangladeshi, Chinese); Black/African/Caribbean/Black British; Mixed/Multiple (White and Black Caribbean, White and Black African, Any other Mixed/Multiple ethnic background);

Other (Arab, Any other ethnic group). For the religion variable, participants were asked to select one option from the following: No religion; Christian; Muslim; Jewish; Hindu; Sikh; Buddhist; Other. Age was a categorical variable in 10-year age groups.

2.5. Statistical Analysis

We used descriptive statistics to summarise the characteristics of transplant recipients and their reported reasons for non-donation from family members. Black, Asian and minority ethnic group participants comprised "Asian/Asian-British", "Black/African/Caribbean/Black British", "Mixed/Multiple ethnic groups", and "Other Ethnic group". We derived a binary variable of Black, Asian and minority ethnicity (code = 1) versus White ethnicity (code = 0) as our primary exposure. The Chi2 test was used to compare the characteristics of White and Black, Asian and minority ethnic group participants, and the reasons given for non-donation. We used multivariable logistic regression to describe the association between the reporting of each reason for non-donation with respondent self-reported ethnicity. We used two models: (i) unadjusted and (ii) adjusted for potential confounders. We specified, a priori, potential confounders including sex and age. We considered socioeconomic position as a mediator on the causal pathway between ethnicity and living donation, rather than a potential confounder: we did not adjust for it in our model as this would result in potential over-adjustment and attenuation of the effect of ethnicity. We used robust standard errors to account for clustering within kidney centres. We tested for interactions between ethnicity and age and sex. We identified missing data and described patterns of missingness. We performed both a complete case analysis and a sensitivity analysis using multiple imputation using chained equations to derive 40 imputed datasets per group, for the exposure variable and potential confounders and then combined using Rubin's rules. All statistical analyses were undertaken using Stata 15 [28].

2.6. Qualitative Analysis

Individuals were able to provide free-text qualitative data responses to the question "Thinking about those people you think could not donate a kidney to you, what are the reasons for this?". All free-text responses from Black, Asian and minority ethnic group respondents were analysed, so no sampling was required. The written free-text responses were typed onto the REDCap database [25]. Free-text responses and participant demographics were then downloaded from REDCap onto an Excel spreadsheet file. NVivo qualitative software was used to facilitate analysis. Data were analysed using inductive thematic analysis [29], as described by Braun and Clarke [30]. After familiarization with the data, sections of text within the responses were coded by assigning descriptive labels. Codes were collated on the basis of shared properties to create initial potential themes, which were then refined. Themes were revisited and finalised during the preparation of the report for publication. Coding and thematic analysis were undertaken independently by both K.W. and P.B. Coding discrepancies were resolved by discussion to enhance rigour and reliability. All themes were reported using a minimum of three illustrative quotes. After completing analysis for Black, Asian and minority group respondents (n = 56), a matching number of White participants (n = 56) were purposively sampled aiming for diversity in terms of age, sex and socioeconomic status, and qualitative responses analysed for comparison.

The Strengthening The Reporting of OBservational studies in Epidemiology (STROBE) and COnsolidated criteria for REporting Qualitative studies (COREQ) guidelines were used to prepare the manuscript [31,32].

2.7. Ethical Approval and Consent

We received NHS Research Ethics Committee (REC) (REC reference 17/LO/1602) and Health Research Authority (HRA) approval. A consent form formed the first page of the questionnaire. The study was funded by a Kidney Research UK Project Grant (RP_028_20170302). The clinical and research activities being reported are consistent with the Principles of the Declaration of Istanbul as outlined in the "Declaration of Istanbul on Organ Trafficking and Transplant Tourism".

3. Results

3.1. Quantitative Findings

A total of 1240 questionnaires were returned from 3103 patients (40% response). The characteristics of all respondents are described in Table 1. LDKT recipients were more likely to respond than DDKT recipients and women were more likely to respond than men (Table S1). Study participants appeared to be generally similar to the National population of DDKT and LDKT recipients though the study sample had fewer Black, Asian and minority ethnic group participants (largest difference 9% for DDKT) (Table S2). Overall, the proportion of missing data was small (<10% for all demographic variables) (Table S3).

Table 1. Participant demographics.

Characteristics		Participants (n = 1240) n (%)
Sex	Female	514 (41.5)
	Male	705 (56.9)
	Missing	21 (1.7)
Type of transplant	Living-donor kidney transplant	672 (54.2)
	Deceased-donor kidney transplant	565 (45.6)
	Missing	3 (0.2)
Age group (years) [a]	20–29	74 (6.0)
	30–39	137 (11.1)
	40–49	209 (16.9)
	50–59	331 (26.7)
	60–69	299 (24.1)
	70–79	150 (12.1)
	80–89	6 (0.5)
	Missing	34 (2.7)
Self-reported Ethnicity [b]	White	1027 (82.8)
	Asian/Asian-British	79 (6.4)
	Black/African/Caribbean/Black British	58 (4.7)
	Mixed/Multiple ethnic groups	10 (0.8)
	Other Ethnic groups	24 (1.9)
	Missing	42 (3.4)
Religion	Christian	717 (57.8)
	Hindu	27 (2.2)
	Sikh	13 (1.1)
	Muslim	21 (1.7)
	Jewish	6 (0.5)
	No religion	335 (27.0)
	Other	38 (3.1)
	Missing	74 (6.0)

[a] No participants aged <20 years. [b] UK's Office for National Statistics 2011 census categories.

White participants were older than Black, Asian and minority ethnic group participants, and a greater proportion of White participants were LDKT recipients compared to Black, Asian and minority ethnic group respondents. Black, Asian and minority ethnic group participants were more likely to report having a religion than White participants: of those with a religion, the majority of Black, Asian and minority ethnic group participants reported a religion other than Christianity, whereas the majority of White participants reported being Christian (Table S4). Black, Asian and minority ethnic group participants reported a larger number of potential donors compared to White respondents (median number of family members ≥ 18 years: 19 versus 16, Wilcoxon rank-sum test $p = 0.02$).

Most participants had not asked any of their relatives to donate ($n = 848/1181$, 71.8%). In total, 81.8% ($n = 973/1189$) reported that one or more relative had offered to donate, with 85.6% of these actually starting donor assessment (representing 14.4% attrition).

Participant responses to the question "Thinking about those people you think could not donate a kidney to you, what are the reasons for this?" differed by ethnicity (Table 2). Black, Asian and minority ethnic group individuals were more likely than White respondents to indicate that family members lived too far away to donate ($p < 0.001$), were prevented from donating by financial concerns ($p < 0.001$), were unable to take time off work ($p < 0.001$), were not the right blood group ($p = 0.002$), or had no-one to care for them after donation ($p < 0.001$). We found no evidence that the proportion of respondents who indicated that age ($p = 0.96$), donor health ($p = 0.88$), or donor weight ($p = 0.36$) were reasons for non-donation differed between White and Black, Asian and minority ethnic group respondents.

Table 2. Participant reported reasons relatives could not donate a kidney to them.

Reported Reason Potential Donor not Suitable for Donation	White $n = 1027$, n (%)	Black, Asian and Minority Ethnic Group $n = 171$, n (%)	White vs. Black, Asian and Minority Ethnic Group Chi^2 p-Value
Age—too old or too young to donate	562 (54.8)	94 (55.0)	0.96
Health—not healthy enough to donate	648 (63.2)	109 (63.7)	0.88
Weight—too over or underweight to donate	152 (14.8)	30 (17.5)	0.36
Location—they live too far away to be able to donate	188 (18.3)	72 (42.1)	<0.001
Financial/cost—the financial impact of donation would be too much	98 (9.6)	40 (23.4)	<0.001
Job—not able to take the time off work to donate	106 (10.3)	29 (17.0)	<0.001
Blood group—not the right blood group to donate	199 (19.4)	51 (29.8)	0.002
No-one to care for them after donation	63 (6.1)	32 (18.7)	<0.001

There was strong evidence that even after adjustment for potential confounders of sex and age, Black, Asian and minority ethnic group individuals were more likely than White respondents to indicate that family members lived too far away to donate (adjusted odds ratio (aOR) 3.25 (95% Confidence Interval (CI) 2.30–4.58)), were prevented from donating by financial concerns (aOR 2.95 (95% CI 2.02–4.29)), were unable to take time off work (aOR 1.88 (95% CI 1.18–3.02)), were not the right blood group (aOR 1.65 (95% CI 1.35–2.01)), or had no-one to care for them after donation (aOR 3.73 (95% CI 2.60–5.35)) (Table 3). The associations did not differ substantially between the complete cases analysis and the analyses with missing variables imputed (Table S5). In total, 11 individuals who had not selected the "Health – not healthy enough to donate" response indicated in the free-text that potential donors had or might develop the same kidney disease as them. In a sensitivity analysis, when these individuals were recoded as selecting "Health" as a reason for non-donation, there was no change in the direction or the size of associations observed in Table 3.

Table 3. Multivariable logistic regression analysis comparing reasons potential donor unsuitability between White and Black, Asian and minority ethnic participants [a].

Reported Reason Potential Donor Not Suitable for Donation	Black, Asian and Minority Ethnicities vs. White Unadjusted Odds Ratio (OR) [95% Confidence Interval (CI)]	Black, Asian and Minority Ethnicities vs. White Adjusted for Sex and Age OR [95% CI]
Age—too old or too young	1.00 [0.75–1.34]	0.98 [0.73–1.32]
Health—not healthy enough	1.02 [0.78–1.34]	0.96 [0.71–1.31]
Weight—too over or underweight	1.22 [0.84–1.77]	1.13 [0.78–1.65]
Location—live too far away	3.23 [2.23–4.68]	3.25 [2.30–4.58]
Financial/cost—financial impact of donation would be too much	2.89 [2.07–4.03]	2.95 [2.02–4.29]
Job—not able to take time off work	1.77 [1.15–2.71]	1.88 [1.18–3.02]
Blood group—not the right blood group	1.76 [1.43–2.17]	1.65 [1.35–2.01]
No-one to care for them after donation	3.51 [2.47–4.99]	3.73 [2.60–5.35]

[a] Complete case analysis.

There was a modest suggestion of interaction between sex and ethnicity (likelihood ratio test $p = 0.03$) in the reporting of "no-one to care for them after donation" as a reason for non-donation (Supplementary Interactions) so the increased risk seen for Black, Asian and minority ethnic group was only seen in men.

3.2. Qualitative Findings

In total, 56 Black, Asian and minority ethnicity individuals provided free-text reasons for potential donor unsuitability: respondent characteristics are presented in Table S6. Four overall themes were identified (Table 4): (i) Burden of disease within the family, (ii) Differing religious interpretations, (iii) Specific geographical concerns, and (iv) A Culture of Silence.

Table 4. UK Black, Asian and minority ethnic participant qualitative analysis themes and illustrative quotes.

Theme	Representative Quote
Burden of disease within family	"Very healthy but slight amount of protein in urine so not able to donate." (Male, 50–59 years, Asian, Hindu, Living-donor kidney transplant (LDKT) "They all have slight renal problem" (Female, 50–59 years, Black, Deceased-donor kidney transplant (DDKT) "Hereditary illness in the family" (Male, 50–59 years, Asian, DDKT) "Mother and 2 sibling have same condition as mine (1 sister & 1 brother)." (Male, 30–38 years, Black, Christian, DDKT)
Differing religious interpretations	"Their religion/faith forbids them to donate 1. thought they were Christians like me. 2. our culture forbids them to donate ... 3. some forbid blood transfusion and the unbelievable reasons for that." (Female, 60–69 years, Black, LDKT) "Superstition/religion (distorted beliefs). Myth." (Female, 50–59 years, Black, Christian, DDKT) "Their religion would not allow them to donate a kidney." (Female, 40–49 years, Black, Christian, LDKT) "Religious/cultural ... " (Male, 50–59 years, Asian, Hindu, LDKT)
Geographical concerns	"All of my family apart from my spouse live in Ethiopia and other countries and would not have access to healthcare or the means to come to the UK" (Male, 40–49 years, Black, Muslim, LDKT) "All my people are in Nigeria, some of them, lack of transport to help them home is the problem some of them have." (Male, 70–79 years, Black, Christian, DDKT) "I had a word with my mum, wife and my son but they couldn't come to the UK due to financial and other reasons." (Male, 40–49 years, Black, Christian, DDKT)
A culture of silence	"I did not ask for a donation so do not have a reason." (Female, 60–69 years, Asian, Sikh, DDKT) "I would not ask my cousins" (Female, 30–39 years, Asian, Muslim, LDKT) "Other 3 cousins from my mother's half sister do not have PKD but they would not offer, they didn't before, I would certainly not ask." (Female, 60–69 years, Other ethnic group, No religion, LDKT) "Are unaware of my current condition." (Male, 20–29 years, Asian, Hindu, LDKT)

3.2.1. Burden of Disease within the Family

A large number of Black, Asian and minority ethnic group respondents stated that potential donors were unable to donate due to presumed or perceived ill health. Respondents reported a heavy burden of both hereditary and non-hereditary kidney disease precluding donation:

"Family history of PKD [polycystic kidney disease]—all siblings, all children and uncles affected." (Female|50–59 years|Asian|LDKT)

"Too old and unhealthy. Heart problem, Diabetes, high blood pressure, inheritance."(Male|60–69 years|Asian|Sikh|DDKT)

Participants also reported that health problems were identified during donor assessment that prevented donation:

"There were genetic issues that were contra-indications such as a cause of cancer which was discovered during screening . . . " (Male|20–29 years|Asian|Muslim|DDKT)

3.2.2. Differing Religious Interpretations

Several participants reported that a relative's religion or faith had prevented them from donating:

"Their religion would not allow them to donate a kidney." (Female|40–49 years|Black|Christian| LDKT)

However, most participants considered the beliefs as unorthodox, describing what they perceived as a distortion of a religious belief:

"Superstition/religion (distorted beliefs). Myth." (Female|60–69 years|Black|LDKT)

and a discordance between the participants' and their relatives' interpretations of their faith:

"Their religion/faith forbids them to donate . . . thought they were Christians like me."(Female|60–69 years|Black|LDKT)

No participants who reported religion as a barrier to donation for their relatives reported that they shared their relatives' beliefs. All but one of the respondents who reported religion as a reason for non-donation self-identified as Christian and was Black/African/Caribbean/Black British.

3.2.3. Geographical Concerns

Several participants reported relatives being unable to donate due to geographical separation. However, it was not the distance alone that was considered a barrier to donation for some:

"While some are abroad they were willing to travel." (Male|60–69 years|Black|Christian|LDKT)

Rather, participants reported difficulties with immigration rules:

"Immigration rules can be problematic too." (Male|40–49 years|Black|Muslim|LDKT)

prohibitive financial concerns:

"My blood relatives live outside the UK. The financial cost has been a major issue."(Male|50–59 years|Other ethnic group|DDKT)

and concerns about the quality of post-donation healthcare in their potential donor's country of residence:

"I come from Papua New Guinea and health services are poor. People are afraid of death during and after donating of their kidneys. After operations the care given is not very good and people end up dying. We lost two relatives from sepsis." (Female|50–59 years| Other ethnic group|Christian|LDKT)

3.2.4. A culture of Silence

Several participants described a "culture of silence" around their illness, reporting that their family were not aware they had kidney disease:

"Are unaware of my current condition." (Male|20–29 years|Asian|Hindu|LDKT)

This was reported as a result of some participants personally not disclosing this information to relatives:

" ... my reluctance to show how ill I was, to soldier on, accept my fate and manage accordingly." (Male|50–59 years|Asian|Sikh|LDKT)

As well as other family members controlling the disclosure of information to the wider family:

"The majority of my extended family do not 'officially' know that I am unwell/having dialysis or had a transplant as my parents did not want them to know." (Male|30–39 years|Other ethnic group|Other religion|DDKT)

A summary model of barriers identified is presented in Figure 1.

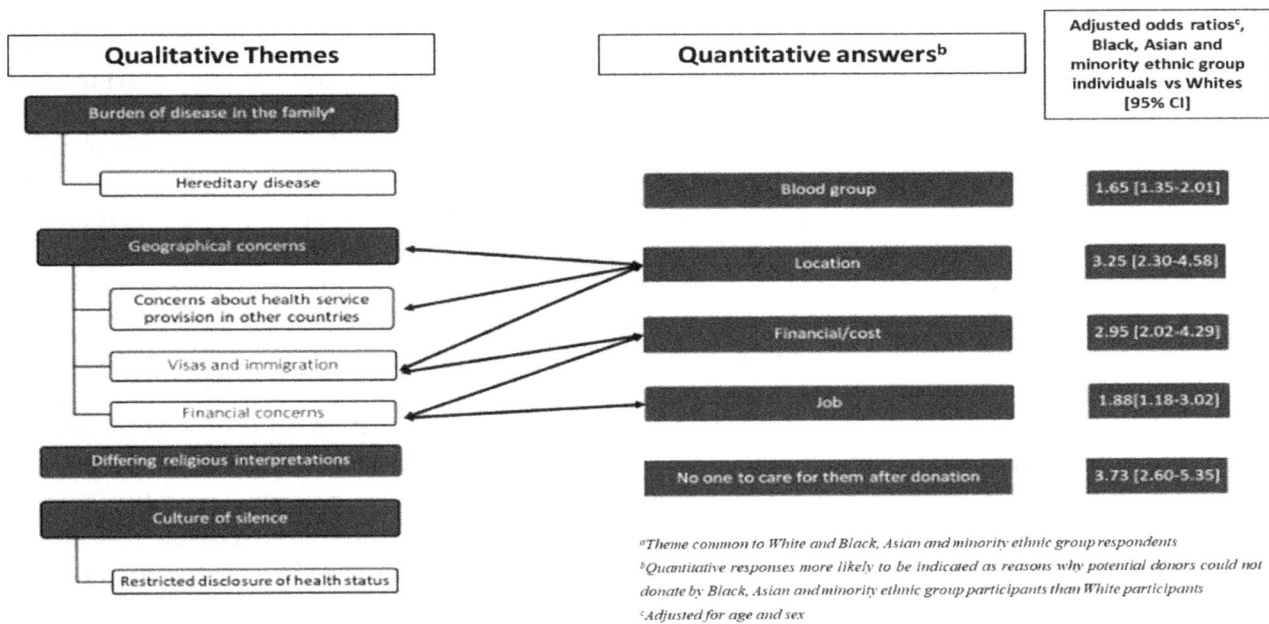

Figure 1. A summary model of barriers to living kidney donation as reported by UK Black, Asian and Minority Ethnic individuals.

3.2.5. Responses from White Participants

Comparing these free-text responses against those from the 56 purposively sampled White participants (Table S7), only one theme proved common to both White and Black, Asian and minority ethnic group respondents—"Burden of disease within the family". Two further themes were identified amongst White respondents that were not evident in the Black, Asian and minority ethnic group dataset: (i) Lack of close family relationships—through relationship breakdown or dysfunction and (ii) Protecting others. These themes and illustrative quotes are presented as Supplementary Material (Table S7).

4. Discussion

The majority of respondents indicated that they had not asked potential donors to donate, suggesting that transplant candidates may make assumptions as to why individuals may or may not be able to donate. Although 81.8% reported that one or more individuals had offered to donate, 14.4% of these participants did not have a potential donor that proceeded to donor assessment. Whilst some of these individuals may have received a DDKT before their potential donor started assessment, others may have been deemed unsuitable for donation by the transplant candidate. These findings highlight the importance of understanding patient-identified reasons as to why individuals are deemed unsuitable as living kidney donors.

Black, Asian and minority ethnic group participants were more likely than White participants to indicate that family members lived too far away to donate, and to report financial concerns in part linked to geographical distance. The qualitative data provided insight into these identified barriers, and as described they would appear to be surmountable. In the UK, NHS England allows potential donors from overseas to be reimbursed for travel, accommodation and visa costs after the event [33]. However these large "up-front" costs may be prohibitive to potential donors, and previous qualitative research has shown that many patients are unaware of the reimbursement policy [26]. Clarifying UK immigration policy and highlighting the reimbursement scheme may help potential Black, Asian and minority ethnic group recipients access their potential donor pool.

Previous research by the authors has suggested that Black, Asian and minority ethnic group ethnicity and non-Christian religious affiliation are associated with greater uncertainty in beliefs about living donation [34]. No respondents in our study reported perceiving a specific religion as forbidding living donation. This may reflect the success of work by faith leaders to clarify positions on living donation within the UK, including a new fatwa clarifying Islamic approval of organ donation and transplantation published in the UK in 2019 [35]. However, the participants' responses indicated that some of their potential donors did perceive religion as a barrier to donation. In particular there were several references to the distortion of religious beliefs being a barrier to donation. This highlights the need to better understand and consider the beliefs of potential donors who belong to non-mainstream religions, who may be outside the remit of denominational faith leaders.

A "culture of silence" about illness was an important theme identified in responses from Black, Asian and minority ethnic group participants. Although not directly comparable to the UK Black, Asian and minority ethnic group population, qualitative research in African-American LDKT recipients and donors has suggested that restricting disclosure and maintaining privacy of health status can protect against feelings of vulnerability [36], help to maintain self-perception and public identity, and is linked with rejection of the sick role which is sometimes associated with better coping skills in patients with kidney disease [37]. Potential African-American donors have also reported negative responses from family and friends regarding donation, and encouraging the recipient not to disclose their health status may be perceived as a protective act in that context [36]. We found that Black, Asian and minority ethnic group participants have larger potential donor pools than White participants, but this "culture of silence" may mean that Black, Asian and minority ethnic group individuals are less able to access their pool and therefore a LDKT. It may also mean that Black, Asian and minority ethnic group individuals are less able to access their social network during time of chronic illness: lack of social support and lack of an informed social network are associated with reduced access to transplantation [26,38–40], and worse transplant outcomes [41]. Interestingly, in White participants, lack of close relationships was identified as reason for non-donation, but this was not reported by Black, Asian and minority ethnic group participants, despite the geographical separation. Strategies to overcome this culture of silence could include interventions that engage with a patient's social network, such as the Dutch home-education model shown to be effective at increasing access to living-donor kidney transplantation for minority ethnic groups [42]. A focus on the potential benefits to family members from the education session (detection of undiagnosed kidney disease, how to optimise own health) could be emphasised. The use of "live donor champions" may also enable discussions to start: in this approach, a friend or family member is trained to undertake an advocate role, sharing information on the patient's behalf with the patient's wider social network [43]. Other approaches that may overcome "cultures of silence" include people with kidney disease, transplant recipients and donors sharing their experiences on an open web-platform such as healthtalk.org (http://healthtalk.org) and the living donation storytelling project (https://explorelivingdonation.org/) [44]. However, such approaches need to be formally evaluated for effectiveness.

Black, Asian and minority ethnic group respondents were more likely to report that potential donors were not the right blood group. Whether this represents true or perceived incompatibility requires further investigation. A single-centre study from the USA in 2002 found that more African-American donors than White donors were prevented from donating due to ABO incompatibility (9.7% vs. 5.6%, $p < 0.01$) [45]; however, to our knowledge this has not been examined in the UK. If found to be true, willingness to participate in the UK Living Kidney Sharing Scheme should be investigated, and participation encouraged.

This was a large, multicentre study utilising both quantitative and qualitative data. The questionnaire was evaluated in cognitive interviews prior to use and then piloted. The proportion of missing data was very small. However, the study has some limitations: (i) There is a risk of self-selection bias given our response rate, although this is comparable to other postal surveys in the UK [46,47] and the 47% response to a survey sent to Dutch and Swedish transplant recipients [48]. There is some evidence that Black, Asian and minority ethnic group individuals may have been under-represented but it is unclear whether the participants in the study would be different in respect to the reported reasons for non-donation. We suspect, if anything they would be more knowledgeable and engaged and so some of our results may underestimate the true associations. We did not have data on the ethnicity of non-responders and so we were unable to ascertain if there was a difference in response rate between the Black, Asian and minority ethnic group and White populations. (ii) Ethnicity can be described as a form of collective identity that draws on notions of ancestry, cultural commonality, geographical origins, and shared physical features. Ethnic identities are social constructs that are fluid across space and time [49]. In this study, ethnicity was coded using the UK's ONS 2011 census categories, but individuals may self-identify with several or none of the ethnic categories used in government statistics [49]. Any ethnic identify categorisation fails to respect the heterogeneity within a group due to differing cultures, religions, languages, HLA-types, whether a person was born in their place of residence or migrated to it, and for migrants, time resident. We analysed all Black, Asian and minority ethnic group respondents as one group as our sample size prevented analysis by more specific ethnic groups (e.g., Asian-Indian, Black British, Chinese). Study findings should be considered an indicator of a signal that requires further detailed investigation. (iii) The questionnaire was only available in English, as several survey tools had only been validated in English. Findings may therefore not be applicable to patients who do not read English, who may be from White or Black, Asian and minority ethnic group groups. (iv) Participants had all received a kidney transplant and findings may not be generalisable to transplant eligible people active on the transplant waiting list. Qualitative responses were limited to hand-written free-text entries and were all in English, which may have restricted participants for whom this was not a first language. In-depth interviews would allow for further investigation of the issues raised. This study describes patient-reported and patient-identified reasons potential donors were not considered suitable for kidney donation. Patients are gatekeepers to the process, making personal judgements as to suitability: both who to approach and whose offers to accept or decline. However, surveying non-donors about their reasons for non-donation would provide a different and important perspective, although such a study would be ethically and practically challenging [50].

5. Conclusions

We have identified multiple patient-identified barriers to living kidney donation in the UK Black, Asian and minority ethnic group population, which should be further investigated and addressed to reduce the ethnic inequity in living-donor kidney transplantation in the UK.

Author Contributions: Conceptualization, P.B., Y.B.-S., C.R.T.; methodology, P.B., Y.B.-S., S.M.; software, K.W., P.B.; formal analysis, K.W., P.B., S.M., A.O.-S.; investigation, K.W., P.B.; data curation, P.B.; writing—original draft preparation, K.W., P.B.; writing—review and editing, K.W., P.B., A.O.-S., S.M., F.J.D., Y.B.-S., C.R.T., F.C., D.I., S.B.; supervision, A.O.-S., Y.B.-S., C.R.T., F.C.; project administration, P.B.; funding acquisition, P.B. All authors have read and agreed to the published version of the manuscript.

Acknowledgments: The authors would like to thank all the study participants, the participating centre research nurses and coordinators (Hugh Murtagh, Nina Bleakley, Mary Dutton, Kulli Kuningas, Cecilio Bing Andujar, Ann-Marie O'Sullivan, Nicola Johnson, Kieron Clark, Thomas Walters, Mary Quashie-Akponeware, Jane Turner, Gillian Curry, Hannah Beer, Lynn.D Langhorne, Sarah Brand, Maria Weetman, Molly Campbell, Megan Bennett, Sharirose Abat, and Agyapong Kwame Ansu) and the local collaborators who facilitated the study (Sarah Heap, Mysore Phanish, Shafi Malik, Aisling Courtney, Adnan Sharif, Nicholas Torpey, Refik Gökmen, Michael Picton, Linda Bisset, Edward Sharples, and Simon Curran).

References

1. Cecka, J.M. Living donor transplants. *Clin. Transpl. Jan.* **1995**, 363–377. [PubMed]
2. Terasaki, P.I.; Cecka, J.M.; Gjertson, D.W.; Takemoto, S. High Survival Rates of Kidney Transplants from Spousal and Living Unrelated Donors. *N. Engl. J. Med.* **1995**, *333*, 333–336. [CrossRef] [PubMed]
3. Laupacis, A.; Keown, P.; Pus, N.; Krueger, H.; Ferguson, B.; Wong, C.; Muirhead, N. A study of the quality of life and cost-utility of renal transplantation. *Kidney Int.* **1996**, *50*, 235–242. [CrossRef] [PubMed]
4. Cecka, J.M. The OPTN/UNOS Renal Transplant Registry. *Clin Transpl.* **2005**, 1–16. [PubMed]
5. Roodnat, J.I.; Van Riemsdijk, I.C.; Mulder, P.G.H.; Doxiadis, I.; Claas, F.H.J.; Ijzermans, J.N.M.; Weimar, W. The superior results of living-donor renal transplantation are not completely caused by selection or short cold ischemia time: A single-center, multivariate analysis. *Transplantation* **2003**, *75*, 2014–2018. [CrossRef]
6. Annual Activity Report—ODT Clinical—NHS Blood and Transplant. Published 2019. Available online: https://www.odt.nhs.uk/statistics-and-reports/annual-activity-report/ (accessed on 19 February 2020).
7. Barnieh, L.; Manns, B.J.; Klarenbach, S.; McLaughlin, K.; Yilmaz, S.; Hemmelgarn, B.R. A description of the costs of living and standard criteria deceased donor kidney transplantation. *Am. J. Transpl.* **2011**, *11*, 478–488. [CrossRef]
8. Smith, C.R.; Woodward, R.S.; Cohen, D.S.; Singer, G.G.; Brennan, D.C.; Lowell, J.A.; Schnitzler, M.A. Cadaveric versus living donor kidney transplantation: A medicare payment analysis. *Transplantation* **2000**, *69*, 311–314. [CrossRef]
9. Maggiore, U.; Budde, K.; Heemann, U.; Hilbrands, L.; Oberbauer, R.; Oniscu, G.C.; Abramowicz, D. Long-term risks of kidney living donation: Review and position paper by the ERA-EDTA DESCARTES working group. *Nephrol. Dial. Transpl.* **2017**, *32*, 216–223. [CrossRef]
10. Muzaale, A.D.; Massie, A.B.; Wang, M.C.; Montgomery, R.A.; McBride, M.A.; Wainright, J.L.; Segev, D.L. Risk of end-stage renal disease following live kidney donation. *JAMA J. Am. Med. Assoc.* **2014**, *311*, 579–586. [CrossRef]
11. Massie, A.B.; Muzaale, A.D.; Luo, X.; Chow, E.K.; Locke, J.E.; Nguyen, A.Q.; Segev, D.L. Quantifying postdonation risk of ESRD in living kidney donors. *J. Am. Soc. Nephrol.* **2017**, *28*, 2749–2755. [CrossRef]
12. Segev, D.L.; Muzaale, A.D.; Caffo, B.S.; Mehta, S.H.; Singer, A.L.; Taranto, S.E.; Montgomery, R.A. Perioperative mortality and long-term survival following live kidney donation. *JAMA J. Am. Med. Assoc.* **2010**, *303*, 959–966. [CrossRef] [PubMed]
13. Lumsdaine, J.A.; Wray, A.; Power, M.J.; Jamieson, N.V.; Akyol, M.; Andrew Bradley, J.; Wigmore, S.J. Higher quality of life in living donor kidney transplantation: Prospective cohort study. *Transpl. Int.* **2005**, *18*, 975–980. [CrossRef] [PubMed]
14. Johnson, E.M.; Anderson, J.K.; Jacobs, C.; Suh, G.; Humar, A.; Suhr, B.D.; Matas, A.J. Long-term follow-up of living kidney donors: Quality of life after donation. *Transplantation* **1999**, *67*, 717–721. [CrossRef] [PubMed]
15. IRODaT—International Registry on Organ Donation and Transplantation. Available online: http://www.irodat.org/?p=database (accessed on 27 February 2020).

16. Udayaraj, U.; Ben-Shlomo, Y.; Roderick, P.; Casula, A.; Dudley, C.; Collett, D.; Caskey, F. Social deprivation, ethnicity, and uptake of living kidney donor transplantation in the United Kingdom. *Transplantation* **2012**, *93*, 610–616. [CrossRef]

17. Wu, D.A.; Robb, M.L.; Watson, C.J.E.; Forsythe, J.L.; Tomson, C.R.; Cairns, J.; Bradley, C. Barriers to living donor kidney transplantation in the United Kingdom: A national observational study. *Nephrol. Dial. Transpl.* **2017**, *32*, 890–900. [CrossRef]

18. Lentine, K.L.; Kasiske, B.L.; Levey, A.S.; Adams, P.L.; Alberú, J.; Bakr, M.A.; Segev, D.L. KDIGO Clinical Practice Guideline on the Evaluation and Care of Living Kidney Donors. *Transplantation* **2017**, *101*, S1–S109. [CrossRef]

19. Rodrigue, J.R.; Kazley, A.S.; Mandelbrot, D.A.; Hays, R.; Rudow, D.L.P.; Baliga, P. Living donor kidney transplantation: Overcoming disparities in live kidney donation in the US—Recommendations from a consensus conference. *Clin. J. Am. Soc. Nephrol.* **2015**, *10*, 1687–1695. [CrossRef]

20. Morgan, M.; Kenten, C.; Deedat, S.; on behalf of the Donation, Transplantation and Ethnicity (DonaTE) Programme Team. Attitudes to deceased organ donation and registration as a donor among minority ethnic groups in North America and the UK: A synthesis of quantitative and qualitative research. *Ethn. Health* **2013**, *18*, 367–390. [CrossRef]

21. Alnaes, A.H. Lost in translation: Cultural obstructions impede living kidney donation among minority ethnic patients. *Cambridge Q. Healthc. Ethics* **2012**, *21*, 505–516. [CrossRef]

22. Bailey, P.K.; Tomson, C.R.V.; MacNeill, S.; Marsden, A.; Cook, D.; Cooke, R.; Ben-Shlomo, Y. A multicenter cohort study of potential living kidney donors provides predictors of living kidney donation and non-donation. *Kidney Int.* **2017**, *92*, 1249–1260. [CrossRef]

23. Barbour, R.S. The case for combining qualitative and quantitative approaches in health services research. *J. Health Serv. Res. Policy* **1999**, *4*, 39–43. [CrossRef] [PubMed]

24. Bailey, P.K.; Tomson, C.R.V.; Ben-Shlomo, Y. What factors explain the association between socioeconomic deprivation and reduced likelihood of live-donor kidney transplantation? A questionnaire-based pilot case-control study. *BMJ Open* **2016**, *6*. [CrossRef]

25. Harris, P.A.; Taylor, R.; Thielke, R.; Payne, J.; Gonzalez, N.; Conde, J.G. Research electronic data capture (REDCap)-A metadata-driven methodology and workflow process for providing translational research informatics support. *J. Biomed. Inform.* **2009**, *42*, 377–381. [CrossRef] [PubMed]

26. Bailey, P.K.; Ben-Shlomo, Y.; Tomson, C.R.V.; Owen-Smith, A. Socioeconomic deprivation and barriers to live-donor kidney transplantation: A qualitative study of deceased-donor kidney transplant recipients. *BMJ Open* **2016**, *6*, e010605. [CrossRef]

27. 2011 Census Analysis: Ethnicity and Religion of the non-UK Born Population in England and Wales—Office for National Statistics. Available online: https://www.ons.gov.uk/peoplepopulationandcommunity/culturalidentity/ethnicity/articles/2011censusanalysisethnicityandreligionofthenonukbornpopulationinenglandandwales/2015-06-18 (accessed on 19 February 2020).

28. StataCorp. *Stata Statistical Software: Release 15*; StataCorp LLC: College Station, TX, USA, 2017.

29. Miles, M.B.; Huberman, A.M.; Saldaña, J. *Qualitative Data Analysis A Methods Sourcebook*, 3rd ed.; SAGE Publications: Thousand Oaks, CA, USA, 2014.

30. Braun, V.; Clarke, V. Using thematic analysis in psychology. *Qual. Res. Psychol.* **2006**, *3*, 77–101. [CrossRef]

31. Von Elm, E.; Altman, D.G.; Egger, M.; Pocock, S.J.; Gøtzsche, P.C.; Vandenbroucke, J.P. Strengthening the reporting of observational studies in epidemiology (STROBE) statement: Guidelines for reporting observational studies. *BMJ* **2007**, *335*, 806–808. [CrossRef]

32. Tong, A.; Sainsbury, P.; Craig, J. Consolidated criteria for reporting qualitative research (COREQ): A 32-item checklist for interviews and focus groups. *Int. J. Qual. Health Care* **2007**, *19*, 349–357. [CrossRef]

33. NHS England. Commissioning Policy: Reimbursement of Expenses for Living Donors. *Reference: NHS England A06/P/a June 2017.* Available online: https://www.england.nhs.uk/publication/commissioning-policy-reimbursement-of-expenses-for-living-donors/ (accessed on 28 September 2020).

34. Bailey, P.K.; Caskey, F.J.; MacNeill, S.; Tomson, C.; Dor, F.J.M.F.; Ben-Shlomo, Y. Beliefs of UK Transplant Recipients about Living Kidney Donation and Transplantation: Findings from a Multicentre Questionnaire-Based Case–Control Study. *J. Clin. Med.* **2019**, *9*, 31. [CrossRef]

35. Zubair, M.; Jurisconsult, B. Organ Donation and Transplantation in Islam An Opinion. Available online: https://nhsbtdbe.blob.core.windows.net/umbraco-assets-corp/16300/organ-donation-fatwa.pdf (accessed on 20 November 2020).

36. Davis, L.A.; Grogan, T.M.; Cox, J.; Weng, F.L. Inter- and Intrapersonal Barriers to Living Donor Kidney Transplant among Black Recipients and Donors. *J. Racial Ethn. Health Disparities* **2017**, *4*, 671–679. [CrossRef]

37. Cerrato, A.; Avitable, M.; Hayman, L.L. The relationship between the sick role and functional ability: One center's experience. *Prog. Transpl.* **2008**, *18*, 192–198. [CrossRef]

38. Bailey, P.; Caskey, F.; MacNeill, S.; Tomson, C.; Dor, F.J.; Ben-Shlomo, Y. Mediators of socioeconomic inequity in living-donor kidney transplantation: Results from a UK multicenter case-control study. *Transpl. Direct.* **2020**, *6*, e540. [CrossRef] [PubMed]

39. Browne, T. The relationship between social networks and pathways to kidney transplant parity: Evidence from black Americans in Chicago. *Soc. Sci. Med.* **2011**, *73*, 663–667. [CrossRef] [PubMed]

40. Clark, C.R.; Hicks, L.S.; Keogh, J.H.; Epstein, A.M.; Ayanian, J.Z. Promoting access to renal transplantation: The role of social support networks in completing pre-transplant evaluations. *J. Gen. Intern. Med.* **2008**, *23*, 1187–1193. [CrossRef] [PubMed]

41. Lpez-Navas, A.; Ros, A.; Riquelme, A.; Martínez-Alarcón, L.; Pons, J.A.; Miras, M.; Parrilla, P. Psychological care: Social and family support for patients awaiting a liver transplant. *Transplant. Proc.* **2011**, *43*, 701–704. [CrossRef]

42. Ismail, S.Y.; Luchtenburg, A.E.; Timman, R.; Zuidema, W.C.; Boonstra, C.; Weimar, W.; Massey, E.K. Home-based family intervention increases knowledge, communication and living donation rates: A randomized controlled trial. *Am. J. Transpl.* **2014**, *14*, 1862–1869. [CrossRef]

43. Garonzik-Wang, J.M.; Berger, J.C.; Ros, R.L.; Kucirka, L.M.; Deshpande, N.A.; Boyarsky, B.J.; Segev, D.L. Live donor champion: Finding live kidney donors by separating the advocate from the patient. *Transplantation* **2012**, *93*, 1147–1150. [CrossRef]

44. Waterman, A.D.; Wood, E.H.; Ranasinghe, O.N.; Lipsey, A.F.; Anderson, C.; Balliet, W.; Salas, M.A.P. A Digital Library for Increasing Awareness About Living Donor Kidney Transplants: Formative Study. *JMIR Form. Res.* **2020**, *4*, e17441. [CrossRef]

45. Lunsford, S.L.; Simpson, K.S.; Chavin, K.D.; Menching, K.J.; Miles, L.G.; Shilling, L.M.; Baliga, P.K. Racial Disparities in Living Kidney Donation: Is There a Lack of Willing Donors or an Excess of Medically Unsuitable Candidates? *Transplantation* **2006**, *82*, 876–881. [CrossRef]

46. Robb, K.A.; Gatting, L.; Wardle, J. What impact do questionnaire length and monetary incentives have on mailed health psychology survey response? *Br. J. Health Psychol.* **2017**, *22*, 671–685. [CrossRef]

47. Harrison, S.; Henderson, J.; Alderdice, F.; Quigley, M.A. Methods to increase response rates to a population-based maternity survey: A comparison of two pilot studies. *BMC Med. Res. Methodol.* **2019**, *19*, 65. [CrossRef]

48. Slaats, D.; Lennerling, A.; Pronk, M.C.; van der Pant, K.A.; Dooper, I.M.; Wierdsma, J.M.; Zuidema, W.C. Donor and Recipient Perspectives on Anonymity in Kidney Donation From Live Donors: A Multicenter Survey Study. *Am. J. Kidney Dis.* **2018**, *71*, 52–64. [CrossRef] [PubMed]

49. Salway, S.; Holman, D.; Lee, C.; McGowan, V.; Ben-Shlomo, Y.; Saxena, S.; Nazroo, J. Transforming the health system for the UK's multiethnic population. *BMJ* **2020**, *368*, m268. [CrossRef] [PubMed]

50. Thiessen, C.; Kulkarni, S.; Reese, P.P.; Gordon, E.J. A Call for Research on Individuals Who Opt Out of Living Kidney Donation. *Transplantation* **2016**, *100*, 2527–2532. [CrossRef] [PubMed]

11

Plasmapheresis Reduces Mycophenolic Acid Concentration: A Study of Full AUC_{0-12} in Kidney Transplant Recipients

Sudarat Piyasiridej [1], Natavudh Townamchai [1,2,3,*], Suwasin Udomkarnjananun [1,2,3], Somratai Vadcharavivad [4], Krit Pongpirul [5,6], Salin Wattanatorn [1,2], Boonchoo Sirichindakul [2,7], Yingyos Avihingsanon [1,3], Kriang Tungsanga [1], Somchai Eiam-Ong [1] and Kearkiat Praditpornsilpa [1]

[1] Division of Nephrology, Department of Medicine, Faculty of Medicine, Chulalongkorn University and King Chulalongkorn Memorial Hospital, Bangkok 10330, Thailand; yam_med16@hotmail.com (S.P.); suwasin.u@gmail.com (S.U.); salin.tob@gmail.com (S.W.); yingyos.a@gmail.com (Y.A.); kriangtungsanga@hotmail.com (K.T.); somchai80754@yahoo.com (S.E.-O.); kearkiat@hotmail.com (K.P.)

[2] Excellence Center for Solid Organ Transplantation, King Chulalongkorn Memorial Hospital, Bangkok 10330, Thailand; boonchoog1@gmail.com

[3] Renal Immunology and Renal Transplant Research Unit, Department of Medicine, Chulalongkorn University, Bangkok 10330, Thailand

[4] Department of Pharmacy Practice, Faculty of Pharmaceutical Sciences, Chulalongkorn University, Bangkok 10330, Thailand; somratai.v@pharm.chula.ac.th

[5] Department of Preventive and Social Medicine, Faculty of Medicine, Chulalongkorn University, Bangkok 10330, Thailand; doctorkrit@gmail.com

[6] Department of International Health, Johns Hopkins Bloomberg School of Public Health, Johns Hopkins University, Baltimore, MD 21205, USA

[7] Department of Surgery, Faculty of Medicine, Chulalongkorn University and King Chulalongkorn Memorial Hospital, Bangkok 10330, Thailand

[*] Correspondence: natavudh.t@chula.ac.th

Abstract: Background: Mycophenolic acid (MPA), a crucial immunosuppressive drug, and plasmapheresis, an effective immunoreduction method, are simultaneously used for the management of various immune-related diseases, including kidney transplantation. While plasmapheresis has been proven efficient in removing many substances from the blood, its effect on MPA plasma levels remains unestablished. Objectives: To evaluate the full pharmacokinetics of MPA by measuring the area under the time–concentration curve (AUC_{0-12}), which is the best indicator for MPA treatment monitoring after each plasmapheresis session, and to compare the AUC_{0-12} measurements on the day with and on the day without plasmapheresis. Methods: A cross-sectional study was conducted in kidney transplantation recipients who were taking a twice-daily oral dose of mycophenolate mofetil (MMF, Cellcept®) and undergoing plasmapheresis at King Chulalongkorn Memorial Hospital, Bangkok, Thailand, during January 2018 and January 2019. The MPA levels were measured by an enzymatic method (Roche diagnostic®) 0, 1/2, 1, 2, 3, 4, 6, 8, and 12 h after MMF administration, for AUC_{0-12} calculation on the day with and on the day without plasmapheresis sessions. Plasmapheresis was started within 4 h after administering the oral morning dose of MMF. Our primary outcome was the difference of AUC_{0-12} between the day with and the day without plasmapheresis. Results: Forty complete AUC measurements included 20 measurements on the plasmapheresis day and other 20 measurements on the day without plasmapheresis in six kidney transplant patients. The mean age of the patients was 56.2 ± 20.7 years. All patients had received 1000 mg/day of MMF for at least 72 h before undergoing 3.5 ± 1.2 plasmapheresis sessions. The mean AUC on the day with plasmapheresis was lower than that on the day without plasmapheresis (28.22 ± 8.21 vs. 36.79 ± 10.29 mg × h/L, $p = 0.001$), and the percentage of AUC reduction was $19.49 \pm 24.83\%$. This was mainly the result of a decrease in AUC_{0-4} of MPA (23.96 ± 28.12% reduction). Conclusions: Plasmapheresis significantly reduces the level of full AUC_{0-12} of MPA. The present study is the first to measure the full AUC_{0-12} in MPA-treated patients undergoing plasmapheresis. Our study suggests that a supplementary dose of MPA is necessary for patients undergoing plasmapheresis.

Keywords: mycophenolic acid; immunosuppression; plasmapheresis; kidney transplantation

1. Introduction

Mycophenolic acid (MPA) is one of the main powerful immunosuppressive drugs widely used for many immunological diseases. There are two MPA compounds available, i.e., mycophenolate mofetil (MMF, Cellcept®) and enteric-coated mycophenolate sodium (EC-MPS, Myfortic®). Both MMF and EC-MPS are similar in terms of efficacy and safety. EC-MPS was developed to improve the side effects of upper gastrointestinal symptoms. The time to reach maximum plasma MPA concentration (t_{max}) of MMF is usually within 1–2 h after an oral dose, while EC-MPS reveals a median lag time from 0.25 to 1.25 h [1]. After absorption from the gastrointestinal tract, 97 to 99% of MPA, which is the active form, will bind to serum albumin. MPA is converted by uridine diphosphate-glucuronosyltransferase (UGT) into inactive mycophenolic acid glucuronide (MPAG), which is mainly excreted by the renal tubules. MPAG can also be excreted in the biliary tract by multidrug-resistant protein (MRP), which can lead to enterohepatic recycling. [1]

Plasmapheresis is one of the most effective methods utilized for rapid immunoglobulin removal in various immunological diseases. Many proteins and protein-bound substances, including medications, can also be removed during plasmapheresis sessions [2,3]. Substances which are likely to be removed during plasmapheresis have the following characters: (1) high blood concentration, (2) high protein bound, (3) low volume of distribution (Vd), and (4) undergoing high-dose/high-efficiency plasmapheresis [4].

Several immunologically mediated diseases can be treated by MPA together with plasmapheresis, i.e., systemic lupus erythematosus (SLE), lupus nephritis, myasthenia gravis, Guillain–Barré syndrome, psoriatic arthritis, relapsed/refractory thrombotic thrombocytopenic purpura (TTP), severe polymyositis/dermatomyositis, inflammatory bowel disease, pemphigus vulgaris, and kidney transplantation [5–7]. Unintentional removal of MPA may result in inadequate immunosuppression and unfavorable outcomes. Of interest, the effect of plasmapheresis on MPA concentration has been studied only in a case series of two patients, one kidney transplant recipient and one patient with myasthenia gravis [8]. MPA removal were measured by considering MPA levels at only two time points—before and after each plasmapheresis session. The MPA removal was calculated on the basis of MPA concentration in plasma effluent. The authors concluded that plasmapheresis of 3 L of plasma did not significantly alter post-plasmapheresis MPA concentration. Currently, there are no available data regarding the effect of plasmapheresis on the area under the concentration–time curve from 0 to 12 h (AUC_{0-12}) of MPA, which is the best indicator of MPA exposure of patients.

The present study was conducted in kidney transplant recipients who were taking stable doses of MMF and had indication for plasmapheresis to examine the effects of plasmapheresis on MPA exposure.

2. Methods

An observational study of patients who were taking MMF (Roche, Basel, Switzerland) in combination with plasmapheresis treatment was conducted in King Chulalongkorn Memorial Hospital, Bangkok, Thailand, during January 2018 and January 2019. The inclusion criteria were kidney transplant recipients older than 18 years, who were under an immunosuppressive regimen of tacrolimus, MMF, low-dose prednisolone and had an indication for plasmapheresis. The dosage of MMF had to be

500 mg orally every 12 h for at least one week. Exclusion criteria were patients with serum albumin concentration lower than 2 g/dL and patients who were coadministered a proton pump inhibitor.

Plasmapheresis sessions were initiated within 4 h after the morning dose of MMF. The plasmapheresis machine was Plasauto EZ®, and the dialyzer was Plasmaflo® with a maximum pore size of 0.3 μm. The total treatment volume was 1.5 plasma volume per session. The blood flow rate was 150 mL/h. The replacement fluid was 5% albumin in the same volume as the treatment volume. The number of sessions required was determined on the basis of the clinical judgment of the attending nephrologists.

Plasmapheresis was performed on an alternate day basis for patients who were prescribed more than one plasmapheresis session.

Patients had to strictly take a stable dose of MMF, i.e., 500 mg orally every 12 h for at least one week, before entering the study. MMF dosage adjustment was not allowed during the study period. Patients were not allowed to have a meal for one hour before and two hours after taking the MMF dose. MPA level was measured by an enzymatic immunoassay method (Roche-diagnostic®). The AUC_{0-12} was calculated with the trapezoidal rule from the MPA levels at nine time points after the morning dose of MMF (C0, C0.5, C1, C2, C3, C4, C6, C8, and C12) (Figure 1). The full AUC_{0-12} was measured on the day just before the day patients underwent plasmapheresis and compared with the AUC_{0-12} of the following day, in which patients received the plasmapheresis treatment. Blood samples were taken via a heparin lock in the arm by using the double-syringe technique.

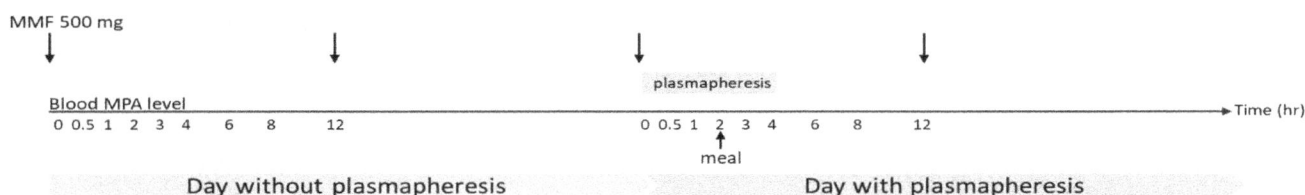

Figure 1. Timing of mofetil (MMF) dosage, plasmapheresis sessions, and meal on the day before and on the day with a plasmapheresis session. MPA: mycophenolic acid.

A complete clinical evaluation including vital signs and body weight was performed. The baseline characteristics including age, cause of end-stage renal disease, type of kidney transplantation, time after kidney transplantation, renal function, indications for plasmapheresis, session of plasmapheresis, and plasma volume per session were recorded.

Absolute and relative frequencies were used for qualitative data. Mean and standard deviation were utilized for numerical data. The chi-squared test was used for comparisons between categorical data. Paired-samples t-test was used to compare the AUC_{0-12} of the day with plasmapheresis and the AUC_{0-12} of the day without plasmapheresis. Data were analyzed using the SPSS statistic version 22 (IBM; New York, NY, USA).

This study was approved by The Research Ethics Review Committee for Research Involving Human Research Participants, Health Sciences Group, Chulalongkorn University (IRB No.CF 333/61). The study was registered with the Thai Clinical Trials Registry (TCTR20190211001).

3. Results

Six kidney transplant recipients were enrolled, with a total of 20 plasmapheresis sessions. There were 40 AUC_{0-12} measurements (each AUC consisted of measurements of MPA levels at 9 time points), 20 of which were recorded on the day just before the day patients underwent plasmapheresis, and the other 20 were recorded on the following day, when patients underwent a plasmapheresis session. The mean (±SD) age of the patients was 56.2 ± 20.7 years, and five patients (83.3%) were men (Table 1). At baseline, the mean (±SD) estimated glomerular filtration rate (eGFR) was 49.7 ± 10.9 mL/min/1.73 m², serum albumin concentration was 3.8 ± 0.4 g/dL, and hemoglobin concentration was 10.3 ± 1.4 g/dL. Indication for plasmapheresis was antibody-mediated rejection (ABMR) for all six patients, who were diagnosed by pathological presentation and donor-specific antibody (DSA) detection. The number of plasmapheresis sessions per patient was 3.5 ± 1.2 (range of 1–4 sessions).

Table 1. Baseline characteristics of the patients.

Characteristics	
Age, year (mean ± SD)	56.2 ± 20.7
(range)	(25–80)
Male (n, %)	5/6, 83%
Cause of ESRD before kidney transplantation	
Unknown (n, %)	6/6, 100%
Type of kidney transplantation	
Living donor kidney transplantation (n, %)	2/6, 33%
History of previous kidney transplantation (n, %)	1/6, 16.7%
HLA mismatch (n, %)	
0	0/6
1–5	6/6, 100%
6	0/6
Panel reactive antibody (n, %)	
0%	4/6, 66.7%
1–80%	0/6
More than 80%	2/6, 33.3%
Induction immunosuppression (n, %)	
Anti-IL2 receptor antibody	4/6, 66.7%
Anti-thymocyte globulin	2/6, 33.3%
Time after transplantation, month (mean ± SD)	97.1 ± 69.5
(range)	(1.97–196.52)
Body weight, kg (mean ± SD)	62.2 ± 12.4
(range)	(42.7–79.3)
eGFR CKD-EPI, mL/min/1.73 m^2 (mean ± SD)	49.7 ± 10.9
Serum albumin, mg/dL (mean ± SD)	3.8 ± 0.4
(range)	(3.0–4.2)
Hemoglobin, mg/dL (mean ± SD)	10.3 ± 1.4
(range)	9.0–12.2
Liver enzyme, U/L (mean ± SD) SGOT	32 ± 42
(range)	(10–117)
SGPT	33 ± 36
(range)	(10–104)
Type of plasmapheresis	
Conventional plasmapheresis (n, %)	6/6, 100%
Indication for plasmapheresis (n, %)	
ABMR	6/6, 100%
Acute ABMR	2/6, 33.3%
Chronic active ABMR	4/6, 66.7%
Plasma volume per session, mL (mean ± SD)	4,041 ± 749
Number of plasmapheresis session in each patient (mean ± SD)	3.5 ± 1.2

ESRD: end-stage renal disease, ABMR: antibody-mediated rejection; eGFR: estimated glomerular filtration rate; CKD-EPI: chronic kidney disease epidemiology collaboration; SGOT: serum glutamic-oxaloacetic transaminase; SGPT: serum glutamate-pyruvate transaminase.

The mean of MPA AUC_{0-12} of the day with plasmapheresis was significantly lower than that of the day without plasmapheresis (28.22 ± 8.21 vs. 36.79 ± 10.29 mg × h/L, $p = 0.001$) (Figure 2). The percentage reduction of AUC_{0-12} was $19.49 \pm 24.83\%$ (Table 2). The early part of the AUC was affected by plasmapheresis sessions. The AUC_{0-4} of the day with plasmapheresis was significantly lower than that of the day without plasmapheresis (15.79 ± 6.46 vs. 21.78 ± 5.66 mg $\times$ h/L, $p < 0.001$), while the AUC_{4-12} was not significantly different between the day with and that without plasmapheresis (12.43 ± 5.02 vs. 15.00 ± 7.56 mg $\times$ h/L, $p = 0.125$).

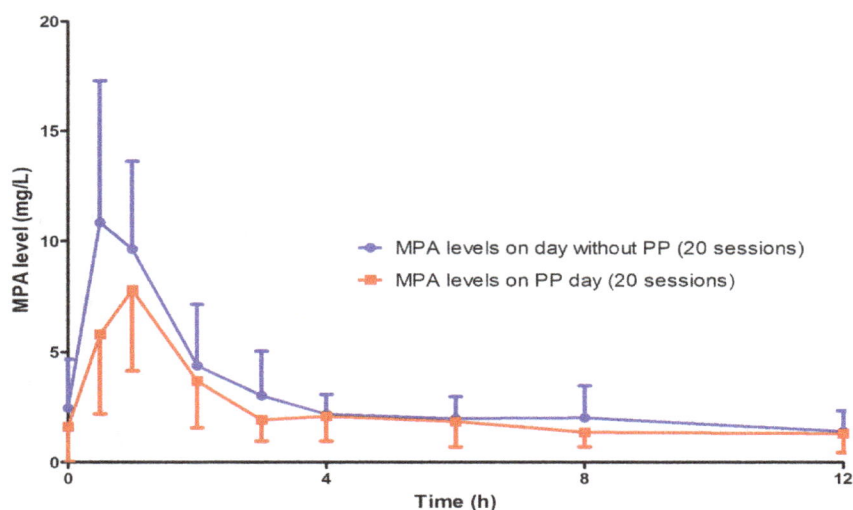

Figure 2. MPA levels on the day with plasmapheresis (20 sessions) compared with those on the day without plasmapheresis (20 sessions). PP: plasmapheresis.

Table 2. Comparison of MPA AUCs recorded on days with and without plasmapheresis, from 0 to 12 h, from 0 to 4 h, and from 4 to 12 h.

Parameters	Day without Plasmapheresis	Day with Plasmapheresis	p-Value
AUC_{0-12} mg $\times$ h/L (mean $\pm$ SD)	36.79 ± 10.29	28.22 ± 8.21	$p = 0.001$
Percentage reduction of AUC_{0-12} (%)	19.49 ± 24.83		-
AUC_{0-4} mg $\times$ h/L (mean $\pm$ SD)	21.78 ± 5.66	15.79 ± 6.46	$p < 0.001$
Percentage reduction of AUC_{0-4} (%)	23.96 ± 28.12		-
AUC_{4-12} mg $\times$ h/L (mean $\pm$ SD)	15.00 ± 7.56	12.43 ± 5.02	$p = 0.125$
Percentage reduction of AUC_{4-12} (%)	3.88 ± 42.89		-
AUC_{0-12} of the first day with plasmapheresis session, mg $\times$ h/L (mean $\pm$ SD)	41.66 ± 10.66	32.26 ± 9.42	$p = 0.001$
Percentage reduction of AUC_{0-12} of the first day with plasmapheresis session (%)	22.86 ± 6.99		-

(AUC; area under the time–concentration curve).

The reduction of MPA AUC_{0-12} was detected as early as the first session of plasmapheresis. The MPA AUC_{0-12} of the day before and of the day of the first session of plasmapheresis were 41.66 ± 10.66 and 32.26 ± 9.42 mg $\times$ h/L, respectively ($p = 0.001$) (Table 2 and Figure 3). The percentage reduction of MPA AUC_{0-12} of the first day of plasmapheresis session was $22.86 \pm 6.99\%$. The AUC_{0-12} of the day before the second to that of the day of the forth plasmapheresis sessions could be rebounded from the AUC_{0-12} of the day with plasmapheresis. However, the rebounded AUC_{0-12} gradually decreased with the number of sessions of plasmapheresis that the patients received (Figure 4). Given that the target therapeutic AUC_{0-12} of MPA is 30 to 60 mg $\times$ h/L for kidney transplantation recipients [9], 17 out of 20 (85%) AUC_{0-12} measured on the day without plasmapheresis achieved the target therapeutic range, compared with only 9 out of 20 (45%) AUC_{0-12} measured on the day with plasmapheresis ($p = 0.008$) (Figure 5).

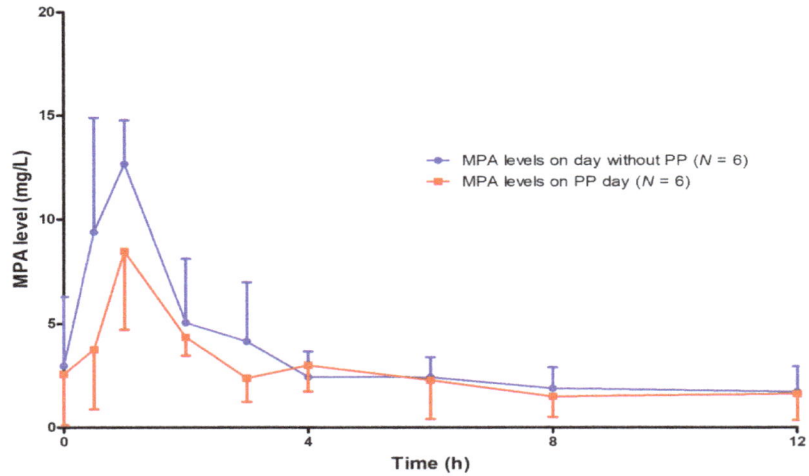

Figure 3. MPA levels on the day before the first plasmapheresis session ($N = 6$) compared with MPA levels on the day with the first plasmapheresis session ($N = 6$).

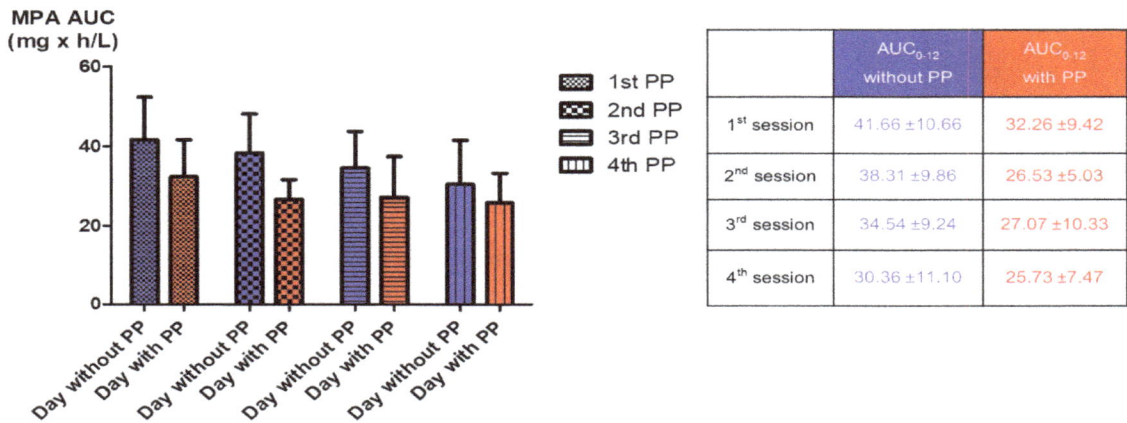

	AUC$_{0-12}$ without PP	AUC$_{0-12}$ with PP
1st session	41.66 ±10.66	32.26 ±9.42
2nd session	38.31 ±9.86	26.53 ±5.03
3rd session	34.54 ±9.24	27.07 ±10.33
4th session	30.36 ±11.10	25.73 ±7.47

Figure 4. Comparison of the mean MPA AUC$_{0-12}$ between the day with and that without plasmapheresis from the first plasmapheresis session to the fourth session.

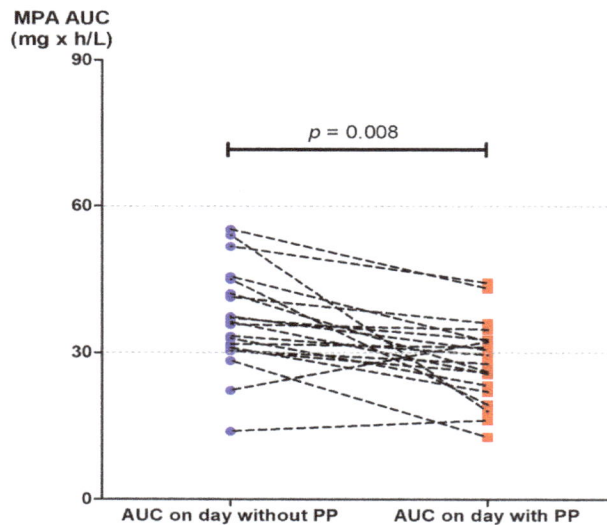

Figure 5. The MPA AUC$_{0-12}$ achieved the target level between the day just before a plasmapheresis session (20 measurements) and the following day, when plasmapheresis was administered (20 measurements).

4. Discussion

The present study is the first to demonstrate the effect of plasmapheresis on MPA exposure by using the full MPA AUC_{0-12}. The AUC_{0-12} of MPA was significantly affected by plasmapheresis. This effect was found starting from the first session of plasmapheresis (Figures 2 and 3). One-fifth of the total AUC_{0-12} was lowered by plasmapheresis. The component of AUC most affected by plasmapheresis was the early part (AUC_{0-4}). Undergoing plasmapheresis treatment immediately after an oral dose of MMF can lower the MPA peak level, leading to exposure to a subtherapeutic level of MPA. Consecutive sessions of plasmapheresis could increase the risk of underimmunosuppression by lowering the rebound of MPA AUC_{0-12} (Figure 4).

MMF is one of the major immunosuppressive agents widely used to treat many immunological diseases. Since overimmunosuppression can lead to many side effects and underimmunosuppression can cause unfavorable treatment outcomes, MPA level monitoring has been recommended to maintain MPA concentration at the therapeutic level [9,10]. Plasmapheresis is one of the most effective methods for rapid immunoglobulin G (IgG) reduction [5]. Many high-molecular-weight substances can also be removed during a plasmapheresis session, especially proteins and albumin, which makes albumin replacement necessary. Since 97 to 99% of MPA is protein-bound, MPA should be theoretically removed from patients during plasmapheresis treatment.

The effect of plasmapheresis on MPA plasma level was reported in only two patients who were administered MMF in combination with plasmapheresis [8]. Plasmapheresis sessions were started 4 h after MMF administration, and MPA removal was assessed at only two time points (pre- and post-plasmapheresis) together with MPA concentration in plasma waste. The authors concluded that a plasmapheresis session starting later than 4 h after the administration of an oral MMF dose did not significantly alter MPA concentration. Since serum proteins can be trapped in the dialyzer and bloodline, monitoring of MPA removal by only measuring MPA in plasma waste may not reflect total MPA removal. Our study monitored MPA exposure by full AUC_{0-12} measurement on the day with a plasmapheresis session as the study arm and on the day without plasmapheresis as the control arm. Alteration in AUC_{0-12} between the day with and the day without plasmapheresis is the best indicator of the effect of plasmapheresis on MPA plasma levels. The early phase of the full MPA AUC (peak level, AUC_{0-4}) is the one mostly affecting MPA exposure and represents more than 50% of AUC_{0-12}. The plasmapheresis sessions designed in the present study started within one hour after oral administration of an MMF dose which is the most crucial period for determining the effects of plasmapheresis on MPA.

MPA together with plasmapheresis is mainly utilized for the treatment of many immunologic conditions and diseases which require potent immunosuppression, such as kidney transplant rejection, severe lupus nephritis, or relapsed/refractory thrombotic thrombocytopenic purpura. The patients enrolled in the present study were kidney transplant recipients who were taking MMF and experienced antibody-mediated rejection, which is indicated for plasmapheresis treatment. The present study reveals that MPA administration without dosage adjustment during consecutive sessions of plasmapheresis can lead to unexpected underimmunosuppression and may increase the failure rate of treatment. The present study demonstrated that MPA AUC_{0-12} is reduced by 20% when a plasmapheresis session is started within 4 h after oral administration of MMF (Table 2, Figure 2). The higher the number of consecutive sessions of plasmapheresis performed, the higher the chance of MPA underexposure (Figure 4). We also further examined the role of MMF dose increments in two patients who underwent plasmapheresis and found that increasing the MMF dose from 1000 mg/day to 1250 mg/day can prevent subtherapeutic AUC_{0-12} during plasmapheresis sessions (unpublished data). An MMF dosage increment of 20% may be required to maintain a therapeutic level of MPA on the day patients undergo plasmapheresis. A further comprehensive study of therapeutic drug monitoring in patients with increased dose of MPA before undergoing plasmapheresis is crucially required. Otherwise, a 4 h delay of the plasmapheresis session after administration of an MMF dose may reduce the effect of plasmapheresis on MPA exposure (Figure 6).

Starting plasmapheresis in patient taking MMF

| Increase MMF dose for 20% before plasmapheresis session | Delay plasmapheresis session for 4 hours after MMF dose |

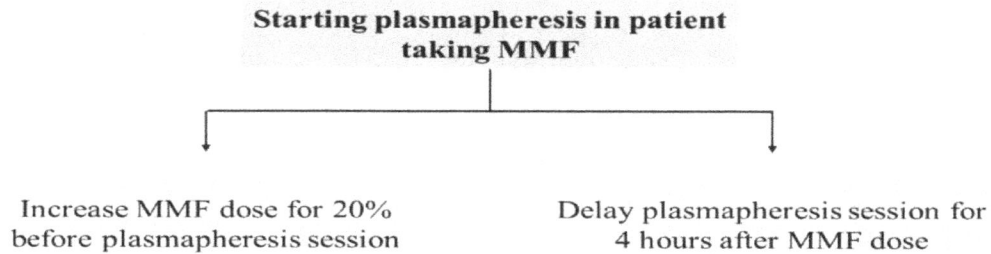

Figure 6. Recommendations for MMF dose or plasmapheresis adjustment in patient receiving concomitant MMF and plasmapheresis treatment.

The MMF dose used in the present study was relatively low. This is because the target population of patients enrolled in this study were kidney transplant recipients who were in the maintenance phase of immunosuppression. Moreover, a study on Asian patients showed that most of the patients achieved the target MPA level with an MMF dose of 1000 mg/day [11]. Besides conventional plasmapheresis, a study of the effects of others apheresis techniques such as double-filtration plasmapheresis and immunoadsorption, which have different kinetics of protein removal, should be carried out.

5. Conclusions

Plasmapheresis significantly reduces MPA plasma levels, particularly in the early phase after oral administration of an MPA dose. This effect should be addressed when combining MPA administration together with plasmapheresis in a treatment protocol.

Author Contributions: Conceptualization, S.P., N.T. and S.U.; methodology, S.P., N.T. and S.V.; formal analysis, N.T. and K.P. (Krit Pongpirul); investigation, S.P. and S.W.; writing-original draft preparation, S.P. and N.T.; writing-review and editing, N.T., B.S., Y.A., K.T., S.E.-O. and K.P. (Kearkiat Praditpornsilpa); visualization, N.T., supervision, N.T.; project administration, N.T.; funding acquisition, S.P. and N.T.

References

1. Staatz, C.E.; Tett, S.E. Clinical pharmacokinetics and pharmacodynamics of mycophenolate in solid organ transplant recipients. *Clin. Pharmacokinet.* **2007**, *46*, 13–58. [CrossRef] [PubMed]
2. Ibrahim, R.B.; Liu, C.; Cronin, S.M.; Murphy, B.C.; Cha, R.; Swerdlow, P.; Edward, D.J. Drug Removal by Plasmapheresis: An Evidence-Based Review. *Pharmacother. J. Hum. Pharmacol. Drug Ther.* **2007**, *27*, 1529–1549. [CrossRef] [PubMed]
3. Katagri, D.; Mogi, K. Double Filtration Plasmapheresis. In *The Concise Manual of Apheresis Therapy*; Springer: Heidelberg, Germany, 2014; pp. 57–64.
4. Ibrahim, R.B.; Balogun, R.A. Medications in Patients Treated with Therapeutic Plasma Exchange: Prescription Dosage, Timing, and Drug Overdose. *Semin. Dial.* **2012**, *25*, 176–189. [CrossRef] [PubMed]
5. Schwartz, J.; Padmanabhan, A.; Aqui, N.; Balogun, R.A.; Delaney, M.; Dunbar, N.M.; Witt, V.; Wu, Y.; Shaz, B.H.; Connelly-Smith, L.; et al. Guidelines on the Use of Therapeutic Apheresis in Clinical Practice-Evidence-Based Approach from the Writing Committee of the American Society for Apheresis: The Seventh Special Issue. *J. Clin. Apher.* **2016**, *31*, 149–338. [CrossRef] [PubMed]
6. Houssiau, F.A.; D'Cruz, D.; Sangle, S.; Remy, P.; Vasconcelos, C.; Petrovic, R.; Fiehn, C.; Garrido, E.D.R.; Gilboe, I.-M.; Tektonidou, M.; et al. Azathioprine versus mycophenolate mofetil for long-term immunosuppression in lupus nephritis: Results from the maintain Nephritis Trial. *Ann. Rheum. Dis.* **2010**, *69*, 2083–2089. [CrossRef] [PubMed]

7. Ekberg, H.; Tedesco-Silva, H.; Demirbaş, A.; Vitko, S.; Nashan, B.; Gürkan, A.; Margreiter, R.; Hugo, C.; Grinyó, J.M.; Frei, U.; et al. Reduced Exposure to Calcineurin Inhibitors in Renal Transplantation. *New Engl. J. Med.* **2007**, *357*, 2562–2575. [CrossRef] [PubMed]

8. Maldonado, A.Q.; Davies, N.M.; Crow, S.A.; Little, C.; Ojogho, O.N.; Weeks, D.L. Effects of Plasmapheresis on Mycophenolic Acid Concentrations. *Transplantation* **2011**, *91*, e3–e4. [CrossRef] [PubMed]

9. Kuypers, D.R.; Le Meur, Y.; Cantarovich, M.; Tredger, M.J.; Tett, S.E.; Cattaneo, D.; Tönshoff, B.; Holt, D.W.; Chapman, J.; Van Gelder, T.; et al. Consensus Report on Therapeutic Drug Monitoring of Mycophenolic Acid in Solid Organ Transplantation. *Clin. J. Am. Soc. Nephrol.* **2010**, *5*, 341–358. [CrossRef]

10. van Gelder, T.; Hilbrands, L.B.; Vanrenterghem, Y.; Weimar, W.; de Fijter, J.W.; Squifflet, J.P.; Hené, R.J.; Verpooten, G.A.; Navarro, M.T.; Hale, M.D.; et al. A randomized double-blind, multicenter plasma concentration controlled study of the safety and efficacy of oral mycophenolate mofetil for the prevention of acute rejection after kidney transplantation. *Transplantation* **1999**, *68*, 261–266. [CrossRef] [PubMed]

11. Pithukpakorn, M.; Tiwawanwong, T.; Lalerd, Y.; Assawamakin, A.; Premasathian, N.; Tasanarong, A.; Thongnoppakhun, W.; Vongwiwatana, A. Mycophenolic acid AUC in Thai kidney transplant recipients receiving low dose mycophenolate and its association with UGT2B7 polymorphisms. *Pharm. Pers. Med.* **2014**, *7*, 379–385. [CrossRef]

12

Optimized Identification of Advanced Chronic Kidney Disease and Absence of Kidney Disease by Combining Different Electronic Health Data Resources and by Applying Machine Learning Strategies

Christoph Weber [1,†], Lena Röschke [1,†], Luise Modersohn [2], Christina Lohr [2], Tobias Kolditz [2], Udo Hahn [2], Danny Ammon [3], Boris Betz [1,*,‡] and Michael Kiehntopf [1,*,‡]

[1] Department of Clinical Chemistry and Laboratory Diagnostics and Integrated Biobank Jena (IBBJ), Jena University Hospital, 07747 Jena, Germany; christoph.weber@med.uni-jena.de (C.W.); lena.marie.roeschke@uni-jena.de (L.R.)

[2] Jena University Language & Information Engineering (JULIE) Lab, Friedrich Schiller University Jena, 07743 Jena, Germany; luise.modersohn@uni-jena.de (L.M.); christina.lohr@uni-jena.de (C.L.); tbs.kldtz@gmail.com (T.K.); udo.hahn@uni-jena.de (U.H.)

[3] Data Integration Center, Jena University Hospital, 07743 Jena, Germany; danny.ammon@med.uni-jena.de

* Correspondence: Boris.Betz@med.uni-jena.de (B.B.); Michael.Kiehntopf@med.uni-jena.de (M.K.);

† Christoph Weber and Lena Röschke contributed equally.
‡ Boris Betz and Michael Kiehntopf contributed equally.

Abstract: Automated identification of advanced chronic kidney disease (CKD ≥ III) and of no known kidney disease (NKD) can support both clinicians and researchers. We hypothesized that identification of CKD and NKD can be improved, by combining information from different electronic health record (EHR) resources, comprising laboratory values, discharge summaries and ICD-10 billing codes, compared to using each component alone. We included EHRs from 785 elderly multimorbid patients, hospitalized between 2010 and 2015, that were divided into a training and a test (n = 156) dataset. We used both the area under the receiver operating characteristic (AUROC) and under the precision-recall curve (AUCPR) with a 95% confidence interval for evaluation of different classification models. In the test dataset, the combination of EHR components as a simple classifier identified CKD ≥ III (AUROC 0.96[0.93–0.98]) and NKD (AUROC 0.94[0.91–0.97]) better than laboratory values (AUROC CKD 0.85[0.79–0.90], NKD 0.91[0.87–0.94]), discharge summaries (AUROC CKD 0.87[0.82–0.92], NKD 0.84[0.79–0.89]) or ICD-10 billing codes (AUROC CKD 0.85[0.80–0.91], NKD 0.77[0.72–0.83]) alone. Logistic regression and machine learning models improved recognition of CKD ≥ III compared to the simple classifier if only laboratory values were used (AUROC 0.96[0.92–0.99] vs. 0.86[0.81–0.91], $p < 0.05$) and improved recognition of NKD if information from previous hospital stays was used (AUROC 0.99[0.98–1.00] vs. 0.95[0.92–0.97]], $p < 0.05$). Depending on the availability of data, correct automated identification of CKD ≥ III and NKD from EHRs can be improved by generating classification models based on the combination of different EHR components.

Keywords: chronic kidney disease (CKD); no known kidney disease (NKD); ICD-10 billing codes; phenotyping; electronic health record (EHR); estimated glomerular filtration rate (eGFR); machine learning (ML); generalized linear model network (GLMnet); random forest (RF); artificial neural network (ANN), clinical natural language processing (clinical NLP); discharge summaries; laboratory values; area under the receiver operating characteristic (AUROC); area under the precision-recall curve (AUCPR)

1. Introduction

Chronic kidney disease (CKD) is a major public health concern characterized by an increasing prevalence and associated with a high level of morbidity and mortality [1,2]. Correct identification of CKD is crucial, e.g., for appropriate dosing of drugs and for early intervention, including the prevention of progression [3]. For clinical research, accurate identification of CKD or absence of kidney disease (NKD = no known kidney disease) is essential for clinical trials and epidemiological studies. In this context, a particular challenge is to store samples from hospitalized patients with known kidney status in clinical biorepositories, as part of Healthcare-Integrated Biobanking (HIB). At the time point of sample selection and storage, only a limited range of information regarding the respective patient phenotype is available.

Administrative data such as ICD-10 billing codes are often used in research trails to identify patients with CKD [4]. However, administrative databases are not maintained with the primary purpose of supporting research; thus, it might be that, e.g., mild impairment of kidney function will be underrepresented because they cannot be billed [5]. Indeed, many studies have demonstrated that ICD-10 billing codes considerably underestimate the prevalence of CKD [6]. Moreover, there is no ICD-10 billing code for NKD, as the purpose of ICD-10 billing codes is to indicate the presence of a disease.

Electronic health records (EHRs) are a promising source for the diagnosis or exclusion of CKD. EHRs contain structured data (laboratory values, epidemiological data) and unstructured data (narrative discharge summaries).

The laboratory assessment of kidney function is based on an equation to estimate the glomerular filtration rate (GFR) [3]. This equation, Chronic Kidney Disease Epidemiology Collaboration (CKD-EPI), includes the blood creatinine level, age, sex and ethnicity [7]. According to the Kidney Disease: Improving Global Outcomes (KDIGO) definition, CKD Stage III and higher can be diagnosed by an eGFR below 60 mL/min/1.73m^2 for a time period of at least 90 days [3]. However, previous laboratory data on hospitalized patients are often not fully available, e.g., they were recorded in other hospitals or in outpatient clinics.

Unstructured data such as discharge summaries can fill the gap of missing medical information. Letters are available in a digital form for every hospitalized patient and often contain complementary information, not only about the current hospital stay, but also about the clinical history of the patient including chronic diseases. Information can be extracted from narrative discharge summaries for example by reusing SNOMED CT codes from EHRs [8], screening the letters for disease-specific keywords [9,10], or using mL based natural language processing (NLP) technology for ICD-10 billing codes [11] or SNOMED CT [12] coding, named entity recognition [13], or relation extraction [14].

Data analysis from EHRs can be performed in a rule-based format for example by strictly adhering to the KDIGO definition of CKD ≥ III. In recent years, various machine learning (ML) methods have been applied to improve the automated recognition of chronic kidney disease, using mainly laboratory values and demographic information [15–20]. However, to the best of our knowledge, no study specifically targeted advanced CKD ≥ III or NKD.

In this study, we hypothesize that combining structured (laboratory values, ICD-10 billing codes) and unstructured (discharge summaries) information from EHRs and applying mL for data analysis can reliably distinguish between patients with advanced CKD (stage ≥ III) and patients with no known kidney disease (NKD) in different scenarios of data availability.

2. Materials and Methods

2.1. Study Population

The dataset of this retrospective study has been derived from the Jena Part of the 3000 PA text corpus of the Smart Medical Information Technology for Healthcare (SMITH) consortium (part of the Medical Informatics Initiative founded by the German Federal Ministry of Education and

Research) [21–23]. The dataset consisted of EHRs from 785 individuals who were from European descent and had an index hospital stay for at least five days on a ward for internal medicine or in an intensive care unit between 2010 and 2015. No individual deceased during the index hospital stay. At the time point of retrospective data collection, all individuals were deceased. The EHRs included discharge summaries, laboratory values and ICD-10 billing codes. The study was approved by the local ethics committee (4639-12/15); data were collected retrospectively and anonymized, individual-level informed consent of participants was waived by the ethics review board. The study was also approved by the data protection officer of Jena University Hospital.

2.2. Classification of CKD and NKD by ICD-10 Billing Codes

For classification of CKD and NKD, ICD-10 billing codes of the index hospital stay, extracted from the hospital accounting system and from hospital discharge summaries, were used. For extraction of kidney diseases from discharge summaries the HEALTH DISCOVERY text mining tool v5.7.0 from AVERBIS (https://health-discovery.io/) was applied using the discharge pipeline with default settings to extract basic medical information (detailed information can be found in the AVERBIS HEALTH DISCOVERY User Manual Version 5.7, 4 December 2018). Subsequently, a Python script was applied to extract the ICD-10 billing codes from these output files. ICD-10 billing codes for CKD classification were used according to ICD-10 billing codes for moderate to severe kidney disease from the Charlson comorbidity index [24] (Supplementary Materials). For the definition of no kidney disease (NKD), none of these codes as well as further ICD-10 billing codes for kidney disease published by the Centers for Disease Control and Prevention (CDC, http://www.cdc.gov/ckd) (Supplementary Materials) should be present.

2.3. Laboratory and Demographic Data

Laboratory values and demographics of the patients were extracted from the laboratory information system (LIS) of the University Hospital of Jena. The following values were considered in the analysis and classification of the study cohort:

- Numerical variables: age, eGFR at admission, eGFR at discharge, eGFR over index hospital stay. Measurements of albumin in urine were available in less than 5% of the cohort and therefore excluded from further analysis.
- Categorical variable: sex.

Descriptive statistics were reported as the mean [SD] or median [I quartile–III quartile] for continuous variables and absolute numbers (percentages) for categorical variables.

2.4. Classification of CKD and NKD by Blood Creatinine and eGFR

In order to define CKD and NKD by laboratory values from the current hospital index stay, we created the following rules. If all eGFR values during the index stay were below 60 mL/min/1.73 m^2, the case was assigned to CKD. If all eGFR values during the index hospital stay were above 60 mL/min/1.73m^2 and there was no presence of AKI (definition see below), the case was assigned to NKD.

2.5. Classification of CKD and NKD by Manual Review

CKD stage III or higher was defined according to the KDIGO guidelines. This included an eGFR, based on the formula CKD-EPI [7], which had to be less than 60 mL/min/1.73 m^2 for at least 3 months (90 days) or by an additional proof of kidney damage [3].

We defined NKD, adapted from James et al. [25], as the complete absence of GFR less than 60 mL/min/1.73m^2, stable serum creatinine measurements, e.g., no fulfillment of acute kidney disease criteria, median absence of proteinuria when multiple measurements were made before and the absence of AKI in patient laboratory history. AKI was present, if serum creatinine had increased by more than 26.5 mmol/L within 48 h or increased more than 1.5-fold over 7 days [26]. In addition, adapted from the publication by Duff et al. [27], we included AKI recovery defined as a decline in creatinine for more than 33% over 7 days.

All cases were reviewed by an advanced medical student and a physician to assess the underlying kidney status based on individual EHRs, including discharge summaries, ICD-10 billing codes and laboratory test results performed before, subsequent to, and during the index hospital stay. Of note, for clarification of difficult cases, the reviewers used information not available to the rule-based or statistical algorithms (e.g., laboratory values after index hospital stay). The review was used as a reference standard for comparison with automated classification.

2.6. Dataset for the Machine Learning Methods

The dataset used for logistic regression and the different mL models is composed of 11 to 19 different categorical and numerical variables. Three of them are derived variables to improve classification.

1. Numerical variables: age; first eGFR of the index hospital stay; last eGFR of the index hospital stay; time difference between the first and last blood measurement of the index hospital stay as an indicator for the length of hospital stay; mean eGFR over index hospital stay; mean eGFR over all available laboratory values.
2. Due to the varying distribution of eGFR measurements, additionally derived numerical variables were defined for usage in mL algorithms: the ratio between the number of hospital visits with eGFR measurements and the number of total visits; the ratio between the number of total eGFR measurements and hospital visits with eGFR measurements; the ratio between the number of eGFR measurements lower than 60 mL/min/1.73 m^2 and hospital visits with eGFR measurements.
3. Categorical variables: sex; occurrence of AKI and AKI recovery over laboratory history; occurrence of AKI and AKI recovery over index stay.

All of these variables were used in all mL models. Further categorical variables, listed below, were added in different combinations, as described in the results.

CKD: eGFR at admission below 60 mL/min/1.73 m^2 (eGFR_admission), eGFR at discharge below 60 mL/min/1.73 m^2 (eGFR_discharge), and all eGFR measurements during index stay below 60 mL/min/1.73 m^2 (eGFR).

NKD: eGFR at admission above 60 mL/min/1.73 m^2 (eGFR_admission), eGFR at discharge above 60 mL/min/1.73 m^2 (eGFR_discharge), eGFR always above 60 mL/min/1.73 m^2 (eGFR_history), all eGFR during index stay above 60 mL/min/1.73 m^2 (eGFR); classification by ICD-10 billing codes (ICD); classification by ICD-10 codes from discharge summaries.

2.7. Classification of CKD and NKD Using Machine Learning Methods

We applied three different mL methods—generalized linear model via penalized maximum likelihood (GLMnet) [28], random forests (RF) [29] and artificial neural network (ANN) [30]. These are all well-established approaches that represent different types of mL methods.

GLMnet is a statistical method in which different models generalize to the concept of a penalty parameter and in which different models have different loss functions. A penalty parameter constrains the size of the model coefficients such that the only way the coefficients can increase is if a comparable decrease in the models loss function is experienced. A loss function essentially calculates how poorly a model is performing by comparing what the model is predicting with the actual value it is supposed to output. If both values are very similar, the loss value will be very low. There are three common penalty parameters (ridge regression, lasso penalty, elastic-net penalty). We used the elastic-net penalty which is controlled by the *alpha* parameter. It bridges the gap between the ridge regression (alpha = 0), which is good for retaining all features while reducing the noise that less influential variables may create and the lasso (alpha = 1) penalty, which actually excludes features from the model.

Like a simple rule-based decision tree, random forests are tree-based models and part of a class of non-parametric algorithms that work by partitioning the feature space into a number of smaller regions. The predictions are obtained by fitting a simpler model in each region. Random forests use the same principles as bagging trees, which grow many trees (*ntree*) on bootstrapped copies of the training data, and extend it with an additional random component through split-variable randomization, where each time a split is to be performed the search for the split variable is limited to a random subset (*mtry*) of the original features.

Artificial neural networks are designed to simulate the biological neural networks of animal brains. They process input examples of a given task and map them against the desired output by forming probability-weighted associations between the two, storing these in the net data structure itself. In its basic form a neural network has three layers. An input layer which consists of all of the original input features, a hidden layer where the majority of the learning process takes place and an output layer [31].

The dataset was randomly split into 80% training and 20% test data. The prevalence for CKD or NKD respectively was similar in the two datasets (Supplementary Materials).

To properly adapt the mL algorithms, we optimized the hyperparameters that are used to control the learning process of a model and cannot be directly estimated from the data. We used a grid search method, which is simply an exhaustive search through a manually specified subset of the hyperparameter space of the learning algorithm. We specified these hyperparameters for every type of model, trailed all combinations and selected the model with the best results (see Supplementary Materials for details). For the GLMnet, the regularization parameter *lambda*, which controls the overall strength of the penalty term and helps to control the model from overfitting to the training data, was calculated during a pre-training of the model. Subsequently the best alpha parameter was determined. It ranges between [0,1] and was divided into steps of 0.1.

Random forest was tuned on the *mtry* parameter in a range between [1,18] depending on the number of features of the model, divided into steps of 1. The *ntree* parameter was set to its default value *ntree* = 100.

The artificial neural network is a fully connected feed-forward network with a single hidden layer. We use a fixed number of units between 11 and 19 in the input layer depending on the number of features of the model and a single unit with a sigmoid activation function for binary classification as the output layer. We optimized the number of units in the hidden layer as a hyperparameter (*size*) for every model in a range between [1,10] divided into steps of 1 (see Supplementary Materials for details).

In addition, all models were evaluated using three separate 10-fold cross-validations as the resampling scheme and were trained to optimize the F1 score. The final F1 score for each model is averaged over the resamples.

Classifications were assessed using sensitivity, specificity, positive predictive value (PPV), negative predictive value (NPV), F1 score, accuracy, area under the receiver operating characteristics (AUROC) and precision-recall curve (AUCPR). For AUROC and AUCPR, the 95% confidence interval was calculated (see Supplementary Materials for formulas and for detailed classification performances regarding the different models).

Area under the precision–recall curve is known to be more informative for class-imbalanced predictive tasks [32], as it is more sensitive to changes in the number of false-positive predictions. Comparison between AUROC was calculated according to DeLong et al. [33].

Analyses were implemented using R STUDIO (version 1.2.5001), the R SOFTWARE (version 3.6.1) [34] and the following packages: *limma* [35] for plots, *rio* [36], *plyr* [37], *nlme* [38], *tidyverse* bundle [39], *pROC* [40], *ROCR* [41] for data management, data analysis and functional programming and *caret* [42] for all mL models. Graphs were generated by GraphPad Prism (version 8.4.2).

3. Results

The study cohort comprises 785 cases, with an average age of 75 years, the majority of individuals were male (61%), and 95% and 49% of the patients had at least one or three severe disease(s) of the Charlson comorbidity index, respectively. Most patients were hospitalized due to cardiovascular disease (40%), gastrointestinal/liver diseases (15%) or oncology disorders (15%). The prevalence of

CKD in this elderly morbid cohort was comparable to other studies that included probably less morbid non-hospitalized patients ([43,44]). The prevalence for patients with no known kidney disease (NKD) was lower than for CKD. NKD was associated with younger age, better kidney function and fewer co-morbidities compared to CKD $\geq$ III. (Table 1).

Table 1. Epidemiological Characteristics from all Individuals and from Individuals with CKD $\geq$ III or NKD Identified by the Reference Standard, Respectively.

Characteristics	Cohort (n = 785)	CKD $\geq$ III (n = 373)	NKD (n = 129)
Age, years, mean [SD]	74.6 [12.2]	77.9 [10]	68.4 [13.7]
Sex, male	476 (60.6%)	215 (57.6%)	79 (61.2%)
eGFR at admission, median, [quartiles], mL/min/1.73 m^2	(n = 780) [1] 49.6 [28.6–77.3] (n = 748)	(n = 372) [1] 28.9 [18.1–41.8]	88.6 [78.5–99.6]
Charlson morbidity category $\geq$1	711 (95.3%)	366 (98.1%)	113 (87.6%)
$\geq$3	387 (49.3%)	224 (60.1%)	36 (27.9%)
Median	2	3	2
Myocardial infarction	128 (16.3%)	75 (20.1%)	11 (8.5%)
Chronic heart failure	419 (54.4)	247 (66.2%)	33 (25.6%)
Peripheral vascular disease	131 (16.7%)	75 (20.1%)	17 (13.2%)
Cerebrovascular disease	51 (6.5%)	28 (7.5%)	7 (5.4%)
Dementia	31 (3.9%)	18 (4.8%)	4 (3.1%)
Chronic pulmonary disease	183 (23.3%)	73 (16.9%)	23 (17.8%)
Rheumatic diseases	13 (1.7%)	4 (1.1%)	3 (2.3%)
Peptic ulcer disease	21 (2.7%)	11 (2.9%)	1 (0.8%)
Hemiplegia or paraplegia	29 (3.7%)	8 (2.1%)	6 (4.7%)
Liver disease	137 (17.5%)	44 (11.8%)	35 (25.1%)
Diabetes mellitus	332 (42.3%)	152 (40.7%)	51 (39.5%)
Any malignancy	137 (17.5%)	32 (8.6%)	38 (29.5%)
Hypertension	567 (72.3%)	270 (72.4%)	93 (72.1%)
Major cause for admission			
Infectious diseases	58 (7.4%)	28 (7.5%)	6 (4.7%)
Oncology disorders	119 (15.2%)	30 (8.0%)	34 (26.4%)
Cardiovascular Diseases	315 (40.1%)	192 (51.5%)	40 (31.0%)
Pulmonary diseases	82 (10.4%)	25 (6.7%)	12 (9.3%)
Gastrointestinal and liver diseases	118 (15.0%)	35 (9.4%)	27 (20.9%)
Kidney diseases	47 (6.0%)	36 (9.7%)	2 (1.6%)
other	46 (5.9%)	27 (7.2%)	8 (6.2%)

[1] eGFR at admission could not be calculated for all individuals because creatinine was massively interfered with by bilirubin or hemoglobin at admission.

In 128 (34%) of patients, the cause of CKD $\geq$ III was further specified by ICD-10 billing codes. In the remaining cohort of 245 patients with CKD $\geq$ III, 90% suffered from diabetes mellitus II and/or hypertension. More than 33% of etiologies for CKD $\geq$ III had been documented only in discharge summaries (Supplementary Materials).

There was a high incidence for AKI (33.6%) and AKI recovery (27.4%) in the CKD $\geq$ III cohort (Supplementary Materials).

Most patients were assigned to CKD status by discharge summaries, followed by eGFR and ICD-10 billing codes (Figure 1a). After manual review, less than 1% of the CKD cases identified by discharge summaries and eGFR and ICD-10 billing codes did not suffer from CKD III–V (Figure 1b). Patients identified by discharge summaries seemed to have a better kidney function at admission, while patients assigned to CKD by eGFR or ICD-10 billing codes had a worse kidney function compared to the reference standard. Similarly, patients identified by eGFR and discharge summaries were less morbid than patients characterized as CKD by ICD-10 billing codes, as indicated by Charlson morbidity categories (Table 2). Of note, 19 patients were identified by manual review only, while each of the three formal criteria failed.

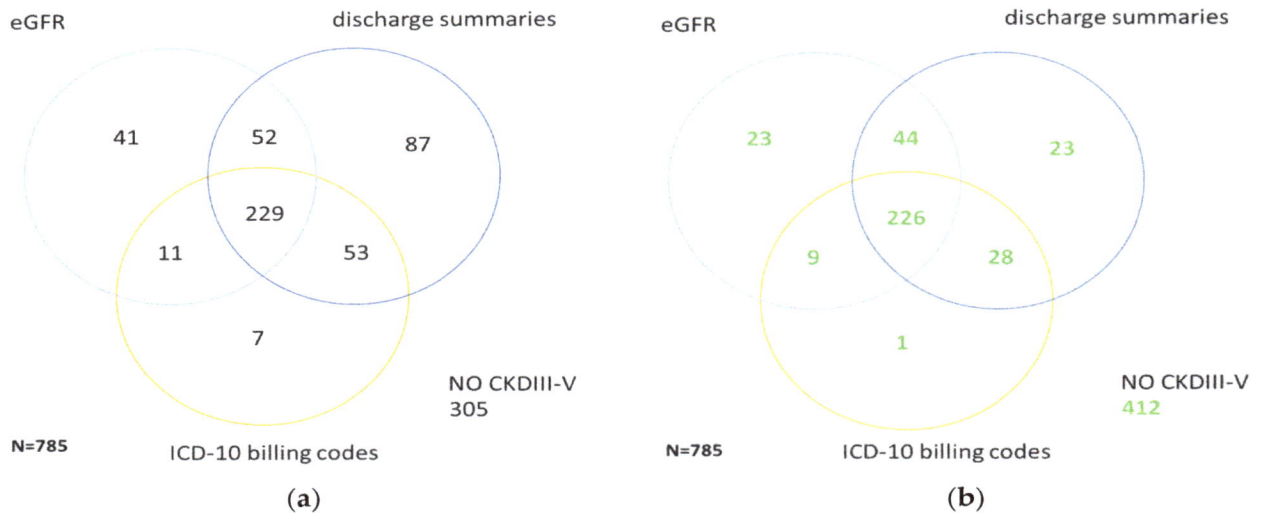

Figure 1. Venn diagrams comparing identification of CKD ≥ III by laboratory results (eGFR values), discharge summaries or ICD -10 billing codes within all patients (**a**) and within patients with CKD ≥ III according to reference standard (**b**). (**a**) Numbers of patients from the study cohort with CKD recognized by laboratory results (eGFR values), discharge summaries or ICD-10 billing codes. (**b**) Numbers of patients from the study cohort with CKD *correctly* recognized by laboratory results (eGFR values), discharge summaries or ICD -10 billing codes. A total of 19 patients were recognized by neither of the three formal criteria, but by manual review only.

Table 2. Epidemiological characteristics from patients with CKD identified by reference standard or recognized by laboratory results (eGFR values), discharge summaries or ICD-10 billing codes.

Characteristics	Reference Standard (n = 373)	eGFR (n = 333)	Discharge Summaries (n = 421)	ICD-10 Billing Codes (n = 300)
Age, years, mean [SD]	77.9 [10]	78.0 [9.7]	76.4 [10.9]	77.2 [10.3]
Sex, male	215 (57.6%)	189 (56.8%)	258 (61.3%)	182 (60.7%)
eGFR at admission, median, [quartiles], mL/min/1.73 m^2	(n = 372) [1] 28.9 [18.1–41.8]	26.8 [17.5–39.4]	(n = 420) [1] 32.9 [19.6–50]	25.7 [15.2–39.6]
Charlson morbidity category ≥1	366 (98.1%)	326 (97.9%)	413 (98.1%)	297 (99%)
≥3	224 (60.1%)	198 (59.5%)	257 (61.1%)	220 (73.3%)
Median	3	3	3	3

[1] eGFR could not be calculated for all individuals because creatinine was massively interfered with by bilirubin or hemoglobin at admission.

Similar to CKD, the patient cohort was investigated for patients with no known kidney disease (NKD). Numbers of patients assigned to NKD by laboratory values, ICD-10 billing codes or discharge summaries are depicted in Figure 2a. Comparison with the reference standard (Figure 2b) confirms 65% of the patients assigned to NKD by all three categories. Patients identified by the laboratory NKD criteria were younger, had a higher eGFR at admission and did therefore better correspond with the reference standard compared to patients assigned to NKD by discharge summaries or ICD-10 billing codes (Table 3).

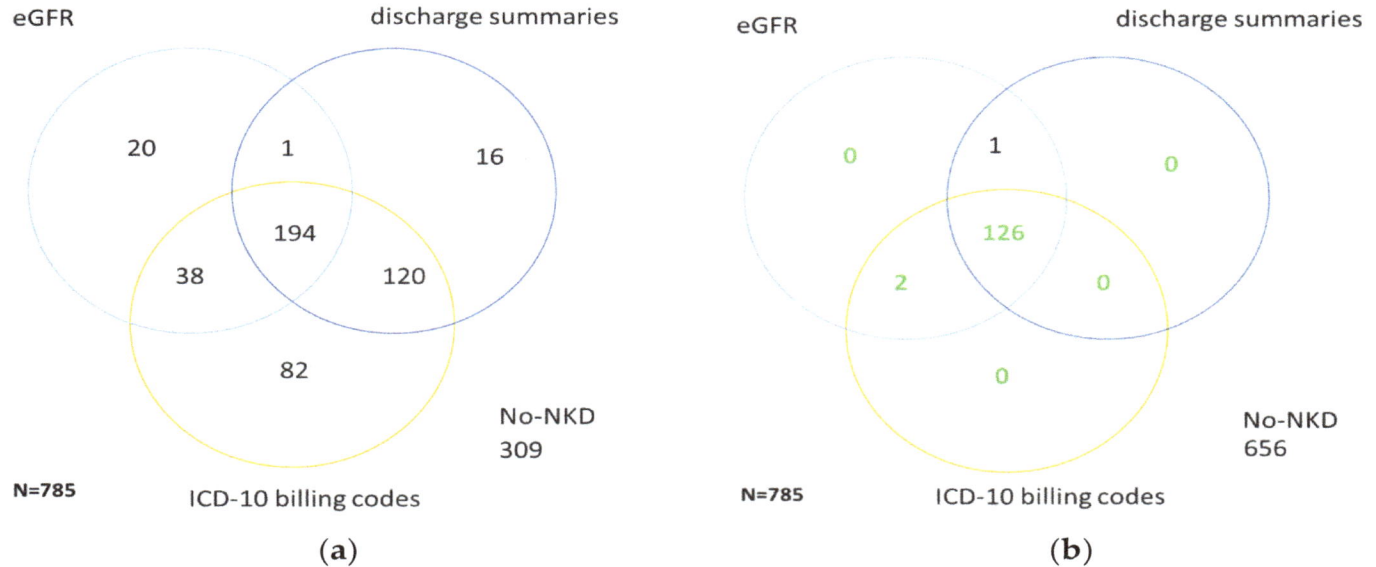

Figure 2. Venn diagrams comparing identification of no known kidney disease (NKD) by laboratory results (eGFR values), discharge summaries or ICD -10 billing codes within all patients (a) and within patients with CKD ≥ III according to reference standard (b). (a) Numbers of patients from the study cohort with NKD recognized via the eHealth sources laboratory results (eGFR values), discharge summaries or ICD-10 billing codes. (b) Numbers of patients from the study cohort with NKD *correctly* recognized via laboratory results (eGFR values), discharge summaries or ICD-10 billing codes.

Table 3. Epidemiological characteristics from patients with NKD identified by reference standard or recognized by sources laboratory results (eGFR values), discharge summaries or ICD-10 billing codes.

Chracteristics	Reference Standard ($n = 129$)	eGFR ($n = 253$)	Discharge Summaries ($n = 334$)	ICD-10 Billing Codes ($n = 437$)
Age, years, mean [SD]	68.4 [13.7]	69.3 [13.3]	72.9 [13.3]	73.3 [13.0]
Sex, male	79 (61.2%)	161 (63.6%)	196 (58.7%)	265 (60.6%)
eGFR at admission, median, [quartiles], mL/min/1.73 m^2	88.6 [78.6–99.3]	84.5 [75.7–96.2]	76.0 *,1 [53.8–89.5]	69.9 *,2 [50.0–87.7]
Charlson morbidity score ≥1	113 (87.6%)	232 (91.7%)	308 (92.2%)	403 (92.2%)
≥3	36 (27.9%)	91 (36.0%)	116 (34.7%)	145 (33.2%)
Median	2	2	2	2

* eGFR could not be calculated for all individuals because creatinine was massively interfered with by bilirubin or hemoglobin at admission. [1] $n = 331$; [2] $n = 434$.

Tables 4 and 5 depict the specificities and sensitivities of the different rules applied for identification of CKD or NKD, respectively. While ICD-10 billing codes show excellent specificity for identification of CKD, the sensitivity was lower compared to discharge summaries and eGFR. Discharge summaries had a better sensitivity, but a reduced specificity compared to ICD-10 billing codes (Table 4). Using eGFR < 60 mL/min/1.73 m^2 during the whole hospital stay results in good sensitivity and specificity. If only the first eGFR at admission or the last eGFR measurement at discharge were used, overall performance (AUROC) did only minimally change compared to the original rule.

Table 4. Performance of different rules for identification of patients with CKD compared to the reference standard.

Category	Sensitivity	Specificity	PPV	NPV	AUROC (CI)	AUCPR (CI)
ICD-10 billing codes	0.71	0.91	0.88	0.78	0.81 (0.78–0.84)	0.86 (0.83–0.90)
Discharge summary	0.86	0.76	0.76	0.86	0.81 (0.78–0.84)	0.84 (0.81–0.88)
eGFR <60 mL/min/1.73 m^2 during Index hospital stay	0.81	0.92	0.91	0.84	0.87 (0.84–0.90)	0.90 (0.87–0.93)
eGFR_at_admission <60 mL/min/1.73 m^2	0.96	0.75	0.77	0.95	0.85 (0.83–0.87)	0.88 (0.84–0.91)
eGFR_at_discharge <60 mL/min/1.73 m^2	0.91	0.82	0.82	0.91	0.86 (0.84–0.89)	0.89 (0.85–0.92)

Table 5. Performance of different rules for identification of patients with NKD compared to the reference standard.

Category	Sensitivity	Specificity	PPV	NPV	AUROC (CI)	AUPR (CI)
ICD-10 billing codes	0.99	0.53	0.29	1	0.76 (0.74–0.78)	0.64 (0.56–0.73)
Discharge summary	0.98	0.68	0.38	1	0.83 (0.81–0.86)	0.68 (0.60–0.76)
eGFR ≥ 60 mL/min/1.73m^2 during Index hospital stay	1.00	0.82	0.52	1	0.91 (0.89–0.92)	0.75 (0.68–0.83)
eGFR_at_admission ≥ 60 mL/min/1.73 m^2	1.00	0.71	0.41	1.00	0.86 (0.84–0.87)	0.70 (0.62–0.78)
eGFR_at_discharge ≥ 60 mL/min/1.73 m^2	1.00	0.64	0.35	1.00	0.82 (0.80–0.84)	0.68 (0.59–0.76)

Regarding NKD, ICD-10 billing codes, discharge summaries and creatinine blood values, at admission, at discharge and during hospital stay, have all excellent sensitivity. However, acceptable specificity (>80%) was achieved only by using eGFR < 60 mL/min/1.73m^2 during the whole hospital stay. However, the PPV was still low at 0.52 (Table 5).

Combining laboratory measurements with discharge summaries and ICD-10 billing codes using logistic regression developed in a training dataset resulted in a better overall performance for identification of CKD (AUROC: 0.96[0.93–0.98]) or NKD (AUROC: 0.94[0.91–0.97]) in the test dataset compared to estimated glomerular filtration rate (eGFR) values (CKD: AUROC 0.85[0.79–0.90]; NKD: AUROC 0.91[0.87–0.94]), discharge summaries (CKD: AUROC 0.87[0.82–0.92], NKD: AUROC 0.84[0.79–0.89]) or ICD-10 billing codes (CKD: AUROC 0.85[0.80–0.91], NKD: AUROC 0.77[0.72–0.83) alone (Figure 3 and Supplementary Materials). Interestingly, the combination of all three categories, however, did not (NKD) or only minimally (CKD ≥ III) increase the performance in comparison with the combination of laboratory results and discharge summaries (CKD: AUROC 0.94[0.9–0.97]; NKD: AUROC 0.95[0.92–0.97]).

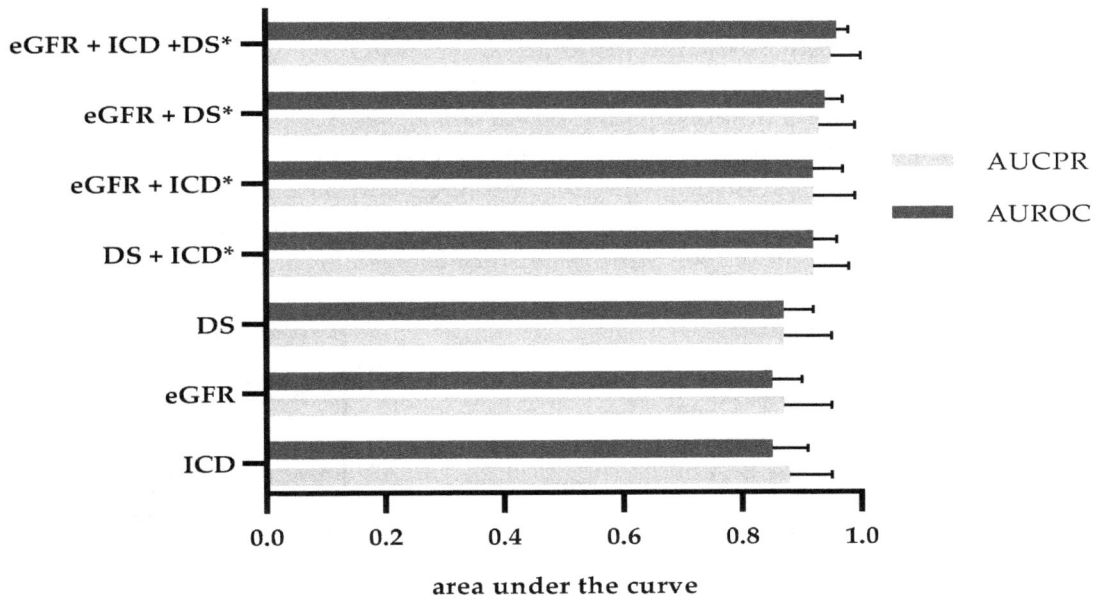

(a)

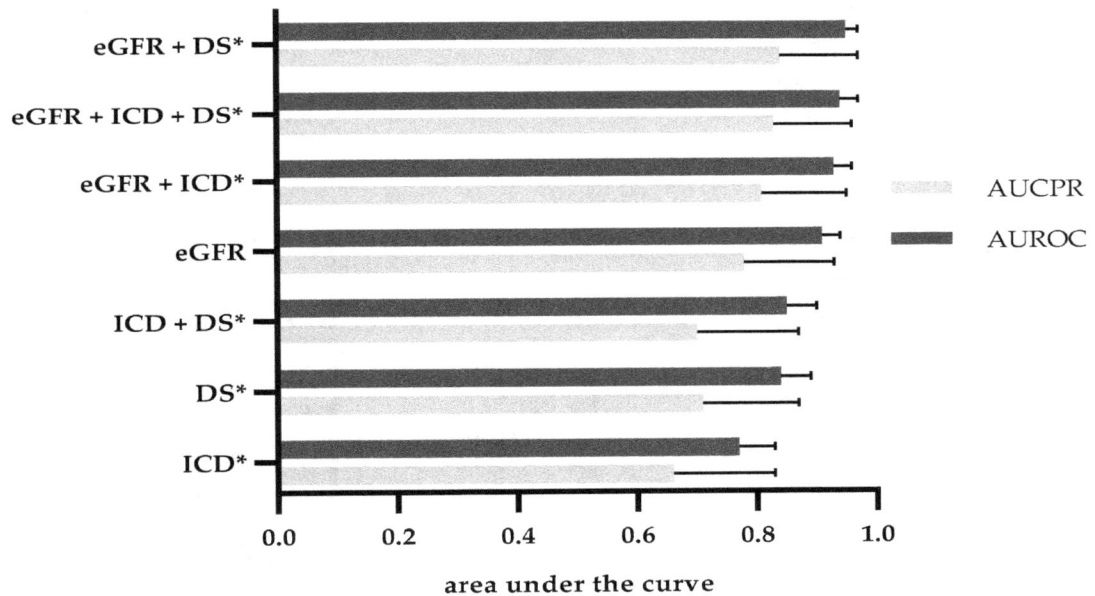

(b)

Figure 3. Area under the receiver operating characteristic (AUROC) and under the precision-recall curve (AUCPR) for simple categorical classifiers based on combinations of EHR components for CKD ≥ III (a) and NKD (b) on the test dataset. eGFR values = "eGFR", discharge summaries = "DS" and ICD-10 billing codes = "ICD". For the complete list of all combinations, see Supplementary Materials. Logistic regression was calculated on the training dataset. Performance is calculated on the test dataset (n = 156). * Indicates $p < 0.05$ for difference in AUROC compared to eGFR.

In NKD, AUROC values were quite high. However, AUCPR values that include sensitivity and PPV were lower. It is therefore helpful to include several parameters, e.g., AUROC and AUCPR for assessing test performance, particularly in imbalanced data [32].

To further improve performance for correct assignment of patients to CKD ≥ III or NKD, we developed a logistic regression and three mL models using (1) all data from the index hospital stay including laboratory values with incidence of AKI and AKI recovery including staging, demographics, ICD-billing codes and ICDs from discharge summaries; (2) laboratory values and demographics from the index hospital stay; (3) and (4) in addition to (1) or (2) includes laboratory values from previous hospital stays, respectively (for a detailed listing of variables, see Supplementary Materials).

Figure 4 shows the AUROCs and AUCPRs of the respective best logistic regression (LR) and best different mL models for identification of CKD ≥ III and NKD compared to the best simple categorical classifier for each scenario. In general, AUROCs of LR and of the different mL models were only slightly different between each other (see Supplementary Materials for more details).

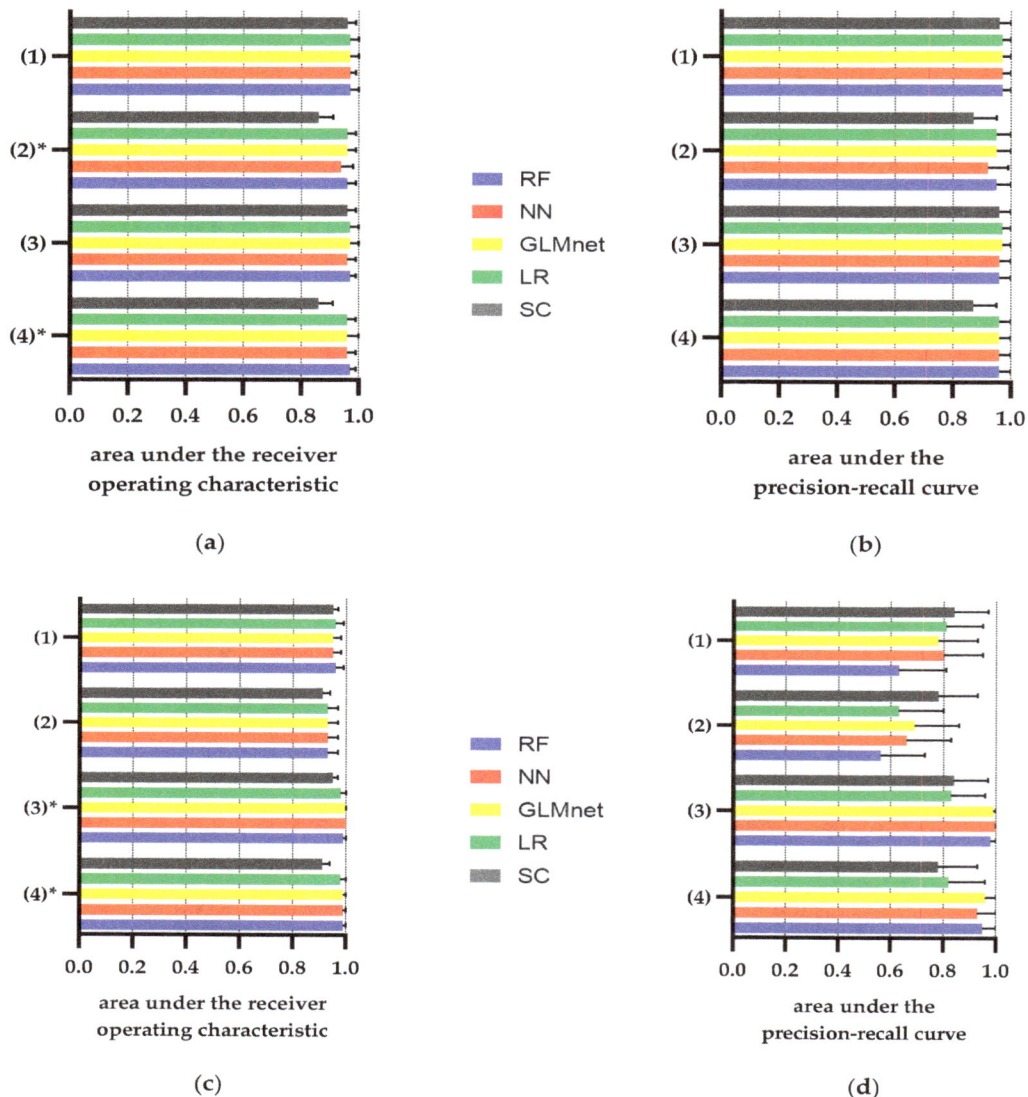

Figure 4. AUROC (**a,c**) and AUCPR (**b,d**) of the simple categorical classifier and of models calculated from logistic regression and the three mL methods for identification of CKD (**a,b**) and NKD (**c,d**) in different scenarios of data availability. (**a**) AUROC and (**b**) AUCPR for identification of CKD ≥ III; (**c**) AUROC and (d) AUCPR for identification of NKD. SC = simple categorical classifier, LR = logistic regression, GLMnet = generalized linear machine network, RF = random forest, NN = Artificial Neuronal Network. N = 156 patients (test dataset). Scenarios: (1) All data from the index hospital stay including laboratory values, demographics, ICD-billing codes and ICDs from discharge summaries; (2) laboratory values and demographics from the index hospital stay; (3) and (4) includes, in addition to (1) or (2), laboratory values from previous hospital stays, respectively. * Indicates $p < 0.05$ for difference in AUROC between SC and all other models.

For identification of CKD ≥ III, the AUROCs of the LR and machine learning models were not significantly better in scenario 1 (LR/ML: 0.97[0.95–1.00]) and scenario 3 (LR/ML: 0.97[0.94–1.00]) compared to the simple classifier in scenario 1 and 3 (0.96[0.94–0.99]), respectively. AUROCs of the LR and mL models significantly ($p < 0.05$) improved in scenario 2 (LR/ML: 0.96[0.92–0.99]) and scenario 4 (LR: 0.96[0.93–0.99]/ML 0.97[0.94–0.99]) compared to the simple classifier in scenario 2 and 4 (0.86[0.81–0.91]), respectively. In scenarios 2 and 4, data were restricted to laboratory values alone.

For identification of NKD, AUROCs of the LR and mL models significantly ($p < 0.05$) improved in scenario 3 (LR: 0.98[0.96–1.00]/ML: 1.00[1.00–1.00]) and scenario 4 (LR: 0.98[0.96–1.00]/ML: 0.99[0.98–1.00]) compared to the simple classifier in scenario 3 (0.95[0.92–0.97]) and scenario 4 (0.91[0.87–0.94]), respectively (Figure 4c). In scenarios 3 and 4, data from previous hospital stays were included. AUCPRs of the logistic regression and mL models for identification of NKD also improved in scenarios 3 and 4 compared to the simple classifier (Figure 4d, see Supplementary Materials for more details). AUROCs of LR and mL models slightly improved in scenario 1 (LR/ML: 0.96[0.93–0.99]) and scenario 2 (LR/ML: 0.93[0.89–0.97]) compared to the simple classifier in scenario 1 (0.95[0.92–0.97]) and scenario 2 (0.91[0.87–0.94]), respectively (Figure 4c). However, AUCPR of LR and mL models decreased in scenario 1 and 2 compared to the simple classifier.

In conclusion, the best LR and mL models slightly improved AUROCs for identification of CKD ≥ III and NKD compared to the best simple categorical classifier in each scenario. However, we observed a significant improvement by models compared to the simple classifier for CKD ≥ III only in scenarios 2 and 4 and for NKD only in scenarios 3 and 4.

4. Discussion

The results of our study demonstrate that laboratory values have the best performance for identifying CKD ≥ III and NKD from EHRs compared to discharge summaries and ICD-10 billing codes in an elderly multimorbid cohort of hospitalized patients. Combining classifiers based on laboratory values (creatinine/eGFR), ICD-10 billing codes or ICD-10 codes extracted from discharge summaries outperformed each component alone for identification of CKD ≥ III and NKD. Classification could be further improved by calculation of logistic regression and mL models if data were restricted to laboratory values (CKD ≥ III) or if additional values from previous hospital stays were added (NKD).

Although each of the mentioned EHR components have been investigated before, we could demonstrate the extent to which the classification is improved by combining laboratory values with ICD-10 billing codes and discharge summaries. Furthermore, we are the first, to our knowledge, to describe classification performance for NKD.

The good sensitivity and specificity of laboratory values for the identification of CKD ≥ III and NKD can be explained by the fact that both entities are mainly defined by blood creatinine and eGFR values [3,26]. However, many epidemiological studies and clinical trials have utilized ICD-10 billing codes for defining CKD status [4]—more than 50% of cardiovascular trials do not report eGFR measurement in respective study populations [45].

Previous studies have demonstrated a high specificity of billing codes. However, many CKD patients will be overlooked by using billing codes alone and the identified cohort is biased towards more advanced CKD stages with higher creatinine values [5,46,47]. These results have been replicated and confirmed in the current study. A sensitivity of 75% indicates that approximately one-quarter of patients with advanced CKD ≥ III had been missed by ICD-10 billing codes. Patients recognized by ICD-10 billing codes had a lower eGFR and showed a higher morbidity in comparison to the reference standard.

However, the sensitivity of ICD-10 billing codes was much better in our study than in a recent study by Diamantidis et al. who reported a very low sensitivity of ICD-10 billing codes for recognizing CKD > III [43]. The discrepancy might be explained by differences in the patient cohorts as the latter study included non-hospitalized patients.

Gomez-Salgado et al., in contrast, recently showed good correlation between ICD-10 billing codes and researchers' judgment based on clinical documentation [48]. A possible explanation for the conflicting results between our study and Gomez-Salgado et al. could be the extent to which laboratory values were considered for identification of CKD.

Our study also confirms previous findings of slight under-documentation of CKD using discharge summaries [49]. Indeed approximately 20% of patients with advanced CKD ≥ III were not identified by discharge summaries. However, in line with the study of Singh et al., we could also show that the sensitivity of discharge summaries is higher than the sensitivity of billing codes for CKD [9]. The reduced specificity of discharge summaries could be explained by the fact that many patients with CKD stage I and II were counted as CKD ≥ III. Differing definitions for chronic kidney disease might also be the reason why a recent study by Hernandez-Boussard et al. observed a better accuracy for unstructured discharge summaries for recognizing CKD compared to our study [50]. Other possible explanations are different information sources and a different study cohort.

In a study by Nadkarni et al., an algorithm was developed and evaluated to identify patients with CKD Stage III caused by hypertension or diabetes, using structured and unstructured information from EHRs [51]. The algorithm based on keywords from medical notes and laboratory values outperformed phenotyping by ICD-10 billing codes by a margin. These results resonate with the outcome of our study that included advanced CKD from any cause in hospitalized patients.

Missing previous health records is a common problem in clinical studies and might affect correct identification of diseases [52]. However, in contrast to the identification of patients with diabetes mellitus [53], we can demonstrate good F1 score (>0.8), although using datasets restricted to the current hospital stay for simple classifiers. For CKD ≥ III, mL models based on laboratory values alone had a similar AUROC as the simple categorical classifiers including discharge summaries and ICD-10 billing codes. This indicates that mL models might be able to—at least partly—compensate for missing information.

The results of our study are encouraging, not only for stratification of patients for clinical and epidemiological studies, but also in the context of, e.g., Healthcare-Integrated Biobanking, where automated classifiers based on minimal clinical information are of great importance for early selection of samples of specific disease entities.

Structured information such as laboratory values and billing codes are often readily available. Results from our study show that a PPV of 0.77, 0.82 or 0.91 can be achieved for the identification of CKD by using eGFR values at admission, at discharge or from the complete hospital stay, respectively. This is in line with other studies demonstrating that a single measurement of eGFR might overestimate the number of CKD cases [54]. The slightly higher PPV when using eGFR values at discharge compared to admission can be explained by the fact that interfering acute kidney injury is more likely to be present at admission than after a successful treatment at discharge.

Suboptimal PPV values associated with false classification can significantly impact the phenotyping process and thus might cause severe bias in the outcomes of subsequent studies. Consequently, there is a need for further optimization of CKD and NKD classification.

Wei et al. combined different sources of information (primary notes, medication and billing codes) to improve phenotyping based on EHR for several chronic diseases (not CKD though) and demonstrated that PPV and F1 score can be increased by combining different information sources [55]. Results from Wei et al. can be confirmed in our study in relation to CKD and NKD with the caveat that eGFR should be included in any combination.

The addition of discharge summaries and/or ICD-10 billing codes to laboratory values not only increases the performance of correct identification of CKD ≥ III but also helped to further specify the cause of the disease in at least one-third of the cohort. There were more etiologies for CKD in the discharge summaries compared to the ICD-10 billing codes.

Another novelty of this study is that, to the best of the authors' knowledge, for the first time the entity of NKD (no known kidney disease) was investigated using EHRs. Identifying NKD is a challenging task because ICD-10 billing codes and discharge summaries are designed to describe the presence of illness rather than its absence. However, the question of NKD might be of particular interest for scientific reasons. The validity of association studies and clinical trials depends on the correct assignment of co-morbidities. If large cohorts of CKD patients are counted as NKD, studies might be biased and results might thus be flawed. Our study demonstrates that single EHR sources had low PPV and AUCPR for NKD assignment. Combining laboratory values with discharge summaries improved PPV and AUCPR. Interestingly, the further addition of ICD-10 billing codes to this combination did not result in a further improvement of PPV and AUCPR. Future epidemiological studies should take these results in consideration for classification of NKD.

Finally, we demonstrated that logistic regression and mL algorithms have the potential to improve recognition of CKD ≥ III and NKD, particularly in certain scenarios of data availability. This might be helpful for the development of clinical decision support systems (CDSS) in the near future that ultimately will allow clinicians and researches almost instantly to evaluate the chronic kidney status of patients.

Direct comparison with other studies applying mL strategies for the detection of CKD is hampered due to different definitions of CKD, different patient cohorts and data variables used. Almansour et al. described an Artificial Neural Network with an accuracy of more than 99% [20]. Salekin et al. used the same cohort and reduced the number of variables down to 12 and achieved an F1 score of 99% by using a wrapper approach to identify the best subset of attributes and a random forest classifier [56]. However, both studies rely on the same data source comprising 24 variables of 400 patients to build a predictive model. In contrast to our study, the dataset does not include series of creatinine measurements or information from discharge summaries or ICD-10 billing codes about CKD. Rashidian et al. used laboratory values, demographics and ICD-10 billing codes to identify patients with CKD achieving a F1 score of approximately 0.8 [57]. In our study, AUROC and AUCPR for identification of CKD from mL algorithms surpassed 0.95 in all scenarios of unrestricted or restricted data availability. One reason for these differences could be that the study by Rashidian et al. did not use discharge letters as source of information. As mentioned before, in our study discharge summaries can add valuable information to the classification process. This is also reflected by the result that mL algorithms did not significantly improve performance of CKD ≥ III identification (AUROC 0.97) compared to a simple classifier based on laboratory values, discharge summaries and ICD-10 billing codes (AUROC 0.96).

The mL algorithms used in our study failed to outperform rule-based classifiers for identification of NKD if data were restricted to the index hospital stay: although AUROC is (non-significantly) increasing, PPV is declining and thus superiority of the models has to be rejected. An explanation for this result could be that the correct assignment of NKD mainly depends on the availability of the complete dataset. Additionally, we cannot exclude that the low prevalence of NKD in our morbid patient cohort affected the efficacy of mL strategies.

To the best of our knowledge, this is the first study trying to detect specifically CKD Stage ≥ III and NKD by mL methods. Therefore, it is mandatory that the proof-of-concept presented here needs further elaboration in larger independent patient cohorts.

The strength of the study is the comprehensive dataset including discharge summaries of the index hospital stay and laboratory values with a reviewed reference standard.

Several limitations need to be acknowledged. The patient cohort included in the study was quite morbid and not representative of a general hospital population or, even more so, an outpatient population. Therefore, the extent of improvement by combining different information sources needs to be prospectively validated in other independent cohorts.

The AVERBIS HEALTH DISCOVERY software tool was used for the extraction of information attributes from discharge summaries that have been predefined by the authors. The use of natural language processing (NLP) methods for information extraction and automated feature selection could have resulted in an increased performance of the data extraction method.

Similarly, the total number of patients was rather small for training mL classifiers. We may guess that, in a larger patient cohort, the performance of the different models might further increase. However, the scope of the present study was to demonstrate the feasibility and potential of using eHealth sources and mL models to improve phenotyping of CKD and NKD.

The models presented in this manuscript focus on the detection of advanced CKD (Stage III or higher) or on the absence of kidney disease. Patients with mild CKD (Stage I and II) are not taken into consideration although the correct identification of this group might be important for clinical treatment and research purpose. Future studies with larger patient cohorts might be able to develop more granular models differentiating between mild and advanced CKD.

Another limitation is that neither a single rule nor a combination of them achieved a sensitivity for identification of CKD $\geq$ III of 100%. This could be explained by the fact that most patients were treated primarily for non-nephrological reasons during the index hospital stay and thus CKD was not mentioned at all in the current discharge summaries or by the ICD-10 billing codes, although they had a documented eGFR < 60 mL/min/1.73m^2 for a period longer than 90 days.

Furthermore, data included in the analysis were incomplete, since laboratory results from primary care or other institutions (for example, from general practitioners or other hospitals) were not available. Most importantly albuminuria was available in less than 5% of the whole cohort and could therefore not included in the analysis.

Missing data, however, reflects "real-world" conditions. Missing data can be, at least partly, compensated for—as shown in our study—by the extraction of unstructured information from the discharge summaries that usually contain a multitude of pre-existing health data from other healthcare providers.

5. Conclusions

In summary, combining laboratory results (creatinine and eGFR) with discharge summaries and ICD-10 billing codes had the best performance in a simple categorical classifier for phenotyping of CKD $\geq$ III and NKD. Logistic regression or mL models had the potential to further improve the correct identification of CKD $\geq$ III if only laboratory values were used and of NKD if data from previous hospital stays were included into models.

Supplementary Materials:

ICD-10 billing codes for definition of CKD; Table S3: ICD-10 billing codes for exclusion of NKD; Table S4: detailed performance characteristics for combinations of simple classifiers for identification of CKD and NKD; Table S5: Detailed AUC-ROC and -PR for combinations of different classifiers for identification of CKD and NKD; Table S6: Cause for CKD in the CKD>III cohort; detailed cause for CKD $\geq$ III and source of information; Table S7: Incidence of AKI and AKI Recovery in the complete study cohort with creati-nine values (n=780) and in CKD>III cohort with creatinine values (n=372); Table S8: Source of information for etiologies of CKD>III; Table S9: Distribution of true positives and true negatives for CKD and NKD, in the training and test datasets; Table S10: Detailed performance characteristics for combinations of different classifiers for identification of CKD and NKD; Table S11: Detailed AUC-ROC and -PR for combinations of different classifiers for identification of CKD and NKD; Table S12: Detailed performance characteristics for different generalized linear model networks for identification of CKD and NKD; Table S13: Detailed AUC-ROC and -PR for different generalized linear model networks for identification of CKD and NKD; Table S14: Detailed performance characteristics for different gen-eralized linear model networks for identification of CKD and NKD; Table S15: Detailed AUC-ROC and -PR for different generalized linear model networks for identification of CKD and NKD; Table S16: Detailed performance characteristics for different random forest models for identification of CKD and NKD; Table S17: Detailed AUC-ROC and -PR for different random forest models for identification of CKD and NKD; Table S18: Detailed performance characteristics for different random forest models for identification of CKD and NKD; Table S19: Detailed AUC-ROC and -PR for different random forest models for identification of CKD and NKD; Table S20: Detailed performance characteristics for different neural networks models for identification of CKD and NKD; Table S21: Detailed AUC-ROC and -PR for for different neural networks models for identification of CKD and NKD; Table S22: Detailed performance characteristics for different neural networks models for identification of CKD and NKD; Table S23: Detailed AUC-ROC and -PR for for different neural networks models for identification of CKD and NKD; Table S24: Detailed performance characteristics for different generalized linear mod-els for identification of CKD and NKD; Table S25: Detailed AUC-ROC and -PR for for different generalized linear models for identification of CKD and NKD; Table S26: Detailed performance characteristics for different generalized linear models for identification of CKD and NKD; Table S27: Detailed AUC-ROC and -PR for for different generalized linear models for identification of CKD and NKD; Table S28: Detailed hyperparameters of different machine learning models; Table S29: Detailed hyperparameters of different machine learning models.

Author Contributions: Conceptualization, U.H., B.B. and M.K.; data curation, C.W. and L.R.; formal analysis, C.W., L.R. and L.M.; funding acquisition, U.H. and M.K.; investigation, C.W., L.R., C.L., T.K., B.B. and M.K.; methodology, C.W., B.B. and M.K.; project administration, M.K.; resources, L.M., C.L., T.K., U.H., D.A. and M.K.; software, C.W.; supervision, U.H. and M.K.; validation, C.W., L.R. and B.B.; visualization, C.W., B.B. and M.K.; writing—original draft, C.W. and B.B.; writing—review & editing, U.H., B.B. and M.K. All authors have read and agreed to the published version of the manuscript.

References

1. Wang, J.; Wang, F.; Saran, R.; He, Z.; Zhao, M.H.; Li, Y.; Zhang, L.; Bragg-Gresham, J. Mortality risk of chronic kidney disease: A comparison between the adult populations in urban China and the United States. *PLoS ONE* **2018**, *13*, e0193734. [CrossRef]

2. Xie, Y.; Bowe, B.; Mokdad, A.H.; Xian, H.; Yan, Y.; Li, T.; Maddukuri, G.; Tsai, C.Y.; Floyd, T.; Al-Aly, Z. Analysis of the Global Burden of Disease study highlights the global, regional, and national trends of chronic kidney disease epidemiology from 1990 to 2016. *Kidney Int.* **2018**, *94*, 567–581. [CrossRef] [PubMed]

3. Kidney Disease: Improving Global Outcomes (KDIGO) CKD Work Group. KDIGO 2012 Clinical Practice Guideline for the Evaluation and Management of Chronic Kidney Disease. *Kidney Int. Suppl.* **2013**, *3*, 1–150.

4. Anderson, J.; Glynn, L.G. Definition of chronic kidney disease and measurement of kidney function in original research papers: A review of the literature. *Nephrol. Dial. Transplant.* **2011**, *26*, 2793–2798. [CrossRef] [PubMed]

5. Jalal, K.; Anand, E.J.; Venuto, R.; Eberle, J.; Arora, P. Can billing codes accurately identify rapidly progressing stage 3 and stage 4 chronic kidney disease patients: A diagnostic test study. *BMC Nephrol.* **2019**, *20*, 260. [CrossRef]

6. Vlasschaert, M.E.; Bejaimal, S.A.; Hackam, D.G.; Quinn, R.; Cuerden, M.S.; Oliver, M.J.; Iansavichus, A.; Sultan, N.; Mills, A.; Garg, A.X. Validity of administrative database coding for kidney disease: A systematic review. *Am. J. Kidney Dis.* **2011**, *57*, 29–43. [CrossRef]

7. Levey, A.S.; Stevens, L.A.; Schmid, C.H.; Zhang, Y.L.; Castro, A.F., 3rd; Feldman, H.I.; Kusek, J.W.; Eggers, P.; Van Lente, F.; Greene, T.; et al. A new equation to estimate glomerular filtration rate. *Ann. Intern. Med.* **2009**, *150*, 604–612. [CrossRef]

8. Bhattacharya, M.; Jurkovitz, C.; Shatkay, H. Co-occurrence of medical conditions: Exposing patterns through probabilistic topic modeling of snomed codes. *J. Biomed. Inform.* **2018**, *82*, 31–40. [CrossRef]

9. Singh, B.; Singh, A.; Ahmed, A.; Wilson, G.A.; Pickering, B.W.; Herasevich, V.; Gajic, O.; Li, G. Derivation and validation of automated electronic search strategies to extract Charlson comorbidities from electronic medical records. *Mayo Clin. Proc.* **2012**, *87*, 817–824. [CrossRef]

10. Upadhyaya, S.G.; Murphree, D.H., Jr.; Ngufor, C.G.; Knight, A.M.; Cronk, D.J.; Cima, R.R.; Curry, T.B.; Pathak, J.; Carter, R.E.; Kor, D.J. Automated Diabetes Case Identification Using Electronic Health Record Data at a Tertiary Care Facility. *Mayo Clin. Proc. Innov. Qual. Outcomes* **2017**, *1*, 100–110. [CrossRef]

11. Lin, C.; Lou, Y.S.; Tsai, D.J.; Lee, C.C.; Hsu, C.J.; Wu, D.C.; Wang, M.C.; Fang, W.H. Projection Word Embedding Model With Hybrid Sampling Training for Classifying ICD-10-CM Codes: Longitudinal Observational Study. *JMIR Med. Inform.* **2019**, *7*, e14499. [CrossRef] [PubMed]

12. Batool, R.; Khattak, A.M.; Kim, T.-S.; Lee, S. Automatic extraction and mapping of discharge summary's concepts into SNOMED CT. In Proceedings of the 35th Annual International Conference of the IEEE Engineering in Medicine and Biology Society, Osaka, Japan, 3–7 July 2013.

13. Tang, B.; Cao, H.; Wu, Y.; Jiang, M.; Xu, H. Recognizing clinical entities in hospital discharge summaries using Structural Support Vector Machines with word representation features. *BMC Med. Inform. Decis. Mak.* **2013**, *13* (Suppl. 1), S1. [CrossRef] [PubMed]

14. Sahu, S.K.; Anand, A.; Oruganty, K.; Gattu, M. Relation extraction from clinical texts using domain invariant convolutional neural network. In Proceedings of the 15th Workshop on Biomedical Natural Language Processing, BioNLP@ACL 2016, Berlin, Germany, 12 August 2016; pp. 206–215.

15. Xiao, J.; Ding, R.; Xu, X.; Guan, H.; Feng, X.; Sun, T.; Zhu, S.; Ye, Z. Comparison and development of machine learning tools in the prediction of chronic kidney disease progression. *J. Transl. Med.* **2019**, *17*, 119. [CrossRef] [PubMed]

16. Polat, H.; Danaei Mehr, H.; Cetin, A. Diagnosis of Chronic Kidney Disease Based on Support Vector Machine by Feature Selection Methods. *J. Med. Syst.* **2017**, *41*, 55. [CrossRef] [PubMed]

17. Chen, Z.; Zhang, Z.; Zhu, R.; Xiang, Y.; Harrington, P.B. Diagnosis of patients with chronic kidney disease by using two fuzzy classifiers. *Chemom. Intell. Lab. Syst.* **2016**, *153*, 140–145. [CrossRef]

18. Alexander Arman, S. Diagnosis Rule Extraction from Patient Data for Chronic Kidney Disease Using Machine Learning. *Int. J. Biomed. Clin. Eng. IJBCE* **2016**, *5*, 64–72. [CrossRef]

19. Elhoseny, M.; Shankar, K.; Uthayakumar, J. Intelligent Diagnostic Prediction and Classification System for Chronic Kidney Disease. *Sci. Rep.* **2019**, *9*, 9583. [CrossRef]

20. Almansour, N.A.; Syed, H.F.; Khayat, N.R.; Altheeb, R.K.; Juri, R.E.; Alhiyafi, J.; Alrashed, S.; Olatunji, S.O. Neural network and support vector machine for the prediction of chronic kidney disease: A comparative study. *Comput. Biol. Med.* **2019**, *109*, 101–111. [CrossRef]

21. Winter, A.; Staubert, S.; Ammon, D.; Aiche, S.; Beyan, O.; Bischoff, V.; Daumke, P.; Decker, S.; Funkat, G.; Gewehr, J.E.; et al. Smart Medical Information Technology for Healthcare (SMITH). *Methods Inf. Med.* **2018**, *57*, e92–e105. [CrossRef]

22. Hahn, U.; Matthies, F.; Lohr, C.; Loffler, M. 3000PA-Towards a National Reference Corpus of German Clinical Language. *Stud. Health Technol. Inform.* **2018**, *247*, 26–30.

23. Lohr, C.; Luther, S.; Matthies, F.; Modersohn, L.; Ammon, D.; Saleh, K.; Henkel, A.G.; Kiehntopf, M.; Hahn, U. CDA-Compliant Section Annotation of German-Language Discharge Summaries: Guideline Development, Annotation Campaign, Section Classification. *AMIA Annu. Symp. Proc.* **2018**, *2018*, 770–779. [PubMed]

24. Quan, H.; Sundararajan, V.; Halfon, P.; Fong, A.; Burnand, B.; Luthi, J.C.; Saunders, L.D.; Beck, C.A.; Feasby, T.E.; Ghali, W.A. Coding algorithms for defining comorbidities in ICD-9-CM and ICD-10 administrative data. *Med. Care* **2005**, *43*, 1130–1139. [CrossRef] [PubMed]

25. James, M.T.; Levey, A.S.; Tonelli, M.; Tan, Z.; Barry, R.; Pannu, N.; Ravani, P.; Klarenbach, S.W.; Manns, B.J.; Hemmelgarn, B.R. Incidence and Prognosis of Acute Kidney Diseases and Disorders Using an Integrated Approach to Laboratory Measurements in a Universal Health Care System. *JAMA Netw. Open* **2019**, *2*, e191795. [CrossRef] [PubMed]

26. Kidney Disease: Improving Global Outcomes AKI Work Group. KDIGO clinical practice guideline for acute kidney injury. *Kidney Int. Suppl.* **2012**, *2*, 1–138.

27. Duff, S.; Murray, P.T. Defining Early Recovery of Acute Kidney Injury. *Clin. J. Am. Soc. Nephrol.* **2020**, *15*. [CrossRef]

28. Friedman, J.; Hastie, T.; Tibshirani, R. Regularization Paths for Generalized Lin, ear Models via Coordinate Descent. *J. Stat. Softw.* **2010**, *33*, 1–22. [CrossRef]

29. Liaw, A.; Wiener, M. Classification and Regression by randomForest. *R News* **2002**, *2*, 18–22.

30. Hagan, M.T.; Demuth, H.B.; Beale, M. *Neural Network Design*, 1st ed.; PWS Pub.: Boston, MA, USA, 1996.

31. Boehmke, B.; Greenwell, B.M. *Hands-on Machine Learning with R*; CRC Press: Boca Raton, FL, USA, 2019.

32. Saito, T.; Rehmsmeier, M. The precision-recall plot is more informative than the ROC plot when evaluating binary classifiers on imbalanced datasets. *PLoS ONE* **2015**, *10*, e0118432. [CrossRef]

33. DeLong, E.R.; DeLong, D.M.; Clarke-Pearson, D.L. Comparing the areas under two or more correlated receiver operating characteristic curves: A nonparametric approach. *Biometrics* **1988**, *44*, 837–845. [CrossRef]

34. RStudio Team. *RStudio: Integrated Development for R*; RStudio, PBC: Boston, MA, USA, 2019; Available online: http://www.rstudio.com/ (accessed on 12 September 2020).

35. Ritchie, M.E.; Phipson, B.; Wu, D.; Hu, Y.; Law, C.W.; Shi, W.; Smyth, G.K. Limma powers differential expression analyses for RNA-sequencing and microarray studies. *Nucleic Acids Res.* **2015**, *43*, e47. [CrossRef]

36. Chan, C.-H.; Chan, G.C.; Leeper, T.J.; Becker, J. *Rio: A Swiss-Army Knife for Data File I/O*; R package version 0.5.16; 2018. Available online: https://cran.r-project.org/web/packages/rio/index.html (accessed on 12 September 2020).

37. Wickham, H. The Split-Apply-Combine Strategy for Data Analysis. *J. Stat. Softw.* **2011**, *40*, 1–29. [CrossRef]

38. Pinheiro, J.; Bates, D.; DebRoy, S.; Sarkar, D.; Team, R.C. *Nlme: Linear and Nonlinear Mixed Effects Models*; R package version 3.1-142; 2019. Available online: https://CRAN.R-project.org/package=nlme (accessed on 12 September 2020).

39. Wickham, H.; Averick, M.; Bryan, J.; Chang, W.; McGowan, L.; François, R.; Grolemund, G.; Hayes, A.; Henry, L.; Hester, J.; et al. Welcome to the Tidyverse. *J. Open Sour. Softw.* **2019**, *4*, 1686. [CrossRef]

40. Robin, X.; Turck, N.; Hainard, A.; Tiberti, N.; Lisacek, F.; Sanchez, J.-C.; Müller, M. pROC: An open-source package for R and S+ to analyze and compare ROC curves. *BMC Bioinform.* **2011**, *12*, 1–8. [CrossRef] [PubMed]

41. Sing, T.; Sander, O.; Beerenwinkel, N.; Lengauer, T. ROCR: Visualizing classifier performance in R. *Bioinformatics* **2005**, *21*, 3940–3941. [CrossRef] [PubMed]

42. Kuhn, M. *Caret: Classification and Regression Training*; R package version 6.0-86; 2020. Available online: https://cran.r-project.org/web/packages/caret/index.html (accessed on 12 September 2020).

43. Diamantidis, C.J.; Hale, S.L.; Wang, V.; Smith, V.A.; Scholle, S.H.; Maciejewski, M.L. Lab-based and diagnosis-based chronic kidney disease recognition and staging concordance. *BMC Nephrol.* **2019**, *20*, 357. [CrossRef]

44. Stevens, L.A.; Li, S.; Wang, C.; Huang, C.; Becker, B.N.; Bomback, A.S.; Brown, W.W.; Burrows, N.R.; Jurkovitz, C.T.; McFarlane, S.I.; et al. Prevalence of CKD and comorbid illness in elderly patients in the United States: Results from the Kidney Early Evaluation Program (KEEP). *Am. J. Kidney Dis.* **2010**, *55*, S23–S33. [CrossRef]

45. Konstantinidis, I.; Nadkarni, G.N.; Yacoub, R.; Saha, A.; Simoes, P.; Parikh, C.R.; Coca, S.G. Representation of Patients With Kidney Disease in Trials of Cardiovascular Interventions: An Updated Systematic Review. *JAMA Intern. Med.* **2016**, *176*, 121–124. [CrossRef]

46. Ronksley, P.E.; Tonelli, M.; Quan, H.; Manns, B.J.; James, M.T.; Clement, F.M.; Samuel, S.; Quinn, R.R.; Ravani, P.; Brar, S.S.; et al. Validating a case definition for chronic kidney disease using administrative data. *Nephrol. Dial. Transplant.* **2012**, *27*, 1826–1831. [CrossRef]

47. Kern, E.F.; Maney, M.; Miller, D.R.; Tseng, C.L.; Tiwari, A.; Rajan, M.; Aron, D.; Pogach, L. Failure of ICD-9-CM codes to identify patients with comorbid chronic kidney disease in diabetes. *Health Serv. Res.* **2006**, *41*, 564–580. [CrossRef]

48. Gomez-Salgado, J.; Bernabeu-Wittel, M.; Aguilera-Gonzalez, C.; Goicoechea-Salazar, J.A.; Larrocha, D.; Nieto-Martin, M.D.; Moreno-Gavino, L.; Ollero-Baturone, M. Concordance between the Clinical Definition of Polypathological Patient versus Automated Detection by Means of Combined Identification through ICD-9-CM Codes. *J. Clin. Med.* **2019**, *8*, 613. [CrossRef]

49. Chase, H.S.; Radhakrishnan, J.; Shirazian, S.; Rao, M.K.; Vawdrey, D.K. Under-documentation of chronic kidney disease in the electronic health record in outpatients. *J. Am. Med. Inform. Assoc.* **2010**, *17*, 588–594. [CrossRef] [PubMed]

50. Hernandez-Boussard, T.; Monda, K.L.; Crespo, B.C.; Riskin, D. Real world evidence in cardiovascular medicine: Ensuring data validity in electronic health record-based studies. *J. Am. Med. Inform. Assoc.* **2019**, *26*, 1189–1194. [CrossRef] [PubMed]

51. Nadkarni, G.N.; Gottesman, O.; Linneman, J.G.; Chase, H.; Berg, R.L.; Farouk, S.; Nadukuru, R.; Lotay, V.; Ellis, S.; Hripcsak, G.; et al. Development and validation of an electronic phenotyping algorithm for chronic kidney disease. *AMIA Annu. Symp. Proc.* **2014**, *2014*, 907–916. [PubMed]

52. Wei, W.Q.; Leibson, C.L.; Ransom, J.E.; Kho, A.N.; Caraballo, P.J.; Chai, H.S.; Yawn, B.P.; Pacheco, J.A.; Chute, C.G. Impact of data fragmentation across healthcare centers on the accuracy of a high-throughput clinical phenotyping algorithm for specifying subjects with type 2 diabetes mellitus. *J. Am. Med. Inform. Assoc.* **2012**, *19*, 219–224. [CrossRef]

53. Wei, W.Q.; Leibson, C.L.; Ransom, J.E.; Kho, A.N.; Chute, C.G. The absence of longitudinal data limits the accuracy of high-throughput clinical phenotyping for identifying type 2 diabetes mellitus subjects. *Int. J. Med. Inform.* **2013**, *82*, 239–247. [CrossRef]

54. Delanaye, P.; Glassock, R.J.; De Broe, M.E. Epidemiology of chronic kidney disease: Think (at least) twice! *Clin. Kidney J.* **2017**, *10*, 370–374. [CrossRef]

55. Wei, W.Q.; Teixeira, P.L.; Mo, H.; Cronin, R.M.; Warner, J.L.; Denny, J.C. Combining billing codes, clinical notes, and medications from electronic health records provides superior phenotyping performance. *J. Am. Med. Inform. Assoc.* **2016**, *23*, e20–e27. [CrossRef]

56. Salekin, A.; Stankovic, J. Detection of Chronic Kidney Disease and Selecting Important Predictive Attributes.
     In Proceedings of the 2016 IEEE International Conference on Healthcare Informatics (ICHI), Chicago, IL,
     USA, 4–7 October 2016; pp. 262–270.
57. Rashidian, S.; Hajagos, J.; Moffitt, R.A.; Wang, F.; Noel, K.M.; Gupta, R.R.; Tharakan, M.A.; Saltz, J.H.;
     Saltz, M.M. Deep Learning on Electronic Health Records to Improve Disease Coding Accuracy. *AMIA
     Summits Transl. Sci. Proc.* **2019**, *2019*, 620–629.

13

Urinary Oxalate Excretion and Long-Term Outcomes in Kidney Transplant Recipients

Alwin Tubben [1],*, Camilo G. Sotomayor [1], Adrian Post [1], Isidor Minovic [2], Timoer Frelink [3], Martin H. de Borst [1], M. Yusof Said [1], Rianne M. Douwes [1], Else van den Berg [1], Ramón Rodrigo [4], Stefan P. Berger [1], Gerjan J. Navis [1] and Stephan J. L. Bakker [1]

[1] Department of Internal Medicine, University Medical Center Groningen, University of Groningen, Hanzeplein 1, 9700 RB Groningen, The Netherlands; c.g.sotomayor.campos@umcg.nl (C.G.S.); a.post01@umcg.nl (A.P.); m.h.de.borst@umcg.nl (M.H.d.B.); m.y.said@umcg.nl (M.Y.S.); r.m.douwes@umcg.nl (R.M.D.); e.van.den.berg@umcg.nl (E.v.d.B.); s.p.berger@umcg.nl (S.P.B.); g.j.navis@umcg.nl (G.J.N.); s.j.l.bakker@umcg.nl (S.J.L.B.)
[2] Department of Laboratory Medicine, University Medical Center Groningen, University of Groningen, Hanzeplein 1, 9700 RB Groningen, The Netherlands; i.minovic@umcg.nl
[3] Metrohm Applikon B.V., 3125 AE Schiedam, The Netherlands; timoer.frelink@metrohm.com
[4] Molecular and Clinical Pharmacology Program, Institute of Biomedical Sciences, Faculty of Medicine, University of Chile, 8380453 Santiago, Chile; rrodrigo@med.uchile.cl
* Correspondence: a.tubben@umcg.nl

Abstract: Epidemiologic studies have linked urinary oxalate excretion to risk of chronic kidney disease (CKD) progression and end-stage renal disease. We aimed to investigate whether urinary oxalate, in stable kidney transplant recipients (KTR), is prospectively associated with risk of graft failure. In secondary analyses we evaluated the association with post-transplantation diabetes mellitus, all-cause mortality and specific causes of death. Oxalate excretion was measured in 24-h urine collection samples in a cohort of 683 KTR with a functioning allograft ≥ 1 year. Mean eGFR was 52 ± 20 mL/min/1.73 m^2. Median (interquartile range) urinary oxalate excretion was 505 (347–732) μmol/24-h in women and 519 (396–736) μmol/24-h in men ($p = 0.08$), with 302 patients (44% of the study population) above normal limits (hyperoxaluria). A consistent and independent inverse association was found with all-cause mortality (HR 0.77, 95% CI 0.63–0.94, $p = 0.01$). Cause-specific survival analyses showed that this association was mainly driven by an inverse association with mortality due to infection (HR 0.56, 95% CI 0.38–0.83, $p = 0.004$), which remained materially unchanged after performing sensitivity analyses. Twenty-four-hour urinary oxalate excretion did not associate with risk of graft failure, post-transplant diabetes mellitus, cardiovascular mortality, mortality due to malignancies or mortality due to miscellaneous causes. In conclusion, in KTR, 24-h urinary oxalate excretion is elevated in 44% of KTR and inversely associated with mortality due to infectious causes.

Keywords: oxalate; hyperoxaluria; kidney transplant recipients; graft failure; post-transplantation diabetes mellitus; all-cause mortality; cardiovascular mortality; infectious mortality

---

1. Introduction

Kidney transplantation is considered the gold standard treatment for end-stage renal disease (ESRD) [1,2]. Short-term survival of kidney transplant recipients (KTR) has improved markedly in the past decades [3,4]. Although a better understanding of modifiable risk factors has been achieved over the recent years [5,6], patients perceive the ever existing threat of premature graft failure (GF) as most compelling, and would like to know whether factors such as lifestyle and diet can contribute to prevention of it [7,8]. Another factor of interest influencing long-term KTR survival is post-transplantation diabetes mellitus (PTDM), which has become increasingly common and may affect patient and graft survival [9]. Further, an increased risk of premature mortality, in particular, increased risk for premature death from cardiovascular and infectious causes remain significant problems in the post-transplantation setting. In KTR, conventional risk factors for cardiovascular mortality are abundantly present, such as hypertension, diabetes mellitus and dyslipidemia. On top of that, KTR had pre-existent renal diseases, which additionally increases the cardiovascular risk [10]. Mortality due to infection is significantly higher in KTR than in the general population due to multiple reasons, to which immunosuppressive therapy is a large contributing factor [11]. Furthermore, KTR are at a two to threefold higher risk of cancer-related mortality compared to the general population [12].

Although different mechanisms underlying these long-term complications of kidney transplantation have been found, substantial unknown mechanisms particular to the post-kidney transplantation setting remain to be identified in order to provide rationale for the markedly high risk of premature mortality in KTR [13]. A recent prospective cohort study in 3123 patients with chronic kidney disease (CKD) stages 2 to 4, found urinary oxalate as a potential risk factor for progression of CKD [14]. In the post-kidney transplantation setting, the study of oxalate remains overlooked. Whether urinary oxalate (reference value ≤455 μmol/24-h) [15] may be prospectively associated with adverse outcomes in KTR remains unknown.

The current study aims to assess the potential association of urinary oxalate excretion with adverse long-term outcomes in a large cohort of extensively phenotyped KTR with a functioning graft ≥1 year. For this purpose, the prospective associations of 24-h urinary oxalate excretion with GF, PTDM, and overall and cause-specific mortality were systematically investigated.

2. Experimental Section

2.1. Study Design and Population

This is a single-center prospective cohort study, initiated in 2008 on with follow-up of endpoints until 2015. KTR with a functioning allograft for at least one year or more who visited the outpatient clinic of the University Medical Center Groningen (Groningen, The Netherlands) between November 2008 and March 2011. Exclusion criteria were no known or apparent systemic illnesses, insufficient knowledge of the Dutch language and history of drug or alcohol addiction according to their patient files. KTR received anti-hypertensive and standard maintenance immunosuppressive therapy. Of the 817 invited KTR, 706 (87%) signed informed consent. Patients missing 24-h urinary oxalate excretion were excluded from the analyses, resulting in 683 KTR eligible for statistical analyses. The study was conducted in concordance with the guidelines formulated in the Declaration of Helsinki and Istanbul, and approved by the Institutional Review Board of the UMCG (METc 2008/186) [16]. The continuous surveillance system according to the American Society of Transplantation was followed for the correct collection of data [17]. When status of patients was unknown, the referring nephrologist or general practitioners were contacted in order to obtain the missing information. There was no loss due to follow-up.

2.2. Study Endpoints

The primary endpoint of this study is death-censored GF. Secondary endpoints are PTDM, all-cause mortality and cause-specific mortality. GF occurrence in this study is defined as ESRD requiring re-transplantation or return to dialysis. A subject was considered to have developed PTDM when the fasting plasma glucose exceeded 7 mmol/L, the HbA1c exceeded 6.5% or use of antidiabetics after transplantation as registered in the patient database [18,19]. Among specific causes of death, we studied cardiovascular mortality, death from infection, death from malignancies, and other causes of death (miscellaneous). Cardiovascular mortality is defined as mortality caused by cardiovascular pathophysiology, coded by ICD-10 codes I10-I52. This information was obtained from linking the patient number to the database of the Central Bureau of Statistics and then, by physicians, reported mortality cause. Infectious mortality and mortality due to malignancies were defined as mortality caused by infectious causes or malignant causes. Miscellaneous causes of mortality have been defined as other causes of death besides the previously described outcomes.

2.3. Baseline Measurements and Definitions

At the outpatient clinic, baseline data was gathered according to a strict and detailed protocol described previously [20]. Anthropometrics were obtained without shoes and heavy garments. Systolic and diastolic blood pressures (SBP and DBP) were measured by means of an automatic device (Philips Suresign VS2+, Andover, MA, USA) according to a standard clinical protocol [16]. Mean arterial pressure (MAP) was automatically calculated by (SBP + DBP × 2)/3. History of cardiovascular disease was searched for in the patient files under ICD-10 code Z86.7.

Body mass index (BMI) was calculated as weight in kilograms divided by height in meters squared (kg/m^2) [21]. Estimated glomerular filtration rate (eGFR) was calculated using the CKD Epidemiology Collaboration (CKD-EPI) creatinine equation as shown in Formula (S1) [22].

2.4. Assesments of Physical Activity and Dietary Intake

Physical activity was quantified using the Short Questionnaire to Assess Health-enhancing physical activity (SQUASH). Activity was expressed in intensity multiplied by the amount of hours [23]. Dietary intake was assessed using a semi-quantitative Food Frequency Questionnaire (FFQ) [24,25]. To obtain the energy of a certain product, the Dutch Food Composition Table of 2016 was used [26]. Micro and macronutrients were adjusted for total energy intake (kCal), because of the potential of correlation and confounding [27].

2.5. Laboratory Measurements

For the collection of 24-h urine samples, the patients were asked to start the collection the day prior to their visit to the outpatient clinic. Collection was done in concordance with a strict protocol, i.e., discarding the first morning urine, collecting the subsequent in 24 h including the next morning's urine [16]. Subsequently, urine samples for oxalate analysis were acidified and stored at −80 °C. Urine oxalate analysis was performed using a validated ion-exchange chromatography assay with conductivity detection (Metrohm, Herisau, Switzerland). Inter-assay precision was monitored using three urine pool samples. Inter-assay precision was 8.2% at 0.17 mmol/L, 7.0% at 0.38 mmol/L and 9.0% at 0.52 mmol/L. Comparison of this method with a routine laboratory GC-MS method showed no systemic difference and no proportional difference. Reverse-phase high performance liquid chromatography (HPLC) was used to measure urinary thiosulfate [28].

2.6. Statistical Analyses

Data was analyzed using IBM SPSS version 23.0 (SPSS Inc., Chicago, IL, USA); Stata version 14.0 (StataCorp., College Station, TX, USA), GraphPad Prism version 7.02 (GraphPad Software, La Jolla, CA, USA), and Rstudio version 3.2.3 (R Foundation for Statistical Computing, Vienna, Austria). A two-sided $p < 0.05$ was considered significant in all following analyses.

Normally distributed variables are expressed as mean ± standard deviation (SD), skewed data as medians (Interquartile range (IQR)), and categorical data as given number and percentage. Baseline characteristics were described for the overall population and by sex-stratified tertiles of 24-h urinary oxalate excretion. Data are presented in tertiles to allow for assessment of linearity of cross-sectional associations of 24-h urinary oxalate excretion with other variables. Sex-stratified tertiles were created by first separately distributing all female subjects according to tertiles and distributing all male subjects according to tertiles, and thereafter combining the tertiles of females and males. We generated sex-specific tertiles because of differences between women and men in oxalate excretion [29–32]. Analyses of difference in baseline characteristics across sex-stratified tertiles of 24-h urinary oxalate excretion were tested by ANOVA for normally distributed continuous variables, Kruskal-Wallis for skewed continuous variables and $\chi2$ test for categorical data. Sex-stratified tertiles of 24-h oxalate excretion were tested for associations with outcomes by Kaplan-Meier analysis, including the log-rank test.

Linear regression analyses were performed to investigate the association of baseline characteristics with 24-h urinary oxalate excretion. Normality was assessed by means of a p–p plot, and a natural log transformation was performed when appropriate. Homoscedasticity was controlled in a scatterplot.

Cox regression analyses were used to investigate the association of 24-h urinary oxalate with primary and secondary outcomes. Model 1 of the Cox proportional-hazards regression analysis was adjusted for demographics, i.e., sex and age. Model 2 was additionally adjusted for transplantation related variables, namely primary renal disease, BMI, donor age, time from transplantation to follow-up, eGFR and proteinuria. In the next models, baseline characteristics which were cross-sectionally associated with 24-h urinary oxalate excretion were subsequently included, and potential confounding of urinary thiosulfate was investigated due to its role in the anion transporters in the proximal renal tubuli (Model 3) [33]. In addition, we also looked for lactate dehydrogenase (LDH) because of its importance in the conversion of glyoxylate (Model 4) [34], for 24-h urinary pH because of its influence on the reaction of oxalate with calcium (Model 5) [35], for fibroblast growth factor 23 (FGF23) because of the relationship with gastrointestinal calcium absorption and oxalate bioavailability [36,37] (Model 6), and for fruits and vegetables as main dietary sources of oxalate [38–40] (Model 7). To allow for detection of a potential threshold effect, which was found in an earlier study on urinary oxalate excretion and CKD [14], Cox regression analyses were also performed according to sex-stratified tertiles with the first tertile as reference.

Spline regression were created to visualize the association of 24-h urinary oxalate excretion for outcomes, for which we consistently found significant associations. Nonlinearity was tested by using the likelihood ratio test, comparing models with linear or linear and cubic spline terms. Restricted cubic splines were knotted at the minimum, median and maximum. The splines were adjusted according to Model 6 of the primary prospective analyses.

Sensitivity Analyses

Several sensitivity analyses were performed to examine the robustness of the associations between 24-h urinary oxalate excretion and outcomes. For that purpose, we reanalyzed the data excluding subjects with potential inadequate 24-h urine collection (i.e., overcollection or undercollection), which was defined as the upper and lower 2.5% of the difference between the estimated and measured volume of a subject's 24-h urine sample. The following formula was used to calculate the estimated 24-h urine volume: $\frac{1}{4}$ ((urine creatinine) * (24-h urine volume)/(serum creatinine)), where creatinine clearance was estimated using the Cockcroft-Gault Formula [41,42]. These analyses were analogous to Model 6 of the primary prospective analyses.

Furthermore, we performed competing risk analyses of outcomes of interest with all-cause mortality as competing event according to Fine and Gray [43]. For that purpose, we performed multivariable Cox regression analyses analogously to Model 6 of the primary prospective analyses.

3. Results

3.1. Baseline Characteristics

In total 683 KTR were included in the analyses (mean age 53 ± 13, 43% female, 99.6% Caucasian ethnicity). Median urinary oxalate excretion was 505 (IQR, 347–732) μmol/24-h in women and 519 (IQR, 396–736) μmol/24-h in men ($p = 0.08$). Forty-four percent of the patients were above the range of clinical hyperoxaluria of ≤455 μmol/24-h. All 227 study subjects in tertile 3 were above the clinical cutoff point for hyperoxaluria, and all 227 subjects in tertile 1 were below the clinical cutoff point. Mean eGFR was 52 ± 20 mL/min/1.73 m^2. Additional baseline characteristics and analyses are shown overall and by sex-stratified tertiles of 24-h urinary oxalate excretion in Table 1.

Table 1. Baseline characteristics of the overall population, and by sex-stratified tertiles of 24-h urinary oxalate excretion. [a]

Baseline Characteristics	Overall KTR n = 683	Sex-Stratified Groups of 24-h Urinary Oxalate Excretion			p
		♀≤ 390; ♂≤ 431 μmol/24-h	♀391-633; ♂432-632 μmol/24-h	♀≥ 633; ♂≥ 632 μmol/24-h	
Oxalate					
Oxalate in 24-h urine, μmol [b]	514 (378-732)	339 (278-278)	514 (461-563)	882 (732-1137)	—
Demographics					
Age, years	53 ± 13	54 ± 13	53 ± 12	51 ± 13	0.04
Sex (female), n (%)	295 (43)	98 (43)	99 (43)	98 (43)	1.00
Ethnicity (Caucasian), n (%)	680 (99.6)	226 (99.6)	228 (99.6)	226 (99.6)	1.00
Body composition					
BSA, m^2	1.94 ± 0.22	1.92 ± 0.21	1.98 ± 0.21	1.94 ± 0.23	0.05
BMI, kg/m^2	26.6 ± 4.8	26.3 ± 4.8	27.0 ± 4.6	26.6 ± 4.8	0.34
Waist circumference, cm	98 (89-108)	97 (89-105)	100 (90-110)	96 (87-106)	0.02
Lifestyle					
Current smoker, n (%)	81 (12)	42 (19)	19 (9)	20 (9)	0.001
Alcohol consumption					0.30
None, n (%)	22 (3)	6 (3)	8 (4)	8 (4)	
0-10 g/day, n (%)	426 (62)	144 (64)	146 (64)	136 (60)	
10-30 g/day, n (%)	137 (20)	44 (19)	44 (19)	49 (22)	
>30 g/dag, n (%)	37 (5)	10 (4)	12 (5)	15 (7)	
SQUASH-score	5070 (2040-7800)	4440 (1680-7240)	5400 (2323-8475)	5580 (2280-7980)	0.10
Cardiovascular					
History of CV disease, n (%)	295 (50)	92 (41)	103 (45)	100 (44)	0.72
SBP, mmHg	136 ± 18	137 ± 17	136 ± 18	135 ± 18	0.42
MAP, mmHg (calculated)	100 ± 12	101 ± 11	100 ± 12	100 ± 13	0.73
LDL cholesterol, mmol/L	3.0 ± 0.9	3.1 ± 0.9	3.0 ± 0.9	2.9 ± 0.9	0.54
Triglycerides, mmol/L	1.7 (1.2-2.3)	1.7 (1.3-2.3)	1.6 (1.2-2.4)	1.7 (1.2-2.2)	0.69
Glucose homeostasis					
Diabetes mellitus, n (%)	162 (24)	52 (23)	58 (25)	53 (23)	0.78
Plasma glucose, mmol/L	5.3 (4.8-6.0)	5.3 (4.8-5.9)	5.2 (4.8-6.2)	5.3 (4.7-6.1)	0.85
Diet					
Av. energy intake, kCal/day	2092 (1720-2536)	2045 (1705-2479)	2104 (1735-2557)	2171 (1759-2589)	0.45
Av. daily fat intake, g/d [c]	84 (65-106)	80 (63-101)	85 (66-106)	86 (64-110)	0.31
Av. daily protein intake, g/d [c]	81 (67-95)	80 (65-95)	81 (66-95)	81 (68-95)	0.82
Glycine, mg/d [c]	3276 ± 806	3228 ± 805	3261 ± 817	3337 ± 794	0.38
Ascorbic acid, mg/d [c]	84 (60-118)	70 (53-101)	82 (60-114)	103 (73-138)	<0.001
Vegetables, g/d	93 ± 58	94 ± 53	90 ± 53	96 ± 66	0.54
Fruits, g/d	123 (65-232)	111 (50-226)	121 (64-228)	165 (81-247)	0.001

Table 1. *Cont.*

Baseline Characteristics	Overall KTR n = 683	Sex-Stratified Groups of 24-h Urinary Oxalate Excretion			p
		♀≤ 390; ♂≤ 431 μmol/24-h	♀391–633; ♂432–632 μmol/24-h	♀≥ 633; ♂≥ 632 μmol/24-h	
Transplantation characteristics					
Age donor, years	43 ± 15	43 ± 15	43 ± 16	43 ± 16	0.85
Sex donor (female), n (%)	322 (47)	108 (49)	99 (44)	15 (52)	0.24
Donor type (living), n (%)	231 (34)	67 (30)	81 (35)	83 (37)	0.24
Serum markers					
Venous pCO2, kPa	5.9 ± 0.8	5.9 ± 0.9	5.9 ± 0.8	5.8 ± 0.8	0.53
Leukocyte count, per 10^9/L	8.2 ± 2.7	8.3 ± 2.6	8.1 ± 2.8	8.1 ± 2.6	0.52
HsCRP, mg/L	1.6 (0.7–4.6)	1.6 (0.8–4.4)	2.0 (0.8–5.3)	1.4 (0.6–3.8)	0.04
Hemoglobin, mmol/L	8.2 ± 1.1	8.1 ± 1.1	8.2 ± 1.1	8.3 ± 1.1	0.11
FGF-23	61 (43–99)	63 (43–107)	61 (42–98)	61 (45–97)	0.66
LDH, U/L	198 (170–232)	195 (169–232)	203 (174–238)	196 (170–223)	0.35
Vitamin B6, nmol/L	29 (18–29)	27 (16–47)	26 (15–44)	36 (22–57)	<0.001
Renal allograft function					
Creatinine, μmol/L	125 (100–160)	126 (99–164)	126 (101–164)	122 (100–157)	0.66
eGFR, mL/min/1.73 m^2	52 ± 20	51 ± 20	52 ± 20	54 ± 20	0.26
Serum cystatin C, mg/L	1.7 (1.3–2.2)	1.7 (1.3–2.5)	1.7 (1.3–2.2)	1.6 (1.3–2.1)	0.25
Proteinuria ≥ 0.5 g/24-h, n (%)	152 (22)	49 (22)	49 (21)	54 (24)	0.59
24-h urine					
pH	6.0 ± 0.5	6.0 ± 0.5	6.0 ± 0.5	6.1 ± 0.5	0.48
UUN excretion, mmol	389 ± 114	349 ± 100	407 ± 111	412 ± 1	<0.001
Phosphate excretion, mmol	25 ± 9	22 ± 8	25 ± 8	27 ± 9	<0.001
Thiosulfate excretion, μmol	7.0 (3.9–12.0)	6.7 (3.7–11.0)	6.9 (4.2–12.5)	7.5 (3.8–12.6)	0.57
Protein excretion, mg	196 (15–367)	163 (15–281)	221 (15–380)	200 (15–417)	0.10

Abbreviations: ♀, female; ♂, male; KTR, kidney transplant recipients; n, number; β, standardized beta; BSA, body surface area; BMI, body mass index; SQUASH, Short Questionnaire to Assess Health-enhancing physical activity; SBP, systolic blood pressure; MAP, mean arterial pressure; LDL, low density lipoprotein; Av., average; hs-CRP, high sensitivity C-reactive protein; LDH, lactate dehydrogenase; eGFR, estimated glomerular filtration rate; UUN, urinary urea nitrogen; FGF-23, fibroblast growth factor 23. [a] Normally distributed variables are expressed as mean ± standard deviation (SD), skewed data as medians (25th–75th inter quartile range (IQR)), categorical data is given as number and percentage, n, (%). Analyses of difference in baseline characteristics across sex-stratified tertiles of 24-h urinary oxalate excretion were tested by ANOVA for normally distributed continuous variables; Kruskal-Wallis for skewed continuous variables; χ^2 test for categorical data. [b] To convert oxalate in μmol/24-h to mg/24-h, multiply by 0.088. [c] Adjusted for energy intake.

3.2. Cross-Sectional Analysis

We found that age ($p = 0.04$), current smoking status ($p = 0.01$), and cystatin C ($p = 0.03$) were inversely associated with 24-h urinary oxalate excretion, whereas plasma glucose ($p = 0.01$), ascorbic acid ($p < 0.001$), fruit consumption ($p < 0.001$), vitamin B6 ($p < 0.001$), urinary urea nitrogen excretion ($p < 0.001$), and phosphate excretion ($p < 0.001$) were positively associated with 24-h urinary oxalate excretion.

3.3. Prospective Analyses

GF and mortality were recorded during a follow-up of 5.3 years (IQR, 4.5–6.0). During follow-up, 83 (12%) patients developed GF, 55 (9%) patients developed PTDM and 149 (22%) patients died, of which 59 deaths (40%) were due to cardiovascular causes, 41 deaths (28%) due to infectious causes, 26 deaths (17%) due to malignancies and 23 deaths (15%) due to miscellaneous causes (Table 2).

Table 2. Association of baseline characteristics with 24-h urinary oxalate excretion. [a]

Baseline Characteristics	β	p
Demographics		
Age, years	−0.08	0.04
Lifestyle		
Current smoker	−0.11	0.01
Plasma glucose, mmol/L	0.10	0.01
Diet		
Ascorbic acid, mg/d [c]	0.24	<0.001
Fruits, g/d	0.16	<0.001
Blood markers		
Vitamin B6 in blood, nmol/L	0.20	<0.001
Renal allograft function		
Cystatin C, blood, mg/L	−0.16	0.03
24-h Urine		
UUN excretion, mmol	0.24	<0.001
Phosphate excretion, mmol	0.25	<0.001

[a] Multivariate linear regression, adjusted for age, sex and eGFR.

3.3.1. GF, PTDM, Cardiovascular Mortality, Mortality due to Malignancies, and Miscellaneous Mortality

A Kaplan-Meier curve for the association of tertiles of 24-h urinary oxalate excretion with GF is shown in Figure 1A ($p = 0.20$, p for trend 0.08). Results of multivariate Cox regression analyses did not show a consistent association of 24-h urinary oxalate excretion with GF (HR 0.71, 95% CI 0.53–0.98) (Table 3). Uni- and multivariate analyses of the associations of 24-h urinary oxalate excretion and potential confounders with GF are shown in Table S1.

A Kaplan-Meier curve for the association of tertiles of 24-h urinary oxalate excretion with PTDM is shown in Figure 1B ($p = 0.24$, p for trend 0.37). Results of multivariate Cox regression analyses showed no association of 24-h urinary oxalate excretion with PTDM (HR 0.95, 95% CI 0.71–1.27) (Table 3).

A Kaplan-Meier curve for the association of tertiles of 24-h urinary oxalate excretion with cardiovascular mortality is shown in Figure 1C ($p = 0.08$, p for trend 0.08). Results of multivariate Cox regression analyses showed cardiovascular mortality is not associated with 24-h urinary oxalate excretion (HR 0.78, 95% CI 0.56–1.10) (Table 4).

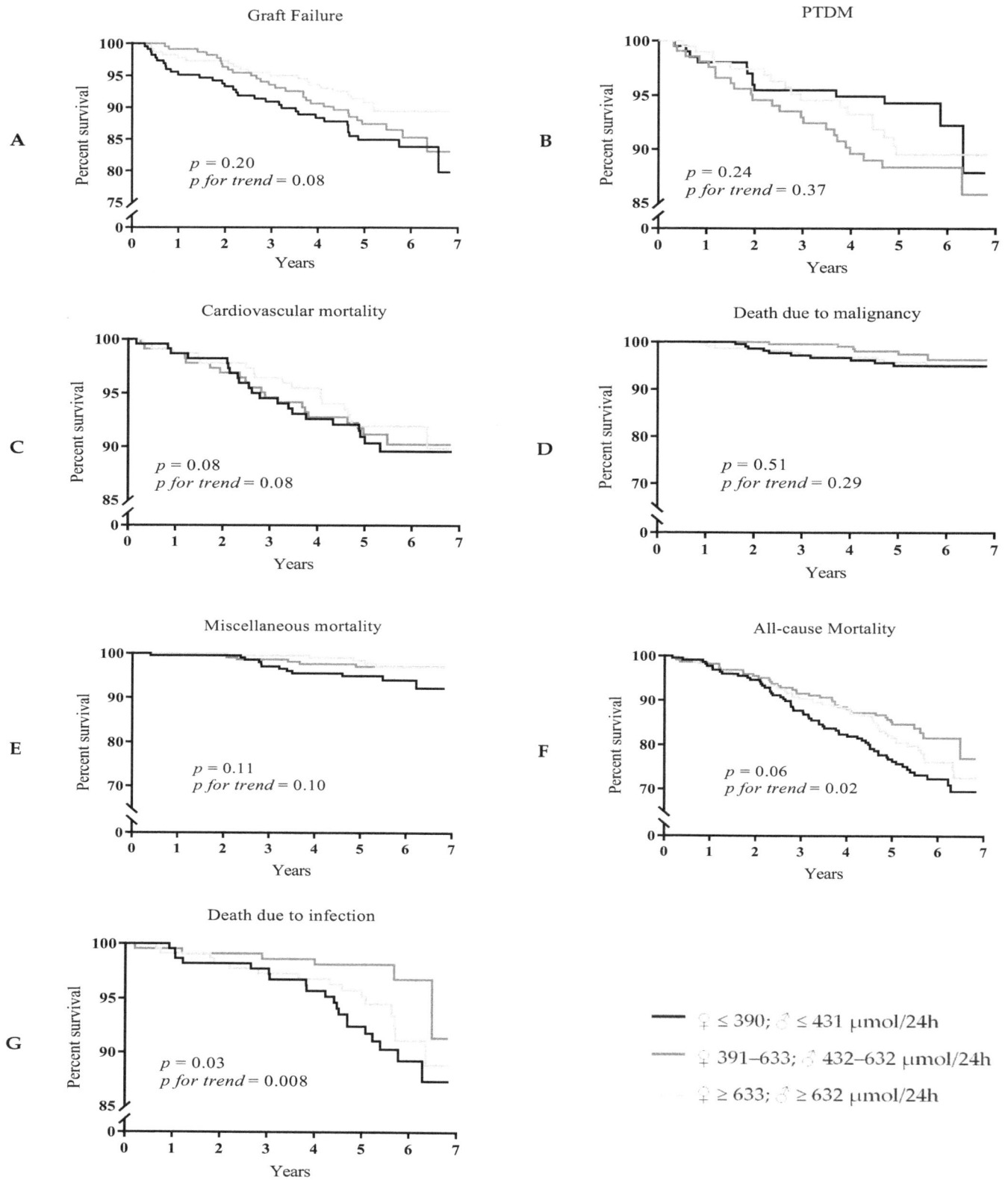

Figure 1. (**A**) Graft failure, (**B**) PTDM, (**C**) cardiovascular mortality, (**D**) death due to malignancy, (**E**) miscellaneous mortality (**F**) all-cause mortality, and (**G**) death due to infection according to sex-stratified tertiles of 24-hour urinary oxalate excretion over approximately 7 years of follow-up.

Table 3. Association of 24-h urine oxalate excretion with graft failure and PTDM.

| | Continuous, per 1–SD | | Tertiles | | | | | |
| | | | Tertile 1 | Tertile 2 | | Tertile 3 | | |
	HR	95%CI	Ref	HR	95% CI	HR	95% CI
Graft Failure							
Model 1	0.80	0.64–1.00	1.00	0.82	0.50–1.36	0.58	0.33–1.00
Model 2	0.78	0.61–1.02	1.00	0.77	0.45–1.32	0.61	0.35–1.08
Model 3	0.72	0.54–0.94	1.00	0.68	0.39–1.17	0.48	0.26–0.86
Model 4	0.71	0.53–0.93	1.00	0.68	0.40–1.18	0.45	0.24–0.82
Model 5	0.71	0.53–0.93	1.00	0.66	0.38–1.15	0.43	0.23–0.80
Model 6	0.71	0.53–0.98	1.00	0.69	0.39–1.20	0.44	0.24–0.83
Model 7	0.75	0.56–1.00	1.00	0.70	0.40–1.25	0.48	0.19–0.77
PTDM							
Model 1	0.93	0.71–1.22	1.00	1.27	0.68–2.37	0.71	0.34–1.46
Model 2	0.91	0.69–1.23	1.00	1.23	0.66–2.32	0.68	0.33–1.41
Model 3	0.91	0.68–1.22	1.00	1.32	0.70–2.50	0.61	0.28–1.33
Model 4	0.94	0.70–1.25	1.00	1.39	0.73–2.68	0.66	0.30–1.44
Model 5	0.95	0.73–1.27	1.00	1.50	0.77–2.91	0.71	0.32–1.57
Model 6	0.95	0.71–1.27	1.00	1.50	0.77–2.91	0.76	0.34–1.73
Model 7	0.99	0.73–1.33	1.00	1.45	0.74–2.83	0.75	0.34–1.69

Multivariate Cox regression were performed for the association of 24-h urinary oxalate excretion with graft failure and PTDM. Model 1: age and sex adjusted. Model 2: Model 1 + adjustment for BMI, primary renal disease, donor age, transplant vintage, eGFR, and proteinuria. Model 3: Model 2 + adjustment for thiosulfate in 24-h urine. Model 4: Model 3 + adjustment for LDH in blood. Model 5: Model 4 + adjustment for pH of 24-h urine. Model 6: Model 5 + adjustment for FGF23. Model 7: Model 6 + adjustment for fruit and vegetables intake.

Table 4. Association of 24-h urine oxalate excretion with all-cause and cardiovascular mortality.

| | Continuous, per 1–SD | | Tertiles | | | | | |
| | | | Tertile 1 | Tertile 2 | | Tertile 3 | | |
	HR	95% CI	Ref	HR	95% CI	HR	95% CI
All-cause mortality							
Model 1	0.83	0.70–0.98	1.00	0.86	0.59–1.25	0.72	0.48–1.74
Model 2	0.81	0.67–0.97	1.00	0.84	0.57–1.23	0.73	0.48–1.14
Model 3	0.76	0.62–0.93	1.00	0.85	0.58–1.25	0.56	0.35–0.88
Model 4	0.76	0.62–0.92	1.00	0.80	0.54–1.18	0.53	0.34–0.83
Model 5	0.77	0.63–0.94	1.00	0.79	0.53–1.17	0.54	0.34–0.86
Model 6	0.77	0.63–0.94	1.00	0.75	0.50–1.13	0.55	0.34–0.86
Model 7	0.83	0.68–1.03	1.00	0.74	0.48–1.15	0.67	0.41–1.11
Cardiovascular mortality							
Model 1	0.90	0.69–1.19	1.00	0.90	0.48–1.69	1.09	0.59–2.00
Model 2	0.87	0.65–1.17	1.00	0.84	0.44–1.62	1.11	0.59–2.08
Model 3	0.78	0.56–1.09	1.00	0.87	0.45–1.69	0.81	0.40–1.63
Model 4	0.77	0.56–1.08	1.00	0.81	0.42–1.57	0.75	0.37–1.53
Model 5	0.79	0.57–1.09	1.00	0.82	0.42–1.59	0.78	0.38–1.57
Model 6	0.78	0.56–1.10	1.00	0.82	0.41–1.62	0.77	0.37–1.59
Model 7	0.79	0.55–1.13	1.00	0.80	0.39–1.66	0.75	0.33–1.70

Multivariate Cox regression were performed for the association of 24-h urinary oxalate excretion with all-cause and cardiovascular mortality. Model 1: age and sex adjusted. Model 2: Model 1 + adjustment for BMI, primary renal disease, donor age, transplant vintage, eGFR, and proteinuria. Model 3: Model 2 + adjustment for thiosulfate in 24-h urine. Model 4: Model 3 + adjustment for LDH in blood. Model 5: Model 4 + adjustment for pH of 24-h urine. Model 6: Model 5 + adjustment for FGF23. Model 7: Model 6 + adjustment for fruit and vegetables intake.

A Kaplan-Meier curve for the association of tertiles of 24-h urinary oxalate excretion with death due to malignancy is shown in Figure 1D ($p = 0.51$, p for trend 0.29). Results of multivariate Cox regression analyses showed mortality due to malignancies is not associated with 24-h urinary oxalate excretion (HR 1.14, 95% CI 0.73–1.77) (Table 5).

A Kaplan-Meier curve for the association of tertiles of 24-h urinary oxalate excretion miscellaneous mortality is shown in Figure 1E ($p = 0.11$, p for trend 0.10). Results of multivariate Cox regression analyses showed miscellaneous death causes are not associated with 24-h urinary oxalate excretion (HR 0.75, 95% CI 0.45–1.26) (Table 5).

Table 5. Association of 24-h urine oxalate excretion with death due to infection, malignancy and other causes.

	Continuous, per 1–SD		Tertile 1	Tertile 2		Tertile 3	
	HR	95% CI	Ref	HR	95% CI	HR	95% CI
Death due to infection							
Model 1	0.67	0.49–0.92	1.00	0.75	0.39–1.47	0.33	0.13–0.83
Model 2	0.58	0.40–0.83	1.00	0.75	0.38–1.49	0.31	0.12–0.79
Model 3	0.54	0.36–0.81	1.00	0.70	0.35–1.40	0.25	0.09–0.68
Model 4	0.56	0.38–0.82	1.00	0.65	0.32–1.30	0.23	0.09–0.63
Model 5	0.57	0.38–0.84	1.00	0.65	0.32–1.32	0.24	0.09–0.66
Model 6	0.56	0.38–0.83	1.00	0.62	0.31–1.26	0.25	0.09–0.67
Model 7	0.58	0.38–0.88	1.00	0.57	0.27–1.21	0.30	0.11–0.83
Death due to malignancy							
Model 1	1.01	0.69–1.50	1.00	1.31	0.54–3.17	0.78	0.28–2.20
Model 2	0.98	0.65–1.47	1.00	1.31	0.54–3.18	0.74	0.26–2.09
Model 3	1.02	0.68–1.53	1.00	1.50	0.60–3.77	0.84	0.29–2.45
Model 4	1.03	0.68–1.55	1.00	1.56	0.62–3.94	0.88	0.30–2.59
Model 5	1.08	0.71–1.62	1.00	1.44	0.56–3.71	0.95	0.32–2.81
Model 6	1.10	0.71–1.71	1.00	1.24	0.45–3.41	1.01	0.33–3.07
Model 7	1.14	0.73–1.77	1.00	1.08	0.36–3.8	1.18	0.37–3.71
Death due to other causes							
Model 1	0.76	0.48–1.21	1.00	0.63	0.23–1.71	070	26–1.89
Model 2	0.82	0.51–1.35	1.00	0.53	0.19–1.47	0.62	0.22–1.74
Model 3	0.77	0.45–1.29	1.00	0.59	0.21–1.65	0.43	0.13–1.41
Model 4	0.76	0.45–1.27	1.00	0.53	0.19–1.51	0.39	0.12–1.29
Model 5	0.76	0.46–1.28	1.00	0.53	0.19–1.51	0.39	0.12–1.29
Model 6	0.75	0.45–1.26	1.00	0.46	0.16–1.35	0.36	0.11–1.20
Model 7	0.96	0.56–1.63	1.00	0.64	0.19–2.19	0.75	0.20–2.74

Multivariate Cox regression were performed for the association of 24-h urinary oxalate excretion with death due to infection, malignancy and other causes. Model 1: age and sex adjusted. Model 2: Model 1 + adjustment for BMI, primary renal disease, donor age, transplant vintage, eGFR, and proteinuria. Model 3: Model 2 + adjustment for thiosulfate in 24-h urine. Model 4: Model 3 + adjustment for LDH in blood. Model 5: Model 4 + adjustment for pH of 24-h urine. Model 6: Model 5 + adjustment for FGF23. Model 7: Model 6 + adjustment for fruit and vegetables intake.

3.3.2. All-Cause and Infectious Mortality

A Kaplan-Meier curve for the association of tertiles of 24-h urinary oxalate excretion with all-cause mortality is shown in Figure 1F ($p = 0.06$, p for trend 0.02). Results of multivariate Cox regression analyses showed, however, that all-cause mortality is independently associated with 24-h urinary oxalate excretion (HR 0.77, 95% CI 0.63–0.94) (Table 4). Uni- and multivariate analyses of the associations of 24-h urinary oxalate excretion and potential confounders with all-cause mortality are shown in Table S2. The association of 24-h urinary oxalate excretion with all-cause mortality demonstrated a nonlinear relationship, as shown by a restricted cubic spline (Figure 2A).

A Kaplan-Meier curve for the association of tertiles of 24-h urinary oxalate excretion with infectious mortality is shown in Figure 1G ($p = 0.03$, p for trend 0.008). Results of multivariate Cox regression analyses showed infectious mortality was independently associated with 24-h urinary oxalate excretion

(HR 0.58, 95% CI 0.38–0.83) (Table 5). The association between 24-h urinary oxalate excretion and infectious mortality demonstrated a nonlinear relationship, as shown by a restricted cubic spline (Figure 2B).

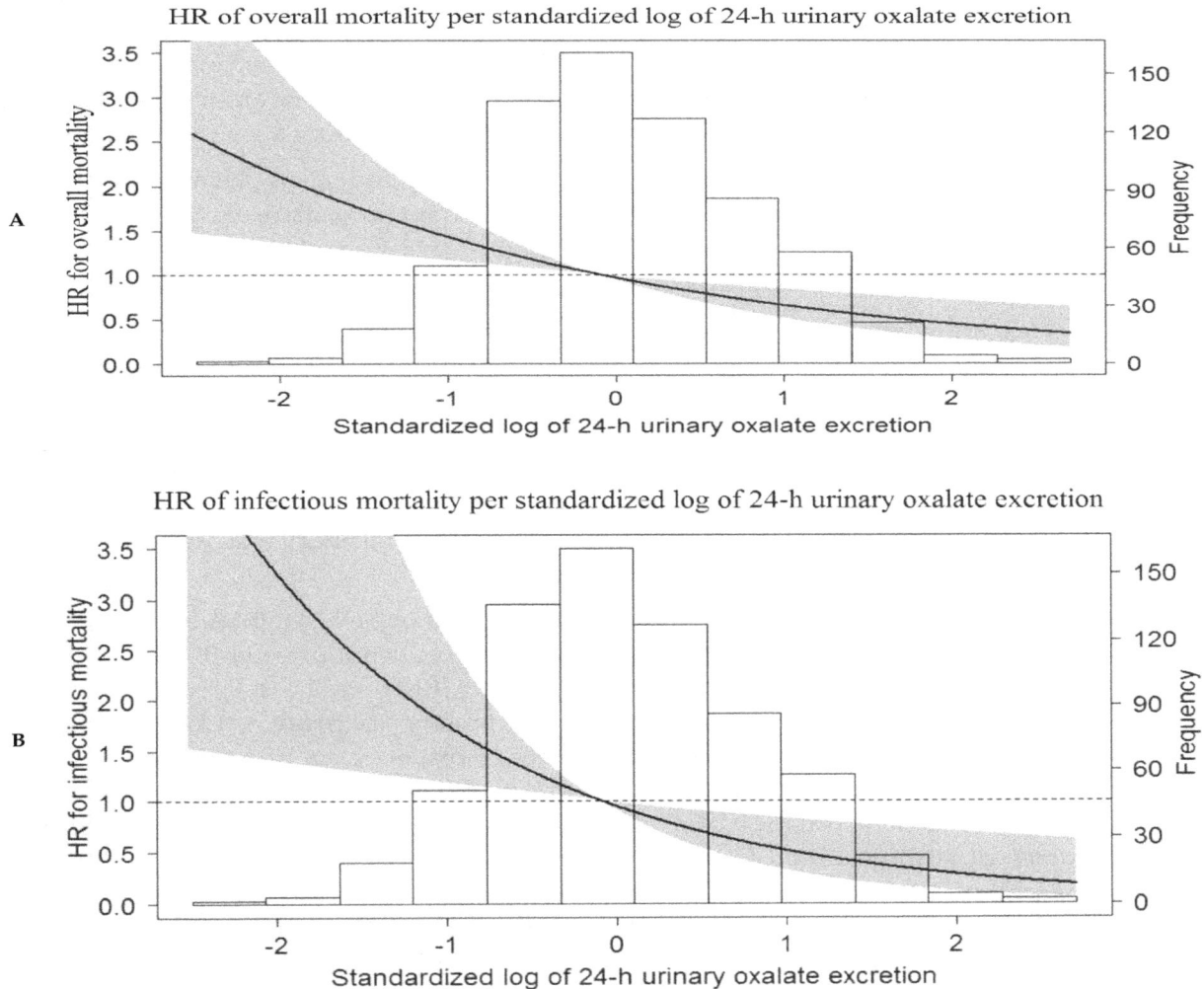

Figure 2. Adjusted association of standardized log 24–hour urinary oxalate excretion with (**A**) all-cause mortality, and (**B**) infectious mortality, based on restricted cubic spline regression, fitted with Model 6. The black line in the graph represents the HR, 95% CI is shown and the gray area.

3.4. Sensitivity Analyses

When we restricted the analyses to subjects with no potential over or undercollection of 24-h urine samples based on differences in expected and observed 24-h urinary creatinine excretions (n = 650), generally similar results were found for GF (HR 0.74, 95% CI 0.55–0.99), PTDM (HR 0.93, 95% CI 0.69–1.26), cardiovascular mortality (HR 0.68, 95% CI 0.47–0.98), mortality due to malignancies (HR 1.10, 95% CI 0.70–1.72), mortality due to miscellaneous causes (HR 0.71, 95% CI 0.41–1.24), all-cause mortality (HR 0.74; 95% CI 0.59–0.92), and infectious mortality (HR 0.58, 95% CI 0.37–0.89).

When competing risk analyses were performed, generally similar results were found for PTDM (HR 1.15, 95% CI 0.91–1.48), cardiovascular mortality (HR 0.82, 95% CI 0.55–1.23), mortality due to malignancies (HR 1.16, 95% CI 0.69–1.95), mortality due to miscellaneous causes (HR 0.84, 95% CI 0.54–1.31), and infectious mortality (HR 0.61, 95% CI 0.45–0.85). The risk of GF was not consistently significant (HR 1.14, 95% CI 0.64–2.26).

4. Discussion

In KTR, median excretion of 24-h oxalate was higher than the clinical cut-off point for hyperoxaluria. No association of 24-h urinary oxalate excretion was found with GF, PTDM, cardiovascular mortality, or mortality due to malignancy or miscellaneous causes, but an independent, inverse association with all-cause mortality and infectious mortality was found. There was respectively a 23% and 44% decrease in hazard ratio per standard deviation increase of 24-h urinary oxalate excretion. The associations remained materially unchanged after adjusting for potential confounders. The association with all-cause and infectious mortality remained materially unchanged after performing sensitivity analyses.

A single-centered prospective study had previously already found an elevated plasma oxalate level in KTR [44]. However, no previous study has provided data on oxalate excretion. The elevated urinary oxalate excretion reflects one of the major findings of this study, being that 44% of the stable KTR are within the clinical range of hyperoxaluria.

To the best of our knowledge, there have not been any previous studies investigating the association of urinary oxalate with GF, PTDM and (cause-specific) mortality in stable KTR. However, a recent study of Waikar et al. with CKD patients stage 2 to 4 found 24-h urinary oxalate excretion to be positively associated with all-cause mortality [14]. With regards to the study of Waikar et al., their first four quintiles can be considered to be below the range of hyperoxaluria of 455μmol/24-h, whereas in our population, only the first tertile can be considered normal with regard to urinary oxalate excretion. This, in part, might explain the difference in association of urinary oxalate excretion with the outcome variables.

The difference between Waikar et al.'s and our study cannot be explained by a higher BMI or diabetes contributing to hyperoxaluria through higher effective renal plasma flow and glomerular hyperfiltration in the Waikar et al. population (respectively, BMI of 32.1 ± 7.7 and 26.6 ± 4.8 and diabetes in 48.9% and 24% of the population) [45]. Low density lipoprotein (LDL) profile was not published in the Waikar et al. report, therefore, difference in oxalate excretion through dyslipidemia cannot be determined [46]. In both studies, the urinary samples were stored at −80 °C. Storage at this temperature can lead to underestimation of oxalate levels through calcium oxalate precipitation [14]. Since the difference of storage time of the samples until measurement is not known, we cannot exclude this as a potential clarification of the found difference. Additionally, spontaneous oxalate generation over the course of the storage might have increased the sample oxalate levels in either studies. Another hypothesis for the interesting difference in 24-h urinary oxalate excretion between the study of Waikar et al. might be found in the possible absence of *Oxalobacter formigenes* in the gut microbiome. KTR have been exposed to antimicrobial prophylactic therapies to lower the risk of opportunistic infections. This greatly affects the diversity of the human microbiome and can cause dysbiosis [47]. Dysbiosis in KTR could contribute to a decrease of *O. formigenes* and therefore, increased gastrointestinal absorption of oxalate, leading to an increased oxalate serum concentration and consequently, elevated urinary excretion.

We found no association with GF, PTDM, mortality due to malignancies, nor mortality due to miscellaneous causes. The results of the proportional hazards models show that the inverse overall association with mortality is mainly driven by infectious mortality. We hypothesized that because 24-h urinary oxalate excretion was positively associated with ascorbic acid, which is inversely associated with overall mortality in RTR through reducing inflammation, an increase in oxalate might contribute to a lower infectious mortality [48]. However, the exact mechanism behind the association of 24-h urinary oxalate excretion with infectious mortality remains to be further investigated, since to our knowledge, there are no studies available showing a potential theoretical explanation.

The strength of this study lays in its prospective design, with a large cohort of stable KTR who were closely monitored according to standardized protocols and continuous surveillance system according to the American Society of Transplantation without loss due to follow-up during a median follow-up of 5.4 years for (specific cause) mortality. The KTR were extensively phenotyped at baseline measurement, providing a broad array of potential confounders to adjust for. The inclusion of the FFQ gives the possibility to assess the associations with dietary intake, rather than just the urinary excretion. Furthermore, urine was collected as 24-h collecting samples, according to a previously described strict protocol, which eliminates possible daily variances in fluid balance and excretion to give a more accurate excretion estimate. Additionally, potential over- or undercollection of the 24-h urine samples was accounted for by means of sensitivity analyses, which showed that the results remained materially unchanged after restricting the study population as described previously.

However, we also acknowledge limitations of the current study. First, we were unable to adjust our results for socioeconomic status at baseline. Next, although the FFQ and SQUASH are validated questionnaires, they are self-reported, which may lead to possible over or underreporting of dietary intake and physical activity. We also acknowledge that our population consists almost entirely of Caucasian ethnicity, therefore, our results call for caution to extrapolate our results to different populations with regard to ethnicity. Finally, data on nephrolithiasis was not documented; therefore, we were unable to assess the association of urinary oxalate with the outcome nephrolithiasis, which remains a rather overlooked topic in KTR. Nevertheless, our results show for the first time a high prevalence of hyperoxaluria in the post-kidney transplant setting, thus emphasizing the need for future studies in which such analyses are performed. Additionally, because the study of the microbiome was beyond the scope of the current study, the hypothesized mechanism of increased gastrointestinal absorption of oxalate to explain the observed levels of hyperoxaluria cannot be further confirmed.

In conclusion, in stable KTR, 24-h urinary oxalate excretion is quantitatively higher than in the general population. Forty-four percent of the current study population showed urinary oxalate levels above the range of clinical hyperoxaluria. This hyperoxaluria might suggest a role of dysbiosis by leading to diminished *O. formigenes* and therefore, higher oxalate absorption and excretion in the current study population. Twenty-four-hour urinary oxalate excretion was not associated with risk of graft failure, post-transplant diabetes mellitus, cardiovascular mortality, mortality due to malignancies, nor death from miscellaneous causes. However, a consistent and independent inverse association was found with infectious mortality. Our data encourages further studies to validate our findings on the associations of oxalate with long-term outcomes in KTR. Future studies are warranted to investigate specific causes of death and the effect of hyperoxaluria post-kidney transplantation.

Author Contributions: Conceptualization, S.J.L.B.; data curation, E.v.d.B.; formal analysis, A.T. and C.G.S.; funding acquisition, C.G.S. and S.J.L.B.; investigation, A.T., C.G.S. and M.Y.S.; methodology, A.T., C.G.S., I.M., T.F., M.H.d.B., M.Y.S., G.J.N. and S.J.L.B.; project administration, S.P.B. and S.J.L.B.; software, M.Y.S.; supervision, C.G.S.; visualization, A.T. and S.J.L.B.; writing—original draft, A.T.; writing—review & editing, C.G.S., A.P., M.Y.S., R.M.D., R.R. and S.J.L.B.

Acknowledgments: This study is based on data of the TransplantLines Food and Nutrition Biobank Cohort Study (ClinicalTrials.gov Identifier: NCT02811835).

References

1. Abecassis, M.; Bartlett, S.T.; Collins, A.J.; Davis, C.L.; Delmonico, F.L.; Friedewald, J.J.; Hays, R.; Howard, A.; Jones, E.; Leichtman, A.B.; et al. Kidney transplantation as primary therapy for end-stage renal disease: A National Kidney Foundation/Kidney Disease Outcomes Quality Initiative (NKF/KDOQI^{TM}) conference. *Clin. J. Am. Soc. Nephrol.* **2008**, *3*, 471–480. [CrossRef] [PubMed]
2. Tonelli, M.; Wiebe, N.; Knoll, G.; Bello, A.; Browne, S.; Jadhav, D.; Klarenbach, S.; Gill, J. Systematic review: Kidney transplantation compared with dialysis in clinically relevant outcomes. *Am. J. Transplant.* **2011**, *11*, 2093–2109. [CrossRef] [PubMed]

3. Kim, W.R.; Lake, J.R.; Smith, J.M.; Schladt, D.P.; Skeans, M.A.; Harper, A.M.; Wainright, J.L.; Snyder, J.J.; Israni, A.K.; Kasiske, B.L. OPTN/SRTR 2016 Annual Data Report: Kidney. *Am. J. Transplant.* **2018**, *18*, 18–113. [CrossRef] [PubMed]

4. Einecke, G.; Sis, B.; Reeve, J.; Mengel, M.; Campbell, P.M.; Hidalgo, L.G.; Kaplan, B.; Halloran, P.F. Antibody-mediated microcirculation injury is the major cause of late kidney transplant failure. *Am. J. Transplant.* **2009**, *9*, 2520–2531. [CrossRef] [PubMed]

5. Eisenga, M.F.; Kieneker, L.M.; Soedamah-Muthu, S.S.; Van Den Berg, E.; Deetman, P.E.; Navis, G.J.; Gans, R.O.B.; Gaillard, C.A.J.M.; Bakker, S.J.L.; Joosten, M.M. Urinary potassium excretion, renal ammoniagenesis, and risk of graft failure and mortality in renal transplant recipients1-3. *Am. J. Clin. Nutr.* **2016**, *104*, 1703–1711. [CrossRef] [PubMed]

6. Minovic, I.; Van Der Veen, A.; Van Faassen, M.; Riphagen, I.J.; Van Den Berg, E.; Van Der Ley, C.; Gomes-Neto, A.W.; Geleijnse, J.M.; Eggersdorfer, M.; Navis, G.J.; et al. Functional Vitamin B-6 status and long-term mortality in renal transplant recipients. *Am. J. Clin. Nutr.* **2017**, *106*, 1366–1374. [CrossRef]

7. Howell, M.; Wong, G.; Rose, J.; Tong, A.; Craig, J.C.; Howard, K. Patient Preferences for Outcomes After Kidney Transplantation: A Best-Worst Scaling Survey. *Transplantation* **2017**, *101*, 2765–2773. [CrossRef]

8. Howell, M.; Tong, A.; Wong, G.; Craig, J.C.; Howard, K. Important outcomes for kidney transplant recipients: A nominal group and qualitative study. *Am. J. Kidney Dis.* **2012**, *60*, 186–196. [CrossRef]

9. Kasiske, B.L.; Snyder, J.J. Diabetes Mellitus after Kidney Transplantation in the United States. *Am. J. Transplant.* **2003**, *3*, 178–185. [CrossRef]

10. Stoumpos, S.; Jardine, A.G.; Mark, P.B. Cardiovascular morbidity and mortality after kidney transplantation. *Transplan. Int.* **2015**, *28*, 10–21. [CrossRef]

11. Chan, S.; Pascoe, E.M.; Clayton, P.A.; McDonald, S.P.; Lim, W.H.; Sypek, M.P.; Palmer, S.C.; Isbel, N.M.; Francis, R.S.; Campbell, S.B.; et al. Infection-Related Mortality in Recipients of a Kidney Transplant in Australia and New Zealand. *Clin. J. Am. Soc. Nephrol.* **2019**, *14*, 1484–1492. [CrossRef] [PubMed]

12. Sprangers, B.; Nair, V.; Launay-Vacher, V.; Riella, L.V.; Jhaveri, K.D. Risk factors associated with post-kidney transplant malignancies: An article from the Cancer-Kidney International Network. *Clin. Kidney J.* **2018**, *11*, 315–329. [CrossRef] [PubMed]

13. Wolfe, R.A.; Roys, E.C.; Merion, R.M. Trends in organ donation and transplantation in the United States, 1999-2008: Special feature. *Am. J. Transplant.* **2010**, *10*, 961–972. [CrossRef] [PubMed]

14. Waikar, S.S.; Srivastava, A.; Palsson, R.; Shafi, T.; Hsu, C.; Sharma, K.; Lash, J.P.; Chen, J.; He, J.; Lieske, J.; et al. Association of Urinary Oxalate Excretion With the Risk of Chronic Kidney Disease Progression. *JAMA Intern. Med.* **2019**, *179*, 542–551. [CrossRef] [PubMed]

15. Williams, H.; Wandzilak, T. Oxalate synthesis, transport and the hyperoxaluric syndromes. *J. Urol.* **1989**, *141*, 742–747. [CrossRef]

16. Eisenga, M.F.; Gomes-Neto, A.W.; Van Londen, M.; Ziengs, A.L.; Douwes, R.M.; Stam, S.P.; Osté, M.C.J.; Knobbe, T.J.; Hessels, N.R.; Buunk, A.M.; et al. Rationale and design of TransplantLines: A prospective cohort study and biobank of solid organ transplant recipients. *BMJ Open* **2018**, *8*, 1–13. [CrossRef]

17. Kasiske, B.L.; Vazquez, M.A.; Harmon, W.E.; Brown, R.S.; Danovitch, G.M.; Gaston, R.S.; Roth, D.; Scandling, J.D. Recommendations for the Outpatient Surveillance of Renal Transplant Recipients. *J. Am. Soc. Nephrol.* **2000**, *11*, 1–86.

18. Abbasi, A.; Peelen, L.M.; Corpeleijn, E.; Van Der Schouw, Y.T.; Stolk, R.P.; Spijkerman, A.M.W.; Van Der A, D.L.; Moons, K.G.M.; Navis, G.; Bakker, S.J.L.; et al. Prediction models for risk of developing type 2 diabetes: Systematic literature search and independent external validation study. *Br. Med. J.* **2012**, *345*, e5900. [CrossRef]

19. 2. Classification and diagnosis of diabetes. *Diabetes Care* **2017**, *40*, S11–S24. [CrossRef]

20. van den Berg, E.; Engberink, M.F.; Brink, E.J.; van Baak, M.A.; Gans, R.O.B.; Navis, G.; Bakker, S.J.L. Dietary protein, blood pressure and renal function in renal transplant recipients. *Br. J. Nutr.* **2013**, *109*, 1463–1470. [CrossRef]

21. Bohlen, A.; Boll, M.; Schwarzer, M.; Groneberg, D.A. Body-Mass-Index. *Diabetologe* **2015**, *11*, 331–345. [CrossRef]

22. Levey, A.S.; Stevens, L.A.; Schmid, C.H.; Zhang, Y.L.; Iii, A.F.C.; Feldman, H.I.; Kusek, J.W.; Eggers, P.; Van Lente, F.; Greene, T. A New Equation to Estimate Glomerular Filtration Rate. *Ann. Intern. Med.* **2009**, *150*, 604–612. [CrossRef] [PubMed]

23. Wendel-Vos, G.C.W.; Schuit, A.J.; Saris, W.H.M.; Kromhout, D. Reproducibility and relative validity of the short questionnaire to assess health-enhancing physical activity. *J. Clin. Epidemiol.* **2003**, *56*, 1163–1169. [CrossRef]

24. Willett, W.C.; Sampson, L.; Stampfer, M.J.; Rosner, B.; Bain, C.; Witschi, J.; Hennekens, C.H.; Speizer, F.E. Reproducibility and validity of a semiquantitative food frequency questionnaire. *Am. J. Epidemiol.* **1985**, *122*, 51–65. [CrossRef]

25. Feunekes, G.I.J.; Van Staveren, W.A.; De Vries, J.H.M.; Burema, J.; Hautvast, J.G.A.J. Relative and biomarker-based validity of a food-frequency questionnaire estimating intake of fats and cholesterol. *Am. J. Clin. Nutr.* **1993**, *58*, 489–496. [CrossRef]

26. Voorlichtingsbureau voor de Voeding Stichting, N. *Nederlands Voedingsstoffen Bestand: NEVO Tabel 2006, Dutch Nutrient Database*; NEVO Foundation: Zeist, The Netherlands, 2006.

27. Willett, W.C.; Howe, R. Adjustmentfor total energyintake in epidemiologic studies. *Am. J. Clin. Nutr.* **1997**, *65*, 1220S–1228S. [CrossRef]

28. Newton, G.L.; Dorian, R.; Fahey, R.C. Analysis of Biological Thiols: Derivatization with Monobromobimane and Separation by Reverse-Phase High-Performacne Liquid Chromatography. *Anal. Biochem.* **1981**, *387*, 383–387. [CrossRef]

29. Ohana, E.; Shcheynikov, N.; Moe, O.W.; Muallem, S. SLC26A6 and NaDC-1 Transporters Interact to Regulate Oxalate and Citrate Homeostasis. *J. Am. Soc. Nephrol.* **2013**, *24*, 1617–1626. [CrossRef]

30. Gee, H.Y.; Jun, I.; Braun, D.A.; Lawson, J.A.; Halbritter, J.; Shril, S.; Nelson, C.P.; Tan, W.; Stein, D.; Wassner, A.J.; et al. Mutations in SLC26A1 Cause Nephrolithiasis. *Am. J. Hum. Genet.* **2016**, *98*, 1228–1234. [CrossRef]

31. Zhao, Z.; Mai, Z.; Ou, L.; Duan, X.; Zeng, G. Serum Estradiol and Testosterone Levels in Kidney Stones Disease with and without Calcium Oxalate Components in Naturally Postmenopausal Women. *PLoS ONE* **2013**, *8*, e75513. [CrossRef]

32. Fan, J.; Chandhoke, P.; Grampsas, S. Role of sex hormones in experimental calcium oxalate nephrolithiasis. *J. Am. Soc. Nephrol.* **1999**, *10*, S376–S380. [PubMed]

33. Hirata, T.; Gallo, C.J.R.; Dow, J.A.T.; Landry, G.M.; Anderson, J.B.; Romero, M.F.; Cabrero, P. Sulfate and thiosulfate inhibit oxalate transport via a dPrestin (Slc26a6)-dependent mechanism in an insect model of calcium oxalate nephrolithiasis. *Am. J. Physiol. Ren. Physiol.* **2015**, *310*, F152–F159.

34. Herman, H.H.; Hagler, L. Oxalate Metabolism I. *Am. J. Clin. Nutr.* **1973**, *26*, 758–765.

35. Wanger, C.A.; Mohebbi, N. Urinary pH and Stone Formation. *J. Nephrol.* **2010**, *23*, 165–169.

36. Jüppner, H. Phosphate and FGF-23. *Kidney Int.* **2011**, *79*, 25–28. [CrossRef]

37. Martin, A.; David, V.; Quarles, L.D. Regulation and Function of the FGF23/Klotho Endocrine Pathways. *Physiol. Rev.* **2012**, *93*, 131–155. [CrossRef]

38. Knight, J.; Madduma-Liyanage, K.; Mobley, J.A.; Assimos, D.G.; Holmes, R.P. Ascorbic acid intake and oxalate synthesis. *Urolithiasis* **2016**, *44*, 289–297. [CrossRef]

39. Taylor, E.N.; Curhan, G.C. Determinants of 24-hour urinary oxalate excretion. *Clin. J. Am. Soc. Nephrol.* **2008**, *3*, 1453–1460. [CrossRef]

40. Meschi, T.; Maggiore, U.; Fiaccardori, E.; Schianchi, T.; Bosi, S.; Giuditta, A.; Ridolo, E.; Guerra, A.; Allegri, F.; Novarine, A.; et al. The effect of fruits and vegetables on urinary stone risk factors. *Kidney Int.* **2004**, *66*, 2402–2410. [CrossRef]

41. Kieneker, L.M.; Bakker, S.J.L.; de Boer, R.A.; Navis, G.J.; Gansevoort, R.T.; Joosten, M.M. Low potassium excretion but not high sodium excretion is associated with increased risk of developing chronic kidney disease. *Kidney Int.* **2016**, *90*, 888–896. [CrossRef]

42. Cockcroft, D.W.; Gault, M.H. Prediction of creatinine clearance from serum creatinine. *Nephron* **1976**, *16*, 31–41. [CrossRef] [PubMed]

43. Fine, J.P.; Gray, R.J. A Proportional Hazards Model for the Subdistribution of a Competing Risk. *J. Am. Stat. Assoc.* **1999**, *94*, 496–509. [CrossRef]

44. Elgstoen, K.B.P.; Johnsen, L.F.; Woldseth, B.; Morkrid, L.; Hartmann, A. Plasma oxalate following kidney transplantation in patients without primary hyperoxaluria. *Nephrol Dial. Transplant.* **2010**, *25*, 2341–2345. [CrossRef] [PubMed]

45. Xue, C.; Zhou, C.; Xu, J.; Zhang, L.; Yu, S. Is urinary oxalate inversely correlated with glomerular filtration rate in chronic kidney disease? *Ren Fail.* **2019**, *41*, 439. [CrossRef]

46.	Masterson, J.H.; Woo, J.R.; Chang, D.C.; Chi, T.; L'Esperance, J.O.; Stoller, M.L.; Sur, R.L. Dyslipidemia is associated with an increased risk of nephrolithiasis. *Urolithiasis* **2014**, *43*, 49–53. [CrossRef]

47.	Bhalodi, A.A.; Van Engelen, T.S.R.; Virk, H.S.; Wiersinga, W.J. Impact of antimicrobial therapy on the gut microbiome. *J. Antimicrob. Chemother.* **2019**, *74*, I6–I15. [CrossRef]

48.	Sotomayor, C.G.; Eisenga, M.F.; Gomes Neto, A.W.; Ozyilmaz, A.; Gans, R.O.B.; De Jong, W.H.A.; Zelle, D.M.; Berger, S.P.; Gaillard, C.A.G.M.; Navis, G.J.; et al. Vitamin C depletion and all-cause mortality in renal transplant recipients. *Nutrients* **2017**, *9*, 568. [CrossRef]

14

Conversion from Standard-Release Tacrolimus to MeltDose® Tacrolimus (LCPT) Improves Renal Function after Liver Transplantation

Johannes von Einsiedel [1,†], Gerold Thölking [2,*,†], Christian Wilms [1], Elena Vorona [1], Arne Bokemeyer [1], Hartmut H. Schmidt [1], Iyad Kabar [1,‡] and Anna Hüsing-Kabar [1,‡]

[1] Department of Medicine B, Gastroenterology and Hepatology, University Hospital Münster, 48149 Münster, Germany; johannes.voneinsiedel@ukmuenster.de (J.v.E.); Christian.Wilms@ukmuenster.de (C.W.); Elena.Vorona@ukmuenster.de (E.V.); Arne.Bokemeyer@ukmuenster.de (A.B.); hepar@ukmuenster.de (H.H.S.); iyad.kabar@ukmuenster.de (I.K.); Anna.Huesing-Kabar@ukmuenster.de (A.H.-K.)

[2] Department of Internal Medicine and Nephrology, University Hospital of Münster Marienhospital Steinfurt, 48565 Steinfurt, Germany

* Correspondence: Gerold.Thoelking@ukmuenster.de

† These authors contributed equally and are both considered first authors.

‡ These authors contributed equally and are both considered last authors.

Abstract: Renal impairment is a typical side effect of tacrolimus (Tac) treatment in liver transplant (LT) recipients. One strategy to avoid renal dysfunction is to increase the concentration/dose (C/D) ratio by improving drug bioavailability. LT recipients converted from standard-release Tac to MeltDose® Tac (LCPT), a novel technological formulation, were able to reduce the required Tac dose due to higher bioavailability. Hence, we hypothesize that such a conversion increases the C/D ratio, resulting in a preservation of renal function. In the intervention group, patients were switched from standard-release Tac to LCPT. Clinical data were collected for 12 months after conversion. Patients maintained on standard-release Tac were enrolled as a control group. Twelve months after conversion to LCPT, median C/D ratio had increased significantly by 50% ($p < 0.001$), with the first significant increase seen 3 months after conversion ($p = 0.008$). In contrast, C/D ratio in the control group was unchanged after 12 months (1.75 vs. 1.76; $p = 0.847$). Estimated glomerular filtration rate (eGFR) had already significantly deteriorated in the control group at 9 months (65.6 vs. 70.6 mL/min/1.73 m^2 at study onset; $p = 0.006$). Notably, patients converted to LCPT already had significant recovery of mean eGFR 6 months after conversion (67.5 vs. 65.3 mL/min/1.73 m^2 at study onset; $p = 0.029$). In summary, conversion of LT recipients to LCPT increased C/D ratio associated with renal function improvement.

Keywords: MeltDose®; LCPT; tacrolimus; renal function; liver transplantation; C/D ratio; metabolism

1. Introduction

The calcineurin inhibitor tacrolimus (Tac) is considered a first-line immunosuppressant in liver transplant (LT) recipients [1–4]. Because of its small therapeutic window, therapy with Tac requires close drug monitoring [5]. In addition, deterioration of renal function induced by acute or chronic calcineurin inhibitor nephrotoxicity (CNIT) is a common side effect [6]. Recent studies have reported characteristics of chronic CNIT in up to 70% of LT recipients [7,8]. Furthermore, up to 8.5% of patients develop end-stage renal disease in long-term follow-up [9].

Several studies have revealed that the risk of CNIT is associated with both high Tac trough concentration and high daily Tac dose [10,11], although CNIT may occur even with low-dose regimens [12]. One potential explanation for this association is the correlation between CNIT and a fast metabolism rate of twice-daily immediate-release Tac (IR-Tac). The Tac blood concentration to daily dose ratio (C/D ratio) has been identified as a simple tool to describe patients' metabolism rate in a steady state, in which a low C/D ratio reflects a high rate of metabolism [13–15]. A low IR-Tac C/D ratio is linked with higher C2 Tac blood concentrations despite comparable trough levels in patients with high C/D ratios [16]. In this regard, a low C/D ratio is strongly associated with an increased risk of CNIT and a faster decline of renal function in both kidney transplant (KT) and LT recipients [13,16–19]. Thus, increasing the C/D ratio by improving Tac bioavailability may result in better nephroprotection. One way of potentially influencing the pharmacokinetics of Tac is to change the formulation of the drug [20].

LCPT is a novel Tac formulation using MeltDose® technology, in which the particle size of the drug is reduced from 10 μm to the smallest possible units (<0.1 μm), resulting in increased dissolution and thus better absorption [21]. This feature, combined with drug release over the entire intestinal tract, results in LCPT having significantly better bioavailability than other Tac formulations. Tremblay et al. showed that the intraday peak-to-trough fluctuation was approximately 30% lower for LCPT than for standard-release Tac (IR-Tac and once- daily extended-release Tac (ER-Tac)) [20]. A dose reduction of up to 30% has been observed in KT and LT recipients on LCPT [22].

Hence, we hypothesize that conversion from standard-release Tac to LCPT increases C/D ratio and thereby preserves renal function.

2. Materials and Methods

2.1. Patients and Study Design

Figure 1 illustrates the enrolment of the subjects in the study. This observational study was performed on patients who had undergone cadaveric liver transplantation at the University Hospital of Münster. LT recipients were included at the time of presentation at our Outpatient Transplant Clinic between March 2017 and August 2018. The study start was defined as the first appointment in this period.

At this time point, the treating physicians made a decision to either leave the patients on their usual immunosuppressive treatment (control group) or to switch them from standard-release Tac (IR- or ER-Tac) to LCPT (intervention group). Data were analysed over a 12-month follow-up. Inclusion criteria were aged over 18 years, intake of standard-release Tac before enrolment, stable graft function and an interval between transplantation and inclusion in the study of at least 1 month. LT recipients were not allowed to receive any medications or agents that could interfere with Tac. The decision about drug conversion was made by treating physicians at their own discretion.

The initial immunosuppressive regimen consisted of Tac (Prograf or Advagraf), mycophenolate mofetil (CellCept, MMF) and prednisolone (Decortin H/Soludecortin H). Tac was given at a dose of 0.1 mg/kg twice daily with a target trough concentration of 8–10 ng/mL during the first month, 6–8 ng/mL from months 2 to 3, and 3–5 ng/mL thereafter. MMF was started at a dose of 1 g twice daily and was adjusted in case of adverse effects. Initial prednisolone was given at a dose of 250 mg once daily intravenously before and immediately after LTx and was tapered stepwise. In most cases, prednisolone had been discontinued within 6–12 months after LTx.

Laboratory data were collected at study onset (at the time of conversion to LCPT or the first presentation during the above-mentioned period in the control group (t_0)) and after 3 (t_3), 6 (t_6), 9 (t_9) and 12 (t_{12}) months. Serum bilirubin, alanine transaminase (ALT) and international normalized ratio (INR) were measured to assess graft function. General demographic data and information on transplantation and diagnoses were obtained from the patient records.

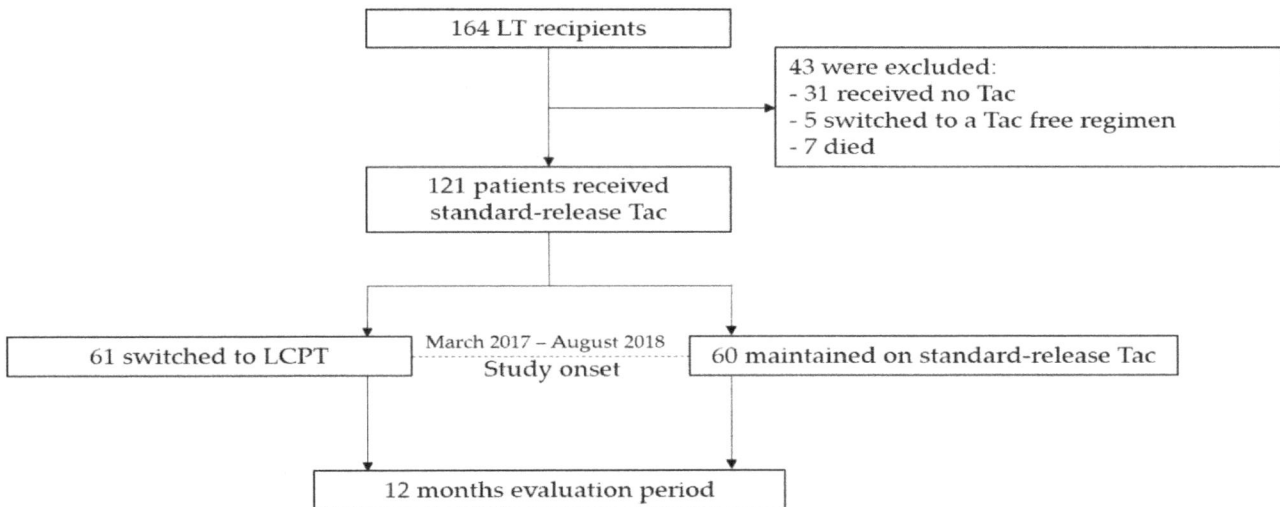

Figure 1. Study design and patient enrolment. A total of 164 liver transplant (LT) recipients were screened for eligibility. Only LT recipients who were started on IR- or ER-Tac (standard-release tacrolimus) and continued taking this drug until the beginning of the study were included. During the enrolment period (March 2017–August 2018), 121 patients met the inclusion criteria and were either switched to LCPT (once-daily MeltDose® tacrolimus (Tac); intervention group) or maintained on standard-release tacrolimus (control group). Clinical data were analysed in a 12-month follow-up. We hypothesized that conversion from standard-release Tac to LCPT increases concentration/dose (C/D) ratio and thereby preserves renal function

The C/D ratio, calculated as the ratio of Tac trough level to the corresponding daily dose, was determined 3 months before study start, at the study start and at subsequent evaluation time points. The t_0 C/D ratio in the intervention group was determined the day before first LCPT intake. Renal function was calculated using the estimated glomerular filtration rate (eGFR) in accordance with the Chronic Kidney Disease Epidemiology Collaboration equation at the corresponding time points. The difference from baseline eGFR (t_0) was determined at the time points of t_3, t_6, t_9 and t_{12}. A negative value indicates deterioration of eGFR, while a positive value indicates improvement.

The study was conducted in accordance with current medical guidelines and the Declarations of Istanbul and Helsinki. The study was also approved by the local ethics committee (Ethik Kommission der Ärztekammer Westfalen-Lippe und der Medizinischen Fakultät der Westfälischen Wilhelms-Universität Münster, No. 2016-046-f-S). Collected patient data were anonymized and written consent for collection and use of the clinical data was obtained.

2.2. Statistical Analysis

Statistical analysis was performed with IBM SPSS® Statistics 25 for Windows (IBM Corporation, Somers, NY, USA). Normally distributed data are shown as mean ± standard deviation; non-normally distributed data are shown as median (minimum–maximum). For unrelated groups, normally distributed data were compared with a t-test, non-normally distributed data with the Mann–Whitney U-test and categorical variables with Fisher's exact test. Comparison of continuous variables within a connected group was performed with the Wilcoxon signed-rank test. Pearson's test was used to describe normally distributed data, whereas Spearman's test was applied to non-normally distributed data. In all statistical evaluations, two-sided tests were used; a p-value of ≤ 0.05 was considered significant for all tests performed.

The study onset was defined as the baseline (t_0). In the first approach, eGFR changes (t_3-t_{12}) from baseline were compared between the intervention group and the control group. In the next step, eGFR changes from every time point to baseline were compared within each group (eGFR slope).

A negative value indicates deterioration in eGFR, whereas a positive value indicates an improvement in renal function.

Multivariable analysis was performed to identify independent predictors of alterations in renal function (ΔeGFR) after 12 months compared with that at baseline. For this purpose, univariable analysis with factors known to potentially influence renal function was initially performed. Variables that showed a p-value < 0.15 in univariable analysis were included in the multivariable analysis. Variables with a significance of <0.05 in multivariable analysis were considered significant.

3. Results

3.1. Study Population

A total of 121 patients were included in this study: 61 in the intervention group and 60 in the control group. An overview of patient characteristics, underlying diagnoses for LTx, comorbidities and immunosuppression is shown in Tables 1 and 2. There were only small differences in the demographic data between the study groups. The control group had a more extended warm ischemic time ($p = 0.005$). As coimmunosuppression, patients received mycophenolate mofetil (MMF) at a daily dose of 1000 (500–2000) mg (LCPT) and 1500 (500–2000) mg (control), everolimus at 2.0 (0.5–5.0) mg (LCPT) and 2.0 (2.0–4.0) mg (control), prednisolone at 5.0 (5.0–7.5) mg (LCPT and control) and sirolimus at 1.0 mg (control). In the intervention group, 45 patients suffered from chronic kidney disease (CKD, categories 2–4). The control group showed a similar distribution in 39 LT recipients. No patients were in CKD category 5 or on dialysis. In the absence of kidney biopsies, the underlying renal disease remained unclear. The median interval between transplantation and study onset was 2.8 (0.1–20.8) years in the intervention group and 6.6 (0.2–16.5) years in the control group ($p < 0.001$). The reasons for a conversion from standard-release Tac to LCPT were CNIT (n = 7), neurotoxicity (n = 5) and prevention of side effects via better bioavailability of LCPT (n = 49).

Table 1. Patient characteristics.

	LCPT (n = 61)	Standard-Release Tac (n = 60)	p-Value
Age at LTx (years)	46.3 ± 16.7	48.8 ± 12.4	0.348 [a]
Age at study onset (years)	51.0 ± 15.9	56.1 ± 12.7	0.054 [a]
Height (m)	1.72 ± 0.087	1.73 ± 0.094	0.714 [a]
Weight (kg)	79.4 ± 20.8	76.7 ± 16.5	0.420 [a]
BMI (kg/m^2)	26.7 ± 6.1	25.6 ± 5.0	0.310 [a]
Sex (male/female)	29 (47.5%)/32 (52.5%)	38 (63.3%)/22 (36.7%)	0.101 [b]
CIT (h)	11.3 ± 2.6	10.5 ± 2.4	0.065 [a]
WIT (min)	38.9 ± 9.2	43.8 ± 8.7	0.005 [a]
Number of grafts			0.255 [b]
One	56 (91.8%)	49 (81.7%)	
Two	4 (6.6%)	8 (13.3%)	
Three	1 (1.6%)	3 (5.0%)	
Blood type			0.545 [b]
A	28 (47.5%)	30 (50.0%)	
B	6 (10.2%)	6 (10.0%)	
AB	6 (10.2%)	2 (3.3%)	
O	19 (32.2%)	22 (36.7%)	
Hepatitis B antigen (positive)	5 (8.2%)	7 (11.9%)	0.556 [b]
Hepatitis C antibody (positive)	9 (14.8%)	8 (13.6%)	1.000 [b]
Recipient CMV IgG (positive)	34 (57.6%)	27 (45.0%)	0.201 [b]
Donor CMV IgG (positive)	32 (56.1%)	37 (63.8%)	0.450 [b]

Statistics: Values shown as mean ± standard deviation or number (percentage). [a] t-test, [b] Fisher's exact test. LCPT, once-daily MeltDose® tacrolimus; Tac, tacrolimus; LTx, liver transplantation; BMI, body mass index; CIT, cold ischemic time; WIT, warm ischemic time; CMV, cytomegalovirus.

Table 2. Underlying diagnoses for LTx, comorbidities and immunosuppression at study start.

	LCPT (n = 61)	Standard-Release Tac (n = 60)	p-Value
Principal diagnosis			0.455
Alcoholism	9 (14.8%)	16 (26.7%)	
Viral hepatitis	15 (24.6%)	15 (25.0%)	
Genetically related metabolic disease	7 (11.5%)	5 (8.3%)	
Toxic: nutritional or NASH	3 (4.9%)	1 (1.7%)	
Autoimmune liver disease	11 (18.0%)	13 (21.7%)	
Other	16 (26.2%)	10 (16.7%)	
Arterial hypertension	36 (59.0%)	37 (61.7%)	0.853
Diabetes mellitus	18 (29.5%)	17 (28.3%)	1.000
Hyperlipidaemia	19 (31.1%)	14 (23.3%)	0.415
CKD at study start			0.598
CKD 2	18 (29.5%)	21 (35.0%)	
CKD 3a	16 (26.2%)	10 (16.7%)	
CKD 3b	9 (14.8%)	7 (11.7%)	
CKD 4	2 (3.3%)	1 (1.7%)	
Tac formulation at study onset			<0.001
Immediate-release Tac	43 (70.5%)	22 (36.7%)	
Extended-release Tac	18 (29.5%)	38 (63.3%)	
Co-immunosuppression			0.060
MMF	34 (55.7%)	35 (58.3%)	
Everolimus	13 (21.3%)	5 (8.3%)	
Prednisolone	3 (4.9%)	10 (16.7%)	
Sirolimus	0	1 (1.7%)	
None	11 (18.0%)	9 (15.0%)	
Reasons for a switch to LCPT			
CNIT	7		
Neurotoxicity	5		
Preventions of side effects	49		

Statistics: Values shown as number (percentage). All p-values from Fisher's exact tests. LCPT, once-daily MeltDose® tacrolimus; Tac, tacrolimus; LTx, liver transplantation; NASH, nonalcoholic steatohepatitis; CKD, chronic kidney disease (categories set with reference to [23]). MMF, mycophenolate mofetil; CNIT, calcineurin inhibitor nephrotoxicity.

3.2. C/D Ratio

At study start (baseline), the C/D ratio in the intervention group was comparable to that in the control group (1.68 (0.30–13.45) vs. 1.76 (0.38–7.40) ng/mL×1/mg, respectively; $p = 0.362$, Table 3). During the 12-month evaluation period, no significant changes in the C/D ratio were observed in the control group. After 12 months, the median C/D ratio was approximately at the baseline level (1.75 (0.49–6.40) ng/mL × 1/mg; $p = 0.847$). In the control group, there was a slight decrease in both the daily Tac dose at study end compared with that at baseline (2.5 (0.5–10.0) vs. 2.8 (0.5–10.0) mg, respectively; $p = 0.084$), as well as in the median Tac trough level (4.7 (1.5–14.3) ng/mL at study onset to 4.1 (1.6–15.6) ng/mL after 12 months; $p = 0.082$). However, the differences in both cases were not significant.

In contrast, the C/D ratio in patients switched to LCPT was 50% higher 12 months after conversion than that at baseline (2.52 (0.58–6.40) vs. 1.68 (0.30–13.45) ng/mL × 1/mg, respectively; $p < 0.001$). A significant increase in the C/D ratio was already observed in this group 3 months after study onset (2.03 (0.33–13.60) ng/mL × 1/mg; $p = 0.008$). Regarding the daily Tac dose, a significant reduction of 33.3% was observed after 12 months compared with that at baseline (2.0 (0.4–7.8) vs. 3.0 (1.0–22.0) mg, respectively; $p < 0.001$)). Moreover, the Tac trough level was significantly reduced at study end (4.4 (2.2–11.8) vs. 6.0 (1.5–26.9) ng/mL at study onset; $p < 0.001$).

To confirm that conditions were stable before study onset, C/D ratios, Tac doses and trough level 3 months before enrolment were also obtained. There were no significant differences between the groups at t_3 (Table 3) nor between study start and 3 months earlier within a group. Patients in the intervention group showed similar median C/D ratio compared with that at baseline (1.44 (0.24–6.20) vs. 1.68 (0.30–13.45) ng/mL × 1/mg, respectively; $p = 0.204$). Daily Tac dose differed significantly due to single outlier values shortly after transplant (3.0 (0.5–12.0) (t_{-3}) vs. 3.0 (1.0–22.0) (t_0) mg; $p = 0.049$), while Tac trough level showed no considerable differences (5.0 (2.4–15.3) (t_{-3}) vs. 6.0 (1.5–26.9) (t_0) ng/mL; $p = 0.722$).

No significant differences were detectable in the control group between baseline and 3 months before: C/D ratio (1.69 (0.40–9.20) vs. 1.76 (0.38–7.40) ng/mL × 1/mg, respectively; $p = 0.626$), Tac daily dose (2.5 (0.5–9.0) vs. 2.8 (0.5–10.0) mg, respectively; $p = 0.362$) and Tac trough level (4.4 (1.5–14.7) vs. 4.7 (1.5–14.3) ng/mL, respectively; $p = 0.742$).

Table 3. Tacrolimus concentration/dose (C/D) ratio, daily dose and blood trough concentration.

	LCPT	Standard-Release Tac	p-Value
Tac C/D ratio (ng/mL × 1/mg)			
3 months before (n = 54 vs. 58)	1.44 (0.24–6.20) on s-r-Tac	1.69 (0.40–9.20)	0.344
At study onset (n = 61 vs. 60)	1.68 (0.30–13.45) on s-r-Tac	1.76 (0.38–7.40)	0.362
After 3 months (n = 61 vs. 60)	2.03 (0.33–13.60)	1.83 (0.41–7.00)	0.735
After 6 months (n = 61 vs. 60)	2.33 (0.77–8.47)	1.63 (0.68–7.40)	0.011
After 9 months (n = 61 vs. 60)	2.13 (0.60–9.33)	1.70 (0.54–7.20)	0.136
After 12 months (n = 61 vs. 60)	2.52 (0.58–6.40)	1.75 (0.49–6.40)	0.009
Tac daily dose (mg)			
3 months before (n = 54 vs. 58)	3.0 (0.5–12.0) on s-r-Tac	2.5 (0.5–9.0)	0.056
At study onset (n = 61 vs. 60)	3.0 (1.0–22.0) on s-r-Tac	2.8 (0.5–10.0)	0.044
After 3 months (n = 61 vs. 60)	2.0 (0.8–8.0)	2.5 (0.5–9.0)	0.330
After 6 months (n = 61 vs. 60)	2.0 (0.8–5.0)	2.5 (0.5–7.0)	0.248
After 9 months (n = 61 vs. 60)	2.0 (0.4–6.0)	2.5 (0.5–9.0)	0.060
After 12 months (n = 61 vs. 60)	2.0 (0.4–7.8)	2.5 (0.5–10.0)	0.047
Tac trough level (ng/mL)			
3 months before (n = 54 vs. 58)	5.0 (2.4–15.3) on s-r-Tac	4.4 (1.5–14.7)	0.087
At study onset (n = 61 vs. 60)	6.0 (1.5–26.9) on s-r-Tac	4.7 (1.5–14.3)	0.005
After 3 months (n = 61 vs. 60)	4.6 (0.5–13.1)	4.4 (2.2–10.4)	0.863
After 6 months (n = 61 vs. 60)	4.7 (1.5–12.7)	4.1 (2.0–10.9)	0.022
After 9 months (n = 61 vs. 60)	4.3 (1.5–15.1)	4.0 (1.9–10.1)	0.867
After 12 months (n = 61 vs. 60)	4.4 (2.2–11.8)	4.1 (1.6–15.6)	0.283

To confirm that conditions were stable before enrolment, values 3 months prior to study onset are given for all patients who had already undergone liver transplantation (n = 54 vs. 58). In the intervention group (LCPT), values 3 months before and the day before the first LCPT intake (study onset) were determined when s-r-Tac was administered. LCPT, once-daily MeltDose® tacrolimus; Tac, tacrolimus; s-r-Tac, standard-release tacrolimus. p-values from Mann–Whitney U-test.

As shown in Figure 2, the C/D ratio at study end was significantly higher in patients on LCPT than in the control group (2.52 (0.58–6.40) vs. 1.75 (0.49–6.40) ng/mL × 1/mg, respectively; $p = 0.009$). The median Tac trough level and the daily dose were significantly higher in the intervention group at study onset (Table 3). After 12-month follow-up, the Tac dose in the LCPT group was significantly reduced compared with that in the control group (2.0 (0.4–7.8) vs. 2.5 (0.5–10.0) mg, respectively; $p = 0.047$). However, the Tac trough level was comparable in the two groups at study end (4.4 (2.2–11.8) vs. 4.1 (1.6–15.6) ng/mL, respectively; $p = 0.283$).

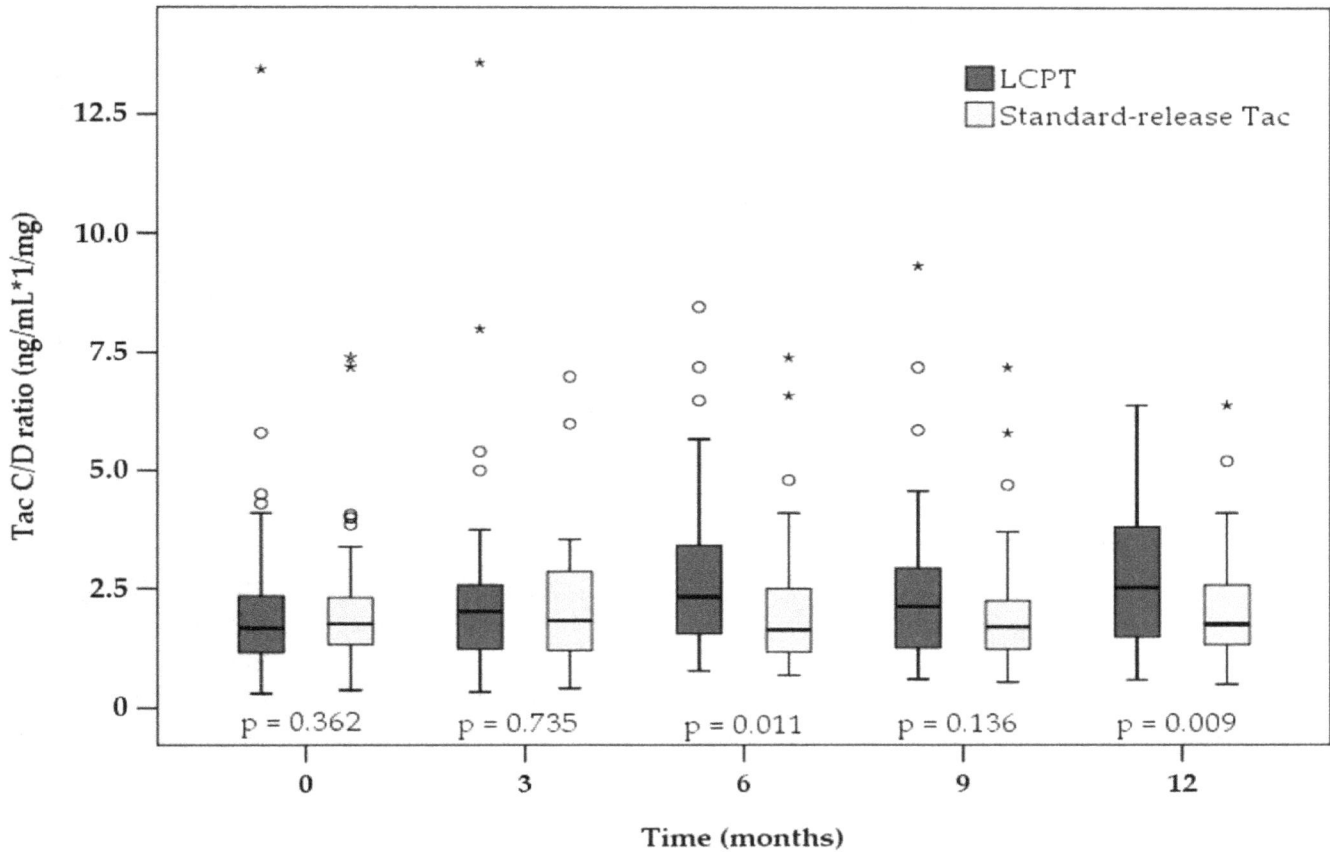

Figure 2. Boxplots of C/D ratio among patients receiving LCPT (dark grey) or standard-release Tac (light brown) at baseline and 3, 6, 9 and 12 months later. There were significant differences between the two study groups at 6 and 12 months after conversion. p-values reflect differences between the groups at each time point.

3.3. Renal Function

At baseline (study onset, t_0), patients in the control group had a higher mean eGFR than patients switched to LCPT (Figure 3), although the difference (ΔeGFR) was not significant ($p = 0.157$). However, mean ΔeGFR in patients on LCPT had significantly improved at 6 months after conversion ($p = 0.029$). In contrast, patients on standard-release Tac showed a significant decline of mean ΔeGFR 9 months after study initiation ($p = 0.006$). Over the 12-month evaluation period, mean ΔeGFR continued to improve significantly in patients receiving LCPT ($p = 0.001$), whereas mean ΔeGFR continued to deteriorate in the control group ($p < 0.001$). In a pairwise comparison between the groups, eGFR values did not differ significantly (Supplementary Table S1).

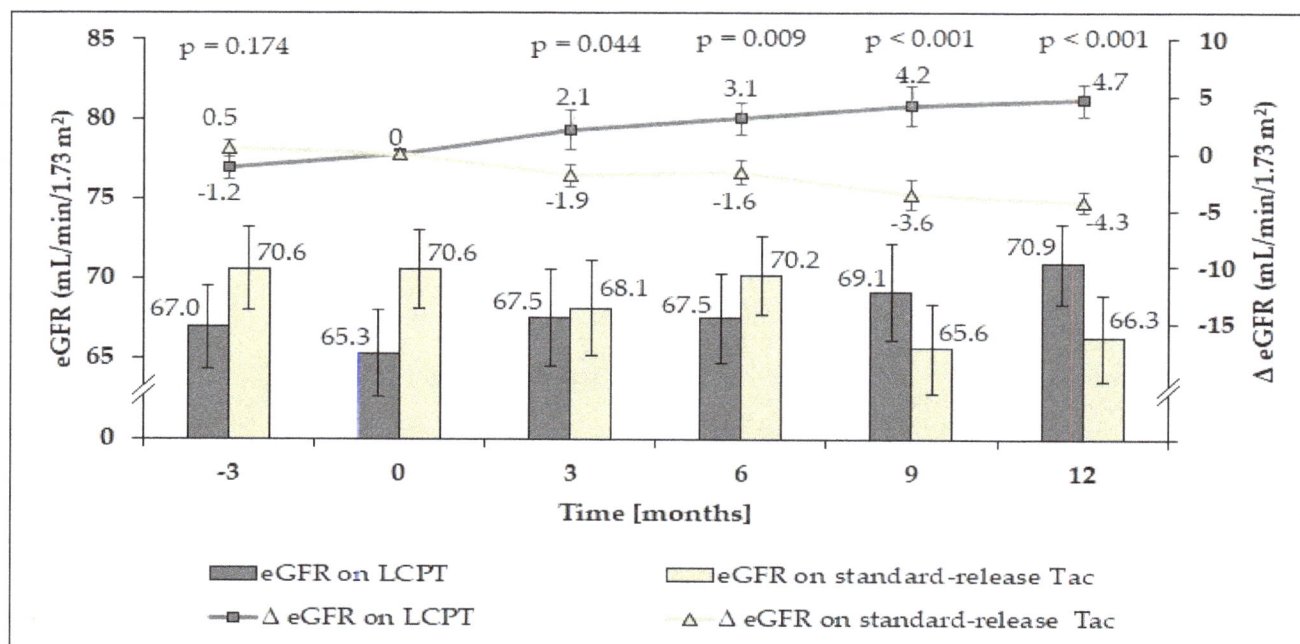

Figure 3. Glomerular filtration rate (eGFR; mL/min/1.73 m^2) over time and the difference from baseline at each time point (ΔeGFR ± SEM) in each study group. Improved renal function with a significantly increased mean ΔeGFR was already observed 3 months after conversion to LCPT (dark grey). *p*-values reflect comparison of ΔeGFR between the study groups.

While absolute eGFR values are meaningful to only a limited extent, eGFR slope (ΔeGFR) relative to the baseline can be used as additional empirical support (Table 4). Three months before study onset, there were no significant differences within the study groups relative to baseline. In the intervention group, renal function increased 6 months after conversion ($p = 0.029$). In contrast, LT recipients in the control group showed a significant decline of eGFR 9 months after study initiation ($p = 0.006$). Over the 12-month evaluation period, renal function continued to significantly improve in patients receiving LCPT ($p = 0.001$), whereas eGFR continued to deteriorate in the control group ($p < 0.001$).

Table 4. Slope analysis (ΔeGFR) of glomerular filtration rate (eGFR; mL/min/1.73 m^2).

Time Point	Estimate	95% Confidence Limit		*p*-Value
		Lower	Upper	
LCPT				
−3 months vs. baseline	−1.2	−3.2	0.8	0.223
3 months vs. baseline	2.1	−1.3	5.5	0.219
6 months vs. baseline	3.1	0.3	6.0	0.029
9 months vs. baseline	4.2	0.8	7.6	0.015
12 months vs. baseline	4.7	1.9	7.5	0.001
Standard-release Tac				
−3 months vs. baseline	0.5	−1.0	1.9	0.547
3 months vs. baseline	−1.9	−3.9	0.0	0.053
6 months vs. baseline	−1.6	−3.8	0.6	0.154
9 months vs. baseline	−3.6	−6.1	−1.1	0.006
12 months vs. baseline	−4.3	−6.2	−2.3	<0.001

The "estimate" value describes the difference between the respective time point and the baseline (ΔeGFR). A negative value shows a decline and a positive value an improvement of eGFR. LCPT, once-daily MeltDose® tacrolimus; Tac, tacrolimus; *p*-values within a group are relative to the baseline.

In further analysis, the eGFR values of the patients suffering from diabetes mellitus and arterial hypertension were compared between the groups.

At every time point, patients with diabetes mellitus had significantly lower eGFR than patients without it, regardless of the study group (Table 5). However, eGFR among diabetic patients recovered in a manner similar to that of nondiabetics upon switching to LCPT. In contrast, renal function deteriorated in patients maintained on standard-release Tac in a similar fashion, regardless of diabetes.

Table 5. Glomerular filtration rate (eGFR; mL/min/1.73 m^2) in diabetic and nondiabetic patients.

Time Point	LCPT			Standard-Release Tac		
	Diabetics (n = 18)	Non-Diabetics (n = 43)	p-Value	Diabetics (n = 17)	Non-Diabetics (n = 43)	p-Value
t_0	52.6 ± 21.3	70.3 ± 19.0	0.003	56.0 ± 20.3	76.3 ± 15.6	<0.001
t_3	56.2 ± 21.2	72.3 ± 20.0	0.013	51.2 ± 17.6	74.9 ± 18.1	<0.001
t_6	56.3 ± 19.2	73.0 ± 18.4	0.004	56.5 ± 20.3	75.5 ± 15.1	<0.001
t_9	57.1 ± 22.1	74.4 ± 17.7	0.007	53.2 ± 22.2	71.5 ± 16.5	0.002
t_{12}	56.3 ± 19.5	77.2 ± 13.4	<0.001	49.9 ± 22.5	72.7 ± 16.6	<0.001

LCPT, once-daily MeltDose® tacrolimus; Tac, tacrolimus; t_0 to t_{12}, time points (months). eGFR values shown as mean ± standard deviation. p-values from t-test.

Patients with arterial hypertension in both study groups had a lower mean eGFR than patients with normal blood pressure at each time point (Table 6). However, renal function recovered in patients treated with LCPT and deteriorated in those maintained on standard-release Tac over the course of the study, regardless of the presence of arterial hypertension.

Table 6. Glomerular filtration rate (eGFR; mL/min/1.73 m^2) in patients with and without arterial hypertension.

Time Point	LCPT			Standard-Release Tac		
	Arterial Hypertension (n = 36)	Normal Blood Pressure (n = 25)	p-Value	Arterial Hypertension (n = 37)	Normal Blood Pressure (n = 23)	p-Value
t_0	59.3 ± 20.7	74.3 ± 18.7	0.006	66.8 ± 21.0	76.6 ± 14.5	0.056
t_3	63.4 ± 22.4	73.1 ± 19.2	0.111	64.6 ± 22.4	74.2 ± 16.7	0.121
t_6	62.6 ± 20.1	74.2 ± 18.5	0.038	65.5 ± 20.4	77.6 ± 12.7	0.015
t_9	65.1 ± 19.9	74.7 ± 20.7	0.120	63.2 ± 21.8	70.4 ± 16.3	0.222
t_{12}	66.7 ± 17.0	76.9 ± 18.3	0.042	61.2 ± 22.4	74.5 ± 15.6	0.015

LCPT, once-daily MeltDose® tacrolimus; Tac, tacrolimus; t_0 to t_{12}, time points (months). eGFR values shown as mean ± standard deviation. p-values from t-test.

Multivariable analysis was performed to identify independent predictors of alterations in renal function expressed as ΔeGFR (Supplementary Table S2). Conversion to LCPT was the only identified independent predictor of significant changes in eGFR.

3.4. Liver Function

During the entire follow-up, we monitored the graft function (Table 7). LT recipients in the LCPT group showed significantly lower serum bilirubin concentrations than the control group at all time points. However, the median values in both study groups remained within the lower part of the normal range throughout the course of the study. Regarding the parameters ALT and INR, no differences were observed between the groups.

Table 7. Assessment of liver function over time in each study group.

	LCPT (n = 61)	Standard-Release Tac (n = 60)	p-Value
Bilirubin (mg/dL)			
At study onset	0.4 (0.2–1.3)	0.6 (0.2–2.0)	0.001
After 3 months	0.4 (0.2–2.2)	0.5 (0.2–4.0)	0.006
After 6 months	0.4 (0.2–1.2)	0.6 (0.2–2.1)	0.010
After 9 months	0.4 (0.2–1.2)	0.5 (0.2–1.9)	0.001
After 12 months	0.5 (0.2–1.2)	0.6 (0.2–2.7)	0.011
ALT (U/L)			
At study onset	20 (8–102)	21 (9–117)	0.431
After 3 months	24 (8–78)	22 (10–140)	0.348
After 6 months	20 (6–92)	18 (8–448)	0.406
After 9 months	20 (7–202)	20 (7–138)	0.997
After 12 months	20 (9–104)	20 (7–380)	0.696
INR			
At study onset	1.0 (0.9–2.2)	1.0 (0.9–1.6)	0.765
After 3 months	1.0 (0.9–2.3)	1.0 (0.9–1.3)	0.871
After 6 months	1.0 (0.9–1.3)	1.0 (0.9–1.6)	0.969
After 9 months	1.0 (0.9–1.3)	1.0 (0.9–1.5)	0.634
After 12 months	1.0 (0.9–1.3)	1.0 (0.9–1.5)	0.217

LCPT, once-daily MeltDose® tacrolimus; Tac, tacrolimus; ALT, alanine transaminase; INR, international normalized ratio; p-values from Mann–Whitney U-test.

4. Discussion

The present study shows that the conversion of LT recipients from standard-release Tac to LCPT was beneficial in regard to renal function. This may be due to the improved bioavailability of LCPT which led to a significant increase in C/D ratio.

Notably, the median daily Tac dose declined by 33.3% among LT recipients after conversion. A dose reduction of approximately 30% with a comparable area under the curve (AUC) was reported in recent studies of KT and LT recipients [20,24,25]. In those studies, this finding was also attributed to the greater bioavailability of LCPT.

In our cohort, the median C/D ratio among LT recipients who switched to LCPT had increased by 50% at 12 months after conversion. The C/D ratio among patients maintained on standard-release Tac remained unchanged over the 12-month period. In accordance with these data, Franco et al. described a 35% increase in the C/D ratio among KT recipients after conversion from IR-Tac and a 83.3% increase among those who were switched from ER-Tac to LCPT [26]. In the study by Rostaing et al., KT recipients had a 20% higher C/D ratio 12 months after conversion to LCPT and a 24.4% higher C/D ratio 24 months after conversion [27]. In contrast, Kamińska et al. showed that the C/D ratio of KT recipients converted from IR-Tac to ER-Tac did not change significantly [28]. To our knowledge, the present study is the first to describe a significant increase in the C/D ratio after a switch to LCPT among LT recipients.

In a previous study, we explored the impact of the C/D ratio on renal function after kidney transplantation (KTx) [14]. Fast metabolizers, defined as patients with a C/D ratio < 1.05 ng/mL × 1/mg, showed a strong association with decreased renal function compared with slow metabolizers in a 24-month follow-up. Similar results were confirmed among LT recipients in a 36-month follow-up study [13]. In that cohort, the cut-off value for fast metabolizers was defined as a C/D ratio < 1.09 ng/mL × 1/mg. In a 5-year follow-up, KT recipients with a lower Tac C/D ratio showed a higher risk of renal impairment as well as higher mortality rates [17]. Recently, several studies confirmed these findings [19,29,30] and a further negative impact of fast Tac metabolism on increased kidney allograft rejection rates and BK virus infections was demonstrated [17,18,31].

Given these results, we postulated that a higher C/D ratio after conversion to LCPT is associated with nephroprotection. Surprisingly, we already observed significant improvement of renal function 6 months after conversion. Twelve months after conversion, the mean ΔeGFR was 4.7 mL/min/1.73 m^2 higher than at baseline. In contrast, eGFR had deteriorated significantly in patients maintained on standard-release Tac 9 months after study onset and ΔeGFR had decreased by 4.3 mL/min/1.73 m^2 at 12 months.

After conversion to LCPT, the median trough level declined from 6.0 ng/mL at study onset to 4.6 ng/mL (month 3) without a subsequent decrease until month 12. A lower Tac trough level in the LCPT group has already been reported in a prospective study, although the same target trough level was given [27]. Alongside better bioavailability of LCPT, trough level reduction might be another reason for the increase in renal function. However, median trough levels did not vary considerably between subsequent time points (t_3–t_{12}) while renal function showed further recovery. Notably, median Tac trough levels were also slightly reduced in the control group (t_0–t_{12}), although eGFR showed further decline over the 12-month follow-up. Therefore, we postulate that improvement of bioavailability and a reduced peak Tac level after conversion to LCPT are factors more relevant to the increase in eGFR than the reduction in Tac trough levels alone.

As an explanation for the nephroprotective potential of LCPT, Schütte-Nütgen et al. hypothesized that a lower daily Tac dose results in a lower peak serum concentration (C_{max}), which in turn reduces the side effects of Tac overdosing within the first hours after drug intake [17]. In a review article on LT recipients, Baraldo reported that LCPT had a similar AUC after 24 h and a similar minimal blood concentration (C_{min}), but had a significantly lower C_{max} and a smaller C_{max}/C_{min} fluctuation ratio when compared with IR-Tac [32]. In addition, Bunnadaprist et al. postulated that there is a reduced cumulative Tac dose in KT recipients receiving LCPT [33]. In a recent study, we also showed that fast metabolizers with a C/D ratio < 1.05 ng/mL × 1/mg had significantly higher Tac blood concentrations than slow metabolizers 2 h after Tac intake [16]. In the same study, we showed that a low C/D ratio was significantly associated with acute CNIT. Although renal biopsy is not routinely performed in LT recipients, we can assume that patients converted to LCPT suffered less frequently from CNIT. In contrast, Kamar et al. reported similar renal function in de novo KTx recipients who were randomized to LCPT or ER-Tac in a 4-week follow-up [34]. Notably, C_{min} and AUC_{0-24} were slightly higher in the LCPT group (at days 3, 7 and 14), a fact that might have influenced the results.

In the current study, the control group had an increased warm ischemic time (WIT) compared with the intervention group (~5 min). Prolonged cold and warm ischemic times can be associated with long-term allograft dysfunction [32]. Nevertheless, at the beginning of our study, the liver function parameters ALT and INR did not differ between the groups and median bilirubin was within the normal range. In a study by Laskey et al., increasing WIT during LTx was associated with a lack of renal recovery in the presence of pretransplant subacute kidney injury [35]. It was concluded that minimization of WIT could potentially avoid renal replacement therapy or the need for subsequent kidney transplantation. At the study start in our cohort, the control group showed even higher eGFR values despite increased WIT compared with the intervention group. Notably, the control group had a more extended interval between LTx and study onset than patients switched to LCPT (6.6 (0.2–16.5) vs.2.8 (0.1–20.8) years, respectively).

In regard to the Tac formulations used before study onset, IR-Tac was administered more frequently than ER-Tac in the intervention group and vice versa in the control group. A recent study on pharmacokinetics in a large transplant cohort showed similar Tac trough levels and bioavailability between these two formulations [36]. Notably, C/D ratio as well as C/D intrapatient variability was reported not to change considerably during conversion from IR-Tac to ER-Tac in KT recipients [28]. These findings justify our and others' approach of including patients taking either one of these formulations [19,29].

In the current study, patients suffering from diabetes mellitus or arterial hypertension had reduced renal function. Interestingly, patients who were switched to LCPT (median C/D ratio increased from 1.68 to 2.52 ng/mL × 1/mg) showed considerable recovery of eGFR independent of the presence of both conditions. In accordance with these findings, Bardou et al. showed that slow Tac metabolizers (C/D ratio > 1.8 ng/mL × 1/mg) were less likely to suffer from diabetes and hypertension after LTx [37].

Finally, we recognize that our study has limitations due to its retrospective design and the limited sample size from a single-centre. In addition, in this study, we cannot provide Tac C_{max}, C_2 (2 h after Tac intake) nor AUC, although higher C_{max} or C_2 could potentially induce higher CNIT. Therefore, we can only hypothesize that, after conversion to LCPT, lower C_2 was a more relevant factor to the improvement of renal function than trough level reduction. Further investigations should also include data on the concentrations of different Tac metabolites, which could be responsible for adverse effects, such as CNIT, infections and myelotoxicity [38,39]. Furthermore, given the retrospective design of this study, the study beginning in the control group had a wide range from March 2017 until August 2018 and the time period from LTx to the beginning of the study was significantly increased compared with that in the intervention group. The longer Tac exposure in the control group might have had a negative influence on renal function in this cohort. However, at t_0, the control group showed even higher eGFR values than patients converted to LCPT (70.6 ± 19.3 vs. 65.3 ± 21.1, respectively).

Another limitation of the study is that the reasons for conversion to LCPT in our study were taken only from the clinical reports from our Outpatient Transplant Clinic. In addition, in contrast to the case for KTx recipients, renal biopsy is not routinely performed in LT recipients which limits our ability to analyse CNIT before study onset.

5. Conclusions

To the best of our knowledge, this is the first study to show that conversion from standard-release Tac to LCPT increases the C/D ratio in LT recipients associated with renal recovery. This finding was independent of known risk factors for renal impairment. Prospective studies are needed to confirm our findings.

Author Contributions: Conceptualization, J.v.E., G.T., I.K. and A.H.-K.; Methodology, J.v.E., G.T., I.K. and A.H.-K.; Formal analysis, J.v.E., G.T., A.B., I.K. and A.H.-K.; Investigation, J.v.E., G.T., I.K. and A.H.-K.; Resources, H.H.S., I.K. and A.H.-K.; Data curation, J.v.E., G.T., I.K., C.W. and A.H.-K.; Writing—original draft preparation, J.v.E., G.T., I.K. and A.H.-K.; writing—review and editing, C.W., E.V., A.B. and H.H.S.; Visualization, J.v.E. and I.K.; Supervision, J.v.E., G.T., I.K. and A.H.-K.; Project administration, H.H.S., I.K. and A.H.-K.; funding acquisition, J.v.E., E.V. and I.K. All authors have read and agreed to the published version of the manuscript.

References

1. Wiesner, R.H.; Fung, J.J. Present state of immunosuppressive therapy in liver transplant recipients. *Liver Transpl.* **2011**, *17* (Suppl. S3), S1–S9. [CrossRef]
2. McAlister, V.C.; Haddad, E.; Renouf, E.; Malthaner, R.A.; Kjaer, M.S.; Gluud, L.L. Cyclosporin versus tacrolimus as primary immunosuppressant after liver transplantation: A meta-analysis. *Am. J. Transplant.* **2006**, *6*, 1578–1585. [CrossRef] [PubMed]
3. European Association for the Study of the Liver. EASL Clinical Practice Guidelines: Liver transplantation. *J. Hepatol.* **2016**, *64*, 433–485. [CrossRef] [PubMed]
4. O'Grady, J.G.; Hardy, P.; Burroughs, A.K.; Elbourne, D.; UK and Ireland Liver Transplant Study Group. Randomized controlled trial of tacrolimus versus microemulsified cyclosporin (TMC) in liver transplantation: Poststudy surveillance to 3 years. *Am. J. Transplant.* **2007**, *7*, 137–141. [CrossRef] [PubMed]
5. Naesens, M.; Kuypers, D.R.; Sarwal, M. Calcineurin inhibitor nephrotoxicity. *Clin. J. Am. Soc. Nephrol.* **2009**, *4*, 481–508. [CrossRef] [PubMed]

6. Beckebaum, S.; Cicinnati, V.R.; Radtke, A.; Kabar, I. Calcineurin inhibitors in liver transplantation - still champions or threatened by serious competitors? *Liver Int.* **2013**, *33*, 656–665. [CrossRef] [PubMed]

7. Ziolkowski, J.; Paczek, L.; Senatorski, G.; Niewczas, M.; Oldakowska-Jedynak, U.; Wyzgal, J.; Sanko-Resmer, J.; Pilecki, T.; Zieniewicz, K.; Nyckowski, P.; et al. Renal function after liver transplantation: Calcineurin inhibitor nephrotoxicity. *Transplant. Proc.* **2003**, *35*, 2307–2309. [CrossRef]

8. Afonso, R.C.; Hidalgo, R.; Zurstrassen, M.P.; Fonseca, L.E.; Pandullo, F.L.; Rezende, M.B.; Meira-Filho, S.P.; Ferraz-Neto, B.H. Impact of renal failure on liver transplantation survival. *Transplant. Proc.* **2008**, *40*, 808–810. [CrossRef]

9. Gonwa, T.A.; Mai, M.L.; Melton, L.B.; Hays, S.R.; Goldstein, R.M.; Levy, M.F.; Klintmalm, G.B. End-stage renal disease (ESRD) after orthotopic liver transplantation (OLTX) using calcineurin-based immunotherapy: Risk of development and treatment. *Transplantation* **2001**, *72*, 1934–1939. [CrossRef]

10. Kuypers, D.R.; de Jonge, H.; Naesens, M.; Lerut, E.; Verbeke, K.; Vanrenterghem, Y. CYP3A5 and CYP3A4 but not MDR1 single-nucleotide polymorphisms determine long-term tacrolimus disposition and drug-related nephrotoxicity in renal recipients. *Clin. Pharmacol. Ther.* **2007**, *82*, 711–725. [CrossRef]

11. Kershner, R.P.; Fitzsimmons, W.E. Relationship of FK506 whole blood concentrations and efficacy and toxicity after liver and kidney transplantation. *Transplantation* **1996**, *62*, 920–926. [CrossRef] [PubMed]

12. Tsuchiya, T.; Ishida, H.; Tanabe, T.; Shimizu, T.; Honda, K.; Omoto, K.; Tanabe, K. Comparison of pharmacokinetics and pathology for low-dose tacrolimus once-daily and twice-daily in living kidney transplantation: Prospective trial in once-daily versus twice-daily tacrolimus. *Transplantation* **2013**, *96*, 198–204. [CrossRef] [PubMed]

13. Tholking, G.; Siats, L.; Fortmann, C.; Koch, R.; Husing, A.; Cicinnati, V.R.; Gerth, H.U.; Wolters, H.H.; Anthoni, C.; Pavenstadt, H.; et al. Tacrolimus Concentration/Dose Ratio is Associated with Renal Function After Liver Transplantation. *Ann. Transplant.* **2016**, *21*, 167–179. [CrossRef] [PubMed]

14. Tholking, G.; Fortmann, C.; Koch, R.; Gerth, H.U.; Pabst, D.; Pavenstadt, H.; Kabar, I.; Husing, A.; Wolters, H.; Reuter, S.; et al. The tacrolimus metabolism rate influences renal function after kidney transplantation. *PLoS ONE* **2014**, *9*, e111128. [CrossRef] [PubMed]

15. Rancic, N.; Dragojevic-Simic, V.; Vavic, N.; Kovacevic, A.; Segrt, Z.; Draskovic-Pavlovic, B.; Mikov, M. Tacrolimus concentration/dose ratio as a therapeutic drug monitoring strategy: The influence of gender and comedication. *Vojnosanit. Pregl.* **2015**, *72*, 813–822. [CrossRef] [PubMed]

16. Tholking, G.; Schutte-Nutgen, K.; Schmitz, J.; Rovas, A.; Dahmen, M.; Bautz, J.; Jehn, U.; Pavenstadt, H.; Heitplatz, B.; Van Marck, V.; et al. A Low Tacrolimus Concentration/Dose Ratio Increases the Risk for the Development of Acute Calcineurin Inhibitor-Induced Nephrotoxicity. *J. Clin. Med.* **2019**, *8*, 1586. [CrossRef]

17. Schutte-Nutgen, K.; Tholking, G.; Steinke, J.; Pavenstadt, H.; Schmidt, R.; Suwelack, B.; Reuter, S. Fast Tac Metabolizers at Risk (-) It is Time for a C/D Ratio Calculation. *J. Clin. Med.* **2019**, *8*, 587. [CrossRef]

18. Egeland, E.J.; Robertsen, I.; Hermann, M.; Midtvedt, K.; Storset, E.; Gustavsen, M.T.; Reisaeter, A.V.; Klaasen, R.; Bergan, S.; Holdaas, H.; et al. High Tacrolimus Clearance Is a Risk Factor for Acute Rejection in the Early Phase After Renal Transplantation. *Transplantation* **2017**, *101*, e273–e279. [CrossRef]

19. Nowicka, M.; Gorska, M.; Nowicka, Z.; Edyko, K.; Edyko, P.; Wislicki, S.; Zawiasa-Bryszewska, A.; Strzelczyk, J.; Matych, J.; Kurnatowska, I. Tacrolimus: Influence of the Posttransplant Concentration/Dose Ratio on Kidney Graft Function in a Two-Year Follow-Up. *Kidney Blood Press. Res.* **2019**, *44*, 1075–1088. [CrossRef]

20. Tremblay, S.; Nigro, V.; Weinberg, J.; Woodle, E.S.; Alloway, R.R. A Steady-State Head-to-Head Pharmacokinetic Comparison of All FK-506 (Tacrolimus) Formulations (ASTCOFF): An Open-Label, Prospective, Randomized, Two-Arm, Three-Period Crossover Study. *Am. J. Transplant.* **2017**, *17*, 432–442. [CrossRef]

21. Grinyo, J.M.; Petruzzelli, S. Once-daily LCP-Tacro MeltDose tacrolimus for the prophylaxis of organ rejection in kidney and liver transplantations. *Expert Rev. Clin. Immunol.* **2014**, *10*, 1567–1579. [CrossRef] [PubMed]

22. Garnock-Jones, K.P. Tacrolimus prolonged release (Envarsus(R)): A review of its use in kidney and liver transplant recipients. *Drugs* **2015**, *75*, 309–320. [CrossRef] [PubMed]

23. Levin, A.; Stevens, P.E. Summary of KDIGO 2012 CKD Guideline: Behind the scenes, need for guidance, and a framework for moving forward. *Kidney Int.* **2014**, *85*, 49–61. [CrossRef] [PubMed]

24. DuBay, D.A.; Teperman, L.; Ueda, K.; Silverman, A.; Chapman, W.; Alsina, A.E.; Tyler, C.; Stevens, D.R. Pharmacokinetics of Once-Daily Extended-Release Tacrolimus Tablets Versus Twice-Daily Capsules in De Novo Liver Transplant. *Clin. Pharmacol. Drug Dev.* **2019**, *8*, 995–1008. [CrossRef] [PubMed]

25. Alloway, R.R.; Eckhoff, D.E.; Washburn, W.K.; Teperman, L.W. Conversion from twice daily tacrolimus capsules to once daily extended-release tacrolimus (LCP-Tacro): Phase 2 trial of stable liver transplant recipients. *Liver Transpl.* **2014**, *20*, 564–575. [CrossRef] [PubMed]

26. Franco, A.; Mas-Serrano, P.; Balibrea, N.; Rodriguez, D.; Javaloyes, A.; Diaz, M.; Gascon, I.; Ramon-Lopez, A.; Perez-Contreras, J.; Selva, J.; et al. Envarsus, a novelty for transplant nephrologists: Observational retrospective study. *Nefrologia* **2019**, *39*, 506–512. [CrossRef]

27. Rostaing, L.; Bunnapradist, S.; Grinyo, J.M.; Ciechanowski, K.; Denny, J.E.; Silva, H.T., Jr.; Budde, K.; Envarsus Study, G. Novel Once-Daily Extended-Release Tacrolimus Versus Twice-Daily Tacrolimus in De Novo Kidney Transplant Recipients: Two-Year Results of Phase 3, Double-Blind, Randomized Trial. *Am. J. Kidney Dis.* **2016**, *67*, 648–659. [CrossRef]

28. Kaminska, D.; Poznanski, P.; Kuriata-Kordek, M.; Zielinska, D.; Mazanowska, O.; Koscielska-Kasprzak, K.; Krajewska, M. Conversion From a Twice-Daily to a Once-Daily Tacrolimus Formulation in Kidney Transplant Recipients. *Transplant. Proc.* **2020**. [CrossRef]

29. Jouve, T.; Fonrose, X.; Noble, J.; Janbon, B.; Fiard, G.; Malvezzi, P.; Stanke-Labesque, F.; Rostaing, L. The TOMATO study (TacrOlimus MetabolizAtion in kidney TransplantatiOn): Impact of the concentration-dose ratio on death-censored graft survival. *Transplantation* **2019**. [CrossRef]

30. Kwiatkowska, E.; Kwiatkowski, S.; Wahler, F.; Gryczman, M.; Domanki, L.; Marchelk-Mysliwiec, M.; Ciechanowski, K.; Drozd-Dabrowska, M. C/D Ratio in Long-Term Renal Function. *Transplant. Proc.* **2019**, *51*, 3265–3270. [CrossRef]

31. Tholking, G.; Schmidt, C.; Koch, R.; Schuette-Nuetgen, K.; Pabst, D.; Wolters, H.; Kabar, I.; Husing, A.; Pavenstadt, H.; Reuter, S.; et al. Influence of tacrolimus metabolism rate on BKV infection after kidney transplantation. *Sci. Rep.* **2016**, *6*, 32273. [CrossRef] [PubMed]

32. Baraldo, M. Meltdose Tacrolimus Pharmacokinetics. *Transplant. Proc.* **2016**, *48*, 420–423. [CrossRef]

33. Bunnapradist, S.; Rostaing, L.; Alloway, R.R.; West-Thielke, P.; Denny, J.; Mulgaonkar, S.; Budde, K. LCPT once-daily extended-release tacrolimus tablets versus twice-daily capsules: A pooled analysis of two phase 3 trials in important de novo and stable kidney transplant recipient subgroups. *Transpl. Int.* **2016**, *29*, 603–611. [CrossRef] [PubMed]

34. Kamar, N.; Cassuto, E.; Piotti, G.; Govoni, M.; Ciurlia, G.; Geraci, S.; Poli, G.; Nicolini, G.; Mariat, C.; Essig, M.; et al. Pharmacokinetics of Prolonged-Release Once-Daily Formulations of Tacrolimus in De Novo Kidney Transplant Recipients: A Randomized, Parallel-Group, Open-Label, Multicenter Study. *Adv. Ther.* **2019**, *36*, 462–477. [CrossRef]

35. Laskey, H.L.; Schomaker, N.; Hung, K.W.; Asrani, S.K.; Jennings, L.; Nydam, T.L.; Gralla, J.; Wiseman, A.; Rosen, H.R.; Biggins, S.W. Predicting renal recovery after liver transplant with severe pretransplant subacute kidney injury: The impact of warm ischemia time. *Liver Transpl.* **2016**, *22*, 1085–1091. [CrossRef] [PubMed]

36. Lu, Z.; Bonate, P.; Keirns, J. Population pharmacokinetics of immediate- and prolonged-release tacrolimus formulations in liver, kidney and heart transplant recipients. *Br. J. Clin. Pharmacol.* **2019**, *85*, 1692–1703. [CrossRef]

37. Bardou, F.N.; Guillaud, O.; Erard-Poinsot, D.; Chambon-Augoyard, C.; Thimonier, E.; Vallin, M.; Boillot, O.; Dumortier, J. Tacrolimus exposure after liver transplantation for alcohol-related liver disease: Impact on complications. *Transpl. Immunol.* **2019**, *56*, 101227. [CrossRef]

38. Zegarska, J.; Hryniewiecka, E.; Zochowska, D.; Samborowska, E.; Jazwiec, R.; Borowiec, A.; Tszyrsznic, W.; Chmura, A.; Nazarewski, S.; Dadlez, M.; et al. Tacrolimus Metabolite M-III May Have Nephrotoxic and Myelotoxic Effects and Increase the Incidence of Infections in Kidney Transplant Recipients. *Transplant. Proc.* **2016**, *48*, 1539–1542. [CrossRef]

39. Vanhove, T.; de Jonge, H.; de Loor, H.; Oorts, M.; de Hoon, J.; Pohanka, A.; Annaert, P.; Kuypers, D.R.J. Relationship between In Vivo CYP3A4 Activity, CYP3A5 Genotype, and Systemic Tacrolimus Metabolite/Parent Drug Ratio in Renal Transplant Recipients and Healthy Volunteers. *Drug Metab. Dispos.* **2018**, *46*, 1507–1513. [CrossRef]

15

Characteristics and Dysbiosis of the Gut Microbiome in Renal Transplant Recipients

J. Casper Swarte [1,2,*], Rianne M. Douwes [1], Shixian Hu [2,3], Arnau Vich Vila [2,3],
Michele F. Eisenga [1], Marco van Londen [1], António W. Gomes-Neto [1], Rinse K. Weersma [2],
Hermie J.M. Harmsen [4] and Stephan J.L. Bakker [1]

[1]   Department of Internal Medicine, Division of Nephrology, University Medical Center Groningen,
     University of Groningen, 9700RB Groningen, The Netherlands; r.m.douwes@umcg.nl (R.M.D.);
     m.f.eisenga@umcg.nl (M.F.E.); m.van.londen@umcg.nl (M.v.L.); a.w.gomes.neto@umcg.nl (A.W.G.-N.);
     s.j.l.bakker@umcg.nl (S.J.L.B.)

[2]   Department of Gastroenterology and Hepatology, University Medical Center Groningen, University of
     Groningen, 9700RB Groningen, The Netherlands; s.hu01@umcg.nl (S.H.); a.vich.vila@umcg.nl (A.V.V.);
     r.k.weersma@umcg.nl (R.K.W.)

[3]   Department of Genetics, University Medical Center Groningen, University of Groningen,
     9700RB Groningen, The Netherlands

[4]   Department of Medical Microbiology, University Medical Center Groningen, University of Groningen,
     9700RB Groningen, The Netherlands; h.j.m.harmsen@umcg.nl

*   Correspondence: j.c.swarte@umcg.nl

Abstract: Renal transplantation is life-changing in many aspects. This includes changes to the gut microbiome likely due to exposure to immunosuppressive drugs and antibiotics. As a consequence, renal transplant recipients (RTRs) might suffer from intestinal dysbiosis. We aimed to investigate the gut microbiome of RTRs and compare it with healthy controls and to identify determinants of the gut microbiome of RTRs. Therefore, RTRs and healthy controls participating in the TransplantLines Biobank and Cohort Study (NCT03272841) were included. We analyzed the gut microbiome using 16S rRNA sequencing and compared the composition of the gut microbiome of RTRs to healthy controls using multivariate association with linear models (MaAsLin). Fecal samples of 139 RTRs (50% male, mean age: 58.3 ± 12.8 years) and 105 healthy controls (57% male, mean age: 59.2 ± 10.6 years) were collected. Median time after transplantation of RTRs was 6.0 (1.5–12.5)years. The microbiome composition of RTRs was significantly different from that of healthy controls, and RTRs had a lower diversity of the gut microbiome ($p < 0.01$). Proton-pump inhibitors, mycophenolate mofetil, and estimated glomerular filtration rate (eGFR) are significant determinants of the gut microbiome of RTRs ($p < 0.05$). Use of mycophenolate mofetil correlated to a lower diversity ($p < 0.01$). Moreover, significant alterations were found in multiple bacterial taxa between RTRs and healthy controls. The gut microbiome of RTRs contained more Proteobacteria and less Actinobacteria, and there was a loss of butyrate-producing bacteria in the gut microbiome of RTRs. By comparing the gut microbiome of RTRs to healthy controls we have shown that RTRs suffer from dysbiosis, a disruption in the balance of the gut microbiome.

Keywords: gut microbiome; renal transplant recipient; diarrhea; immunosuppressive medication; gut microbiota; kidney transplantation; 16S rRNA sequencing; butyrate-producing bacteria; Proteobacteria

1. Introduction

It is becoming increasingly evident that the gut microbiome plays a role in various diseases such as inflammatory bowel disease, diabetes, autoimmune diseases, and cancer [1]. However, less is known about the role of the gut microbiome in the field of renal transplantation. Renal transplantation is the best available treatment for patients with end-stage renal disease (ESRD). Despite improved prognosis and quality of life (QoL) compared to dialysis treatment, renal transplant recipients (RTRs) suffer from many problems in the years after transplantation. After transplantation one out of five RTRs suffers from chronic diarrhea which is associated with a lower QoL, increased abdominal complaints, higher mortality, and gut dysbiosis [2–4]. Furthermore, all RTRs use immunosuppressive drugs and frequently require antibiotics which potentially influence the gut microbiome [5]. Chronic diarrhea and the use of immunosuppressive drugs may change the gut microbiota composition. As a consequence, this can disrupt gut homeostasis leading to a disruption in the balance of the gut microbiome called dysbiosis. This has previously been reported in mice studies. The introduction of prednisolone and tacrolimus to mice resulted in dysbiosis, an overgrowth of *Escherichia coli*, and an increased colonization with opportunistic pathogens [6]. However, the gut microbiome of RTRs has not been studied extensively.

In previous studies among allogenic stem cell transplant recipients and RTRs, a lower diversity of the gut microbiome was observed [7,8]. Furthermore, this lower diversity of the gut microbiome in allogenic stem cell recipients was associated with a higher risk of mortality [9]. In addition, Annavajhala et al. demonstrated that liver transplant recipients with a lower gut microbiome diversity have a higher risk of colonization by multidrug-resistant bacteria [10]. These studies show that the gut microbiome is clinically relevant in the field of transplantation. However, the role of the gut microbiome in renal transplantation has not been adequately studied. Characterization of the gut microbiome in the first three months after renal transplantation showed significant changes in the composition of the gut microbiome and showed that diarrhea was associated with dysbiosis and a loss of diversity [8]. It is currently unknown whether dysbiosis of the gut microbiome remains prevalent more than one year after transplantation and which factors are determinants of the gut microbiota composition in RTRs. The aim of this study was to characterize the gut microbiome of RTRs for at least more than one year post-transplantation. We compared the composition of the gut microbiome between RTRs and healthy controls and identified determinants of the gut microbiome of RTRs.

2. Experimental Section

2.1. Study Population

We included 139 RTRs who were at least one year post-transplantation and 105 healthy donors from the TransplantLines Biobank and Cohort Study (ClinicalTrials.gov Identifier NCT03272841). TransplantLines is a prospective observational cohort study in solid transplant recipients [11]. Donors underwent medical screening in the University Medical Center Groningen (UMCG) and can be considered healthy controls. All participants were included during a study visit at the outpatient clinic of the UMCG between September 2015 and April 2018. RTRs were treated with standard antihypertensive and immunosuppressive therapy. The research protocol of the TransplantLines study was approved by the independent medical ethics committee of UMCG (METC 2014/077) and was performed in adherence to the Declaration of Helsinki and the Declaration of Istanbul. All subjects provided a written informed consent.

2.2. Patient Characteristics

All measurements were performed during a study visit at the outpatient clinic. Weight, length, and waist and hip circumference were measured in duplicate. Body fat percentage was measured using the multifrequency bioelectrical impedance device (BIA, Quadscan 4000, Bodystat, Douglas, British Isles). Blood pressure was measured by qualified nurses according to a standard clinical protocol as described previously [11]. Hypertension was classified as a mean systolic pressure >140 mm Hg, and/or a mean diastolic pressure >90 mm Hg and/or use of antihypertensive medication. Diabetes mellitus was defined according to the guidelines of the American Diabetes Association [12]. Estimated glomerular filtration rate (eGFR) was calculated using the serum creatinine-based chronic kidney disease epidemiology collaboration (CKD-EPI) formula. Proteinuria was defined as urinary protein excretion >0.5 g per 24 h. Glucose and hemoglobin A1c (HbA1c) were determined using standard laboratory methods. Smoking status was recorded using a questionnaire. Medication use was retrieved from medical records and verified with patients during study visits. The study design is described in detail in the TransplantLines design paper [11].

2.3. Sample Collection

Blood samples were collected after an overnight fasting period of 8–12 h and stored at −80 °C. Participants were instructed to collect a fecal sample the day prior to the study visit at home and store the sample on ice. Upon arrival at the UMCG the fecal samples were immediately stored at −80 °C. Participants also collected 24-hour urine samples the day prior to the study visit.

2.4. DNA Extraction and 16S rRNA Sequencing

Deoxyribonucleic acid (DNA) was extracted from 0.25 g feces [13]. The genes for the 16S rRNA V4 and V5 region were amplified by polymerase chain reaction (PCR) using the TaKaRa Taq Hot start version kit (TaKaRa Bio Inc., Kusatsu, Japan). We used the 341F and 806R primers containing a 6-nucleotide Illumina-MiSeq adapter sequence. The PCR product was purified with AMPure XP beads (Beckman Coulter, USA). DNA concentrations were measured with Qubit 2.0 Fluorometer to ensure equal library presentation for each sample, dilutions were made accordingly [14]. The normalized DNA library was sequenced using the MiSeq Benchtop Sequencer.

2.5. Microbiome Profiling

Bacterial taxonomy was assigned using PAired-eND Assembler for DNA sequences (PANDAseq), Quantitative Insights Into Microbial Ecology (QIIME), and ARB [15–17]. QIIME was used to assign taxonomy to the phylum, class, order, family, and genus level. ARB was used to assign taxonomy to the species level. As previously described, PANDAseq was used to increase the quality of sequence reads. Readouts with at quality score lower than 0.9 were discarded according to the protocol followed by Heida et al. [14].

2.6. Statistical Analyses

Data are presented as mean ± standard deviation (SD) for normally distributed data and median with interquartile range (IQR) for non-normally distributed data. Differences between baseline characteristics of RTRs and healthy controls were tested using a t-test or a Mann–Whitney u-test.

Sample richness/evenness was estimated using the Shannon index using QIIME. The microbial dissimilarities matrix (Bray–Curtis) was obtained using *vegdist* from the *vegan* R-package [18]. Principal coordinates were constructed and plotted with the *cmdscale* function. We used permutational multivariate analysis of variance using distance matrices (ADONIS) to analyze the variance in the Bray–Curtis matrix that could be explained by metadata such as age, sex, body mass index (BMI), fat percentage, smoking, eGFR, and medication. Pearson correlation was used to correlate metadata to the Shannon diversity index. p-values <0.01 were considered statistically significant.

Multivariate analysis by linear models (MaAsLin) is a tool to find associations between clinical metadata and bacterial abundance. We used MaAsLin to find associations between microbiome data and clinical phenotype. MaAsLin performs a boosted, additive general linear model between metadata and microbial abundance [19]. Covariates including sex, body mass index (BMI), smoking, use of antihypertensive medication, use of antibiotics, use of statins, use of proton-pump inhibitor (PPI), and read depth were forced into the model. These covariates are known to influence the gut microbiome [20]. All p-values were corrected for multiple testing using false discovery rate (FDR). $p_{FDR} < 0.10$ was considered statistically significant for taxonomic analysis.

3. Results

3.1. Baseline Characteristics

We included 139 RTRs (age 58.3 ± 12.8 years; 50% males) at a median post-transplantation time of 6.0 (1.5–12.5) years and 105 healthy controls (age 59.2 ± 10.6 years; 57% males). Mean BMI was 27.7 ± 5.4 kg/m^2 for RTRs and 27.2 ± 6.0 kg/m^2 for controls. In total 3 (3%) healthy controls and 38 (27%) RTRs had diabetes mellitus ($p < 0.001$). RTRs had a significantly higher HbA1c, 40.0 (37.0–46.0) compared to healthy controls, 37.5 (36.0–40.0) ($p < 0.001$). RTRs had a significantly lower eGFR of 48.3 ± 16.7 mL/min/1.73 m^2 compared with 69.0 ± 19.2 mL/min/1.73 m^2 for controls ($p < 0.001$). In total 7 (5%) RTRs used antibiotics, 115 (83%) RTRs used antihypertensive medication, 96 (69%) RTRs used PPIs, and 66 (47%) RTRs used statins. Cyclosporine was used by 25 (18%) RTRs, tacrolimus by 79 (57%) RTRs, azathioprine was used by 13 (9%) RTRs, mycophenolate mofetil by 100 (72%) RTRs, and prednisolone by 133 (96%) RTRs (Table 1).

Table 1. Baseline characteristics of renal transplant recipients (RTRs) and controls.

Demographics	Control	RTRs	p-Value
Number of Subjects, n (%)	105	139	-
Age (years)	59.2 ± 10.6	58.3 ± 12.8	0.96
Male, n (%)	60 (57)	69 (50)	0.24
BMI (kg/m^2)	27.2 ± 6.0	27.7 ± 5.4	0.60
Diabetes Mellitus, n (%)	3 (3)	38 (27)	<0.001
Hypertension, n (%)	10 (10)	115 (83)	<0.001
Smoking, n (%)	-	12 (9)	-
Years since Transplantation, Median (IQR)	-	6.0 (1.5–12.5)	-
Cardiovascular Parameters			
Glucose, mmol/L, Median (IQR)	5.4 (4.0–5.9)	5.4 (4.9–6.2)	0.06
HbA1c, mmol/L, Median (IQR)	37.5 (36.0–40.0)	40.0 (37.0–46.0)	<0.001
Systolic Blood Pressure (mmHg)	130.4 ± 14.2	136.5 ± 17.7	0.02
Diastolic Blood Pressure (mmHg)	75.8 ± 9.4	78.5 ± 9.6	0.03
Heart Frequency (bpm)	69.7 ± 25.8	72.1 ± 13.1	0.02
Renal Function Parameters			
Serum Creatinine (μmol/L)	97.3 ± 22.1	133.1 ± 42.6	<0.001
eGFR (mL/min/1.73 m^2)	69.0 ± 19.2	48.3 ± 16.7	<0.001
Proteinuria (0.5 g/24 h), n (%)	0 (0)	11 (7.9)	-
Medication, n (%)			
Antibiotics ($n = 1$)	0 (0)	7 (5)	-
Antihypertensive Agents ($n = 8$)	10 (10)	115 (83)	<0.001
Proton-pump Inhibitors	8 (8)	96 (69)	<0.001
Statins	8 (8)	66 (47)	<0.001
Cyclosporine	-	25 (18)	-
Tacrolimus	-	79 (57)	-
Azathioprine	-	13 (9)	-
Mycophenolate mofetil	-	100 (72)	-
Prednisolone	-	133 (96)	-

All characteristics are presented as means ± standard deviation unless otherwise stated. IQR—interquartile range.

3.2. Diversity of the Gut Microbiome

The median Shannon diversity index, a measure for the diversity of the gut microbiome, was significantly lower in RTR samples with 3.4 (3.1–3.8) vs. 3.7 (3.5–4.0) for healthy controls ($p < 0.001$). The median operational taxonomic units (OTUs) per sample was 256 (214–304) for RTRs and 314 (260–351) for healthy controls ($p < 0.001$) (Figure 1). The diversity between samples was further assessed using beta diversity analysis. The gut microbiome was significantly different between RTRs and healthy controls ($p < 0.01$). A separation in gut microbiota composition can be observed between RTRs and healthy controls in the principal coordinate plot (Figure 2). A permutational multivariate analysis of variance using distance matrices (ADONIS) was performed to estimate the variation explained in the gut microbiome by different variables. In total, 5.8% of the variation of the gut microbiome of RTRs and healthy controls was significantly explained by sample type (RTR or healthy control, $p < 0.001$). Furthermore, using ADONIS, baseline characteristics including medication use were tested in the gut microbiome of RTRs. Within the gut microbiome of RTRs age (1.2%), BMI (1.1%), and eGFR (1.0%) significantly explained variation within the gut microbiome. Furthermore, the use of PPIs (1.2%) and the use of mycophenolate mofetil (1.0%) significantly explained variation within the gut microbiome of RTRs. Age was positively correlated to the Shannon diversity index ($p < 0.01$). Use of mycophenolate mofetil and use of antibiotics was negatively correlated to the Shannon diversity index ($p < 0.01$) (Figure 3).

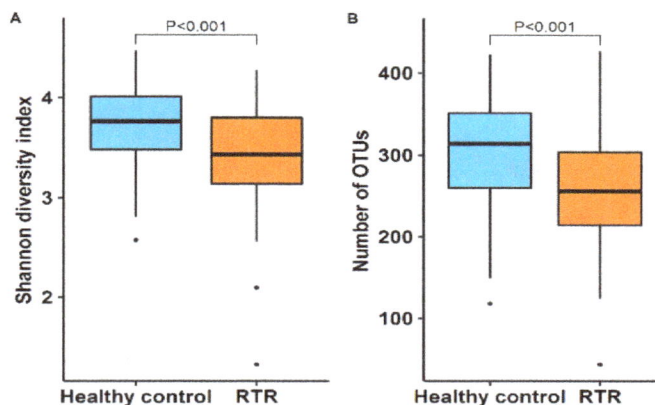

Figure 1. This is a figure showing the diversity of the gut microbiome of renal transplant recipients (RTRs) compared to healthy controls: (**A**) a boxplot depicting the Shannon diversity index, which is a measure for the diversity of the gut microbiome, was significantly lower in RTRs compared to healthy controls ($p < 0.001$); (**B**) a boxplot showing the number of observed operation taxonomic units (OTUs) between RTRs and healthy controls ($p < 0.001$).

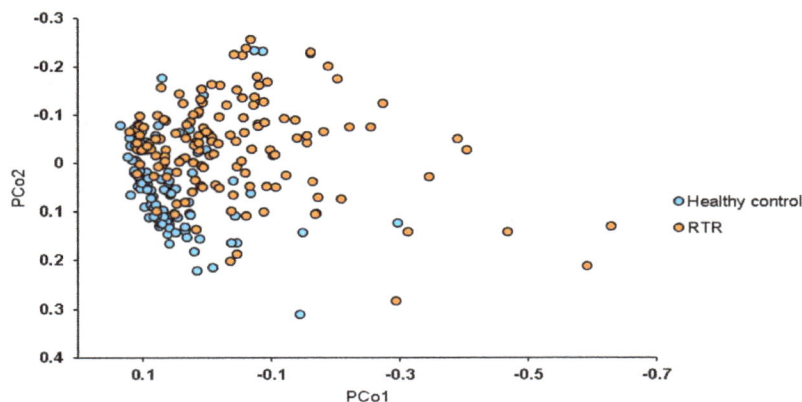

Figure 2. Principal coordinate analysis of 139 RTRs and 105 healthy controls. The principal coordinates plot shows principal coordinates for the Bray–Curtis distance, a measure for the composition of the gut microbiome, for RTRs and healthy controls. Separation in the composition of the gut microbiome between RTRs and healthy controls can be observed. PCo1 is principal coordinate 1 and PCo2 is principal coordinate 2. The gut microbiome of RTRs is significantly different from that of healthy controls in the first coordinate (PCo1 *vs.* PCo2: $p < 0.01$). RTR or healthy control status significantly explained 5.8% of variation in the gut microbiome ($p < 0.001$).

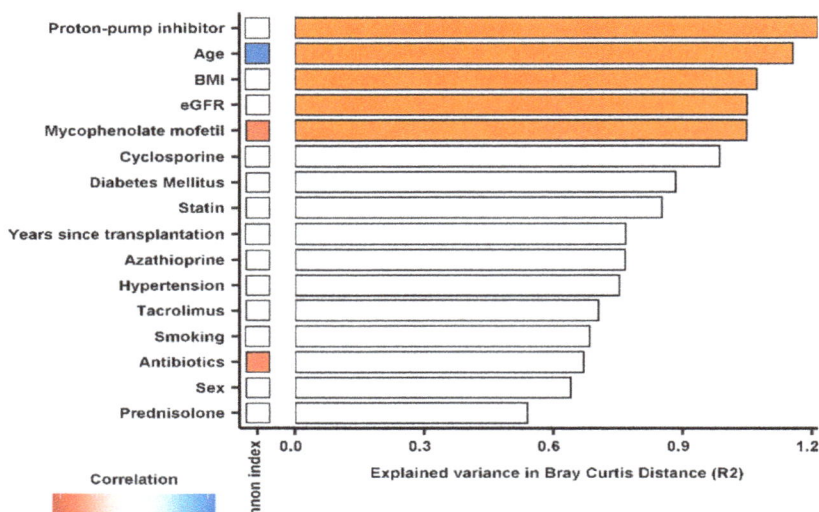

Figure 3. Depiction of variables that are associated with variation in the gut microbiome within RTRs. In the bar plots, the x-axis represents the percentage of explained variance in the gut microbiome of RTRs expressed as the Bray–Curtis distance. The heatmap depicts significant negative correlations (red) and positive correlations (blue) with the Shannon diversity index ($p < 0.01$). These variables were tested only in the gut microbiome of RTRs. Bars in orange represent variables which significantly explain variance in gut microbiota composition ($p < 0.05$).

3.3. Composition of the Gut Microbiome

We analyzed the gut microbiome at different taxonomic levels: phylum, class, order, family, genus, and species. Using MaAsLin, we were able to identify significant differences in taxa abundances between RTRs and healthy controls while correcting for age, sex, BMI, smoking, use of antihypertensive medication, use of antibiotics, use of statins, use of PPIs, and read depth. In total, we found significant alterations in 127 of the 447 bacterial taxa abundances in the gut microbiome of RTRs ($p_{FDR} < 0.10$) (Table 2). On the phylum level we found that RTRs have significantly higher levels of Proteobacteria and lower levels of Actinobacteria ($p_{FDR} < 0.10$) (Figure 4). Within the phylum Proteobacteria, the species *E. coli* was significantly more abundant in the gut microbiome of RTRs ($p_{FDR} < 0.10$). Within the phylum Actinobacteria multiple species had a lower abundance within the gut microbiome of RTRs, especially multiple *Bifidobacterium* species ($p_{FDR} < 0.10$). The predominant phylum Firmicutes was not significantly different in RTRs compared to healthy controls. However, within the phylum Firmicutes there were many significantly different species in the gut microbiome of RTRs compared to healthy controls (Figure 4 and Table S1). An extensive overview of MaAsLin results for complete taxonomy is provided in Table S1.

Table 2. Overview of significantly altered taxa between renal transplant recipients and healthy controls.

Taxonomic Level	Total Number of Taxa [1]	Number of Significant Taxa [2]
Phylum	6	2
Class	17	5
Order	31	8
Family	60	18
Genus	123	27
Species	205	63
Total	442	123

[1] Total number of taxa with an abundance >0.1%; [2] $p_{FDR} < 0.10$.

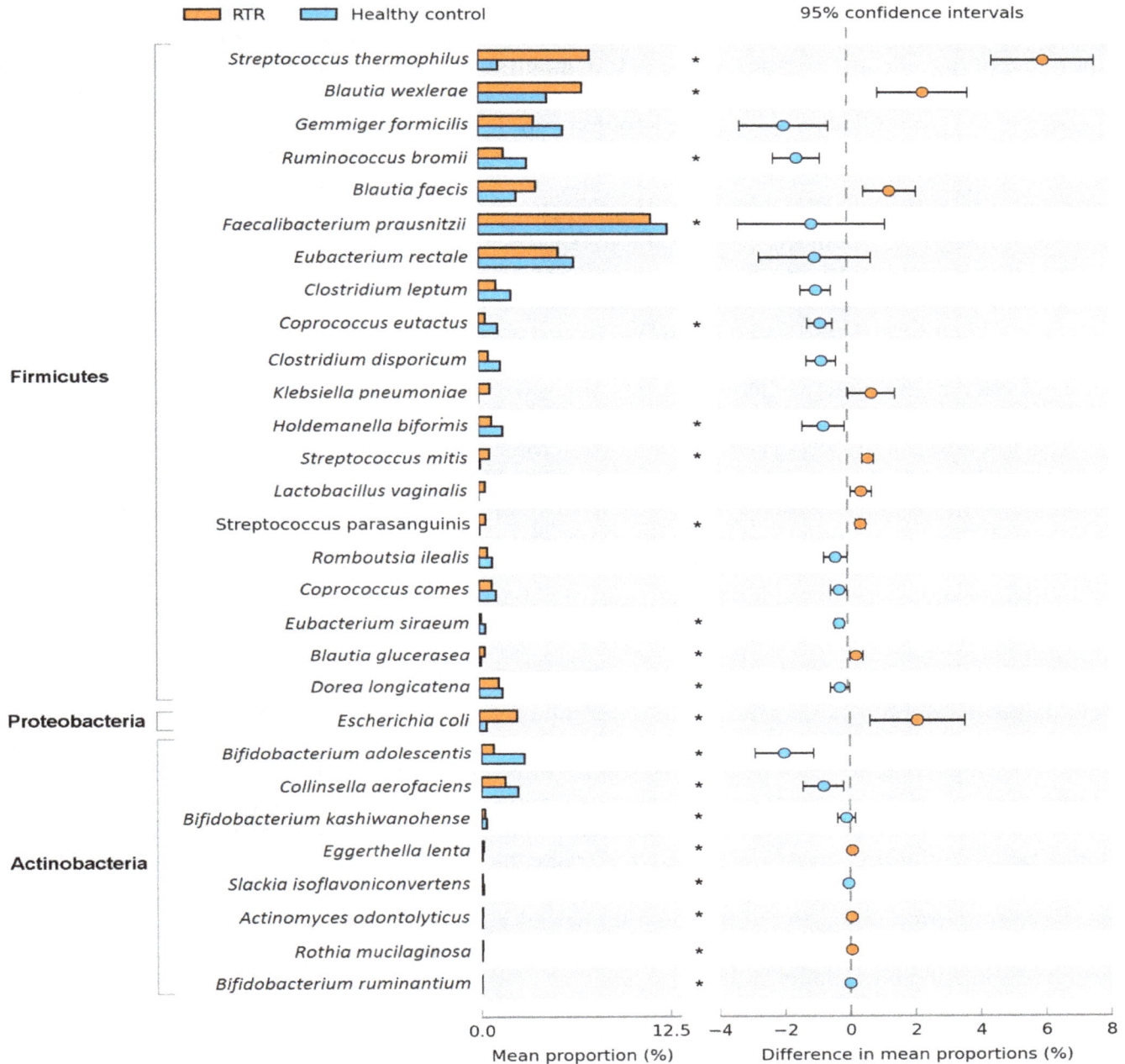

Figure 4. This figure depicts the abundance of phyla and species for RTRs and healthy controls. Bar plots represent the mean proportion and differences in mean proportions with 95% confidence intervals are depicted on the right. Taxa that are depicted were filtered for a difference in mean proportion >0.2%. $p_{FDR} < 0.10$ was considered as statistically significant and indicated in the plot with a star (*).

4. Discussion

We have shown that the gut microbiome of RTRs is different compared to the gut microbiome of healthy controls. Interestingly, we demonstrated that RTRs have dysbiosis characterized by general loss of microbial diversity. We found that RTRs have an increased abundance of Proteobacteria, a decrease in Actinobacteria, and a loss of butyrate-producing bacteria. Finally, we found that age, BMI, eGFR, the use of PPIs, and the use of mycophenolate mofetil are determinants of the gut microbiome of RTRs and that age, BMI, and the use of mycophenolate mofetil correlate to the diversity of the gut microbiome.

In a pilot study of Lee et al., significant changes were seen in the gut microbiome of RTRs when pre-transplantation samples were compared to post-transplantation samples. The diversity, although not significant, was lower after transplantation. Proteobacteria and Enterobacteriales were increased in the gut microbiome post-transplantation [8]. We observed a significant loss of diversity in the composition of the gut microbiome in RTRs with a similar increase in Proteobacteria. It is known that a lower diversity is associated with various diseases such as inflammatory bowel disease (IBD), metabolic disease and cardiovascular disease, as stated by the Human Microbiome Consortium [21]. Previous research in a cohort of allogeneic hematopoietic stem cell transplantation (allo-HSCT) recipients demonstrated that a lower diversity of the gut microbiome was associated with a higher mortality risk [9]. Additionally, allo-HSCT recipients who were deceased had a higher level of Gammaproteobacteria, Enterobacteriales, and Enterobacteriaceae [7]. These findings are strikingly similar to the results of our study. We also observed a lower diversity and higher levels of Proteobacteria, Gammaproteobacteria, Enterobacteriaceae, *Escherichia*, *Streptococcus*, and *Lactobacillus* in the gut microbiome of RTRs. However, it is unknown whether these changes in the composition of the gut microbiome are associated with mortality in RTRs.

The lower diversity observed in the gut microbiome of RTRs suggest that RTRs suffer from dysbiosis. We found increased levels of Proteobacteria which has previously been proposed as a marker for dysbiosis in the gut microbiome [22]. Furthermore, we observed a loss of butyrate-producing bacteria in RTRs. Butyrate is a short-chain fatty acid (SCFA) that plays a key role in maintaining gut health. Butyrate is associated with trans-epithelial fluid transport, reduction of inflammation and oxidative stress, reinforcement of the epithelial barrier, and has potential protective properties against colorectal cancer [23]. In this study, lower levels of *Faecalibacterium prausnitzii*, *Gemmiger formicilis*, *Eubacterium rectale*, *Coprococcus catus*, *Coprococcus comes* and *Roseburia* were observed in the gut microbiome of RTRs. These are all well-known butyrate-producing bacteria [24]. The decrease of butyrate production in RTRs could be detrimental to their gut health. Furthermore, animal studies show that butyrate has immunomodulatory properties through the effect on regulatory T-cells (Treg), which in turn plays a key role in suppressing inflammatory responses. Increasing butyrate in the gut improved renal dysfunction and reduced local and systemic inflammation in mice [25,26]. These results have also been observed in allogeneic bone marrow transplant recipients. Reduced butyrate altered gene regulation and resulted in fewer Treg cells. Restoring butyrate levels led to improved junction integrity, decreased apoptosis, and improved graft versus host disease [27]. Dysbiosis and a loss of butyrate-producing bacteria in the gut microbiome of RTRs could therefore have detrimental effects on gut health. Further research is needed to study the clinical consequences of the loss of butyrate-producing bacteria in RTRs.

In another study of Lee et al., a loss of diversity and a loss of butyrate-producing bacteria was also observed in RTRs with post-transplantation diarrhea. In this study, post-transplantation diarrhea was not associated with common infectious diarrheal pathogens but rather with dysbiosis [4]. RTRs had lower levels of *Ruminococcus*, *Coprococcus*, and *Dorea* in this study. These findings are in accordance with results from our study, which also demonstrated lower levels of *Ruminococcus* in the microbiome of RTRs. However, we did not observe higher levels of *Coprococcus* and *Dorea* in RTRs. One reason for this might be that we included patients more than one year after transplantation while Lee et al. included patients within the first year after transplantation. In addition, we corrected for various factors that influence the composition of the gut microbiome, which was not done in the study by Lee et al. [8].

We found many significant differences in taxa abundance in RTRs compared to healthy controls. Some of these differences in the composition of the gut microbiome might indicate that RTRs suffer from increased inflammation in the gut. For example, the abundance of Proteobacteria was much higher in RTRs compared to healthy controls. This was also observed in patients with severe intestinal inflammation and inflammatory bowel disease (IBD), colorectal cancer, necrotizing enterocolitis, and irritable bowel syndrome (IBS) [28]. Increased oxygen availability in the gut colonocytes could explain these findings, since it is associated with inflammation in the gut and drives the expansion of aerobic Proteobacteria, Enterobacteriaceae, and *E. coli* while lowering the levels of anaerobic bacteria such as *Bifidobacterium* and butyrate-producing bacteria [22,28]. In this study, RTRs indeed had an increased abundance of Proteobacteria, Enterobacteriaceae, and *E. coli*, and lower levels of Clostridia and Bifidobacteria. These similarities in the gut microbiome composition of RTRs and IBD patients suggest that RTRs may be suffering from inflammation in the gut, which could lead to a loss of epithelial barrier function and diarrhea [29].

In this study, we showed that use of PPIs and mycophenolate mofetil was associated with variation within the gut microbiome of RTR. Imhann et al. demonstrated that the use of PPIs changes the gut microbiome, especially an increase of *Streptococcus* species was found in PPI users [30]. We found multiple *Streptococcus* species that had a higher abundance in the gut microbiome of RTRs. This could be due to the use of PPIs. The influence of immunosuppressive medication on the gut microbiome is not yet well studied in RTRs. In a previous murine study, prednisolone, tacrolimus, and mycophenolate mofetil changed the gut microbiome [6]. Mycophenolate mofetil has multiple side effects including diarrhea [31]. In our study, the use of mycophenolate mofetil was significantly correlated to a lower diversity of the gut microbiome. A lower diversity of the gut microbiome is more prevalent in less healthy individuals. More research is needed to investigate the interplay between the use of mycophenolate mofetil, the gut microbiome, and clinical outcomes.

Improving the observed dysbiotic state of RTRs might have clinical implications concerning long-term outcome after renal transplantation. Important issues are that many RTRs suffer from cognitive decline and development of skin cancer [32,33]. Dysbiosis might contribute to cognitive decline due to an effect of the gut microbiome on the gut–brain axis [34]. The same mechanism might apply to the occurrence of skin cancer, due to an effect of the gut microbiome on the gut–skin axis [33,35]. Improving the dysbiotic state of the gut microbiome in RTRs may therefore be a modifiable factor that allows for inhibition of cognitive decline and skin cancer after renal transplantation. Changing the diet of RTRs might be an intervention that allows for improvement of the gut dysbiosis of RTRs. Diet has been identified as an important potentially modifiable factor influencing the gut microbiome [20]. After transplantation, many RTRs adhere to the diet that was prescribed prior to transplantation [36]. This diet includes a protein restriction, which is meant to limit and prevent uremic symptoms and progression of decline of renal function [37]. It also includes a phosphorus restriction to prevent hypophosphatemia, and a potassium restriction to prevent occurrence of hyperkaliemia, cardiac arrhythmias, and acute cardiac death [37]. Improving diet and eating habits may have a positive effect on the composition of the gut microbiome, which could ultimately translate into a beneficial effect on cognitive function [38]. Future, larger cohort studies could focus on the influence of diet on the gut microbiome in RTRs, and on potential sex differences therein. Potential sex differences in the gut microbiome might be of interest, but cohorts to allow for determining those likely need to be large, because previously reported sex differences in the gut microbiome are small [20,39].

We showed that there are many differences in the gut microbiome of RTRs compared to healthy controls. However, the current study should be interpreted within its limitations. The main indication for renal transplantation is chronic kidney disease (CKD). Alterations in the gut microbiome of patients with CKD are already present before transplantation. Patients with CKD also suffer from a lower diversity of the gut microbiome and dysbiosis. A lower colonization by Bifidobacteria and an increase in Enterobacteriaceae was observed in patients with CKD [26]. These findings are similar to our findings which suggest that the dysbiosis observed in RTRs may already be present pre-transplantation and does not recover post-transplantation [8]. Moreover, we measured the composition of the gut microbiome using 16S rRNA sequencing instead of metagenomic sequencing. Therefore, we were unable to analyze metabolic pathways of bacteria. Furthermore, SCFA were not measured in the current study. Therefore, it remains unknown whether the observed loss of butyrate-producing bacteria also leads to a decreased production of butyrate. Future studies should include pre-transplantation patients and study how the gut microbiome develops after transplantation. Focus should be on the metagenome of RTRs to study the effects of dysbiosis, the metabolism genes, and metabolites. Furthermore, current studies of the gut microbiome mainly focus on bacteria. However, at the kingdom level of the gut microbiome, there are many more micro-organisms such as archaea, fungi, eukaryotes, as well as viruses which could also play an important role in the gut microbiome of immunosuppressed patients [40].

In conclusion, the gut microbiome of RTRs more than one year post-transplantation is significantly different from that of healthy controls. The gut microbiome of RTRs contains more Proteobacteria and less Actinobacteria and there is a loss of butyrate-producing bacteria which could be detrimental to gut health. The use of mycophenolate mofetil and antibiotics is associated with variation in the gut microbiome of RTRs and correlated to a lower diversity. The results of this study are preliminary and require replication in a larger cohort. Nevertheless, we demonstrate that RTRs suffer from dysbiosis more than one year post-transplantation and that the use of mycophenolate mofetil correlates to a lower diversity.

Author Contributions: Conceptualization, J.C.S., H.J.M.H., and S.J.L.B.; data curation, J.C.S., M.F.E., M.v.L., and A.W.G.-N.; formal analysis, J.C.S., S.H., and S.J.L.B.; investigation, J.C.S.; methodology, J.C.S., S.H., A.V.V., H.J.M.H., and S.J.L.B.; resources, H.J.M.H. and S.J.L.B.; software, J.C.S. and S.H.; supervision, R.K.W., H.J.M.H., and S.J.L.B.; writing—original draft, J.C.S.; writing—review and editing, J.C.S., R.M.D., S.H., M.F.E., A.V.V., M.v.L., A.W.G.-N., R.K.W., H.J.M.H., and S.J.L.B. All authors have read and agreed to the published version of the manuscript.

Acknowledgments: The authors thank Rebekka van den Bosch, Rudi Tonk, Carien Bus-Spoor, and Ranko Gacesa for technical assistance.

References

1. Thursby, E.; Juge, N. Introduction to the human gut microbiota. *Biochem. J.* **2017**, *474*, 1823–1836. [CrossRef]
2. Ekberg, H.; Kyllönen, L.; Madsen, S.; Grave, G.; Solbu, D.; Holdaas, H. Clinicians underestimate gastrointestinal symptoms and overestimate quality of life in renal transplant recipients: A multinational survey of nephrologists. *Transplantation* **2007**, *84*, 1052–1054. [CrossRef] [PubMed]
3. Bunnapradist, S.; Neri, L.; Wong, W.; Lentine, K.L.; Burroughs, T.E.; Pinsky, B.W.; Takemoto, S.K.; Schnitzler, M.A. Incidence and Risk Factors for Diarrhea Following Kidney Transplantation and Association with Graft Loss and Mortality. *Am. J. Kidney Dis.* **2008**, *51*, 478–486. [CrossRef] [PubMed]
4. Lee, J.R.; Magruder, M.; Zhang, L.; Westblade, L.F.; Satlin, M.J.; Robertson, A.; Edusei, E.; Crawford, C.; Ling, L.; Taur, Y.; et al. Gut microbiota dysbiosis and diarrhea in kidney transplant recipients. *Am. J. Transplant.* **2019**, *19*, 488–500. [CrossRef] [PubMed]
5. Zimmermann, M.; Zimmermann-Kogadeeva, M.; Wegmann, R.; Goodman, A.L. Mapping human microbiome drug metabolism by gut bacteria and their genes. *Nature* **2019**, *570*, 462–467. [CrossRef] [PubMed]
6. Tourret, J.; Willing, B.P.; Dion, S.; MacPherson, J.; Denamur, E.; Finlay, B.B. Immunosuppressive treatment alters secretion of ileal antimicrobial peptides and gut microbiota, and favors subsequent colonization by uropathogenic Escherichia coli. *Transplantation* **2017**, *101*, 74–82. [CrossRef] [PubMed]
7. Taur, Y.; Jenq, R.R.; Perales, M.A.; Littmann, E.R.; Morjaria, S.; Ling, L.; No, D.; Gobourne, A.; Viale, A.; Dahi, P.B.; et al. The effects of intestinal tract bacterial diversity on mortality following allogeneic hematopoietic stem cell transplantation. *Blood* **2014**, *124*, 1174–1182. [CrossRef] [PubMed]
8. Lee, J.R.; Muthukumar, T.; Dadhania, D.; Toussaint, N.C.; Ling, L.; Pamer, E.; Suthanthiran, M. Gut microbial community structure and complications after kidney transplantation: A pilot study. *Transplantation* **2014**, *98*, 697–705. [CrossRef]
9. Taur, Y.; Jenq, R.R.; Ubeda, C.; Van Den Brink, M.; Pamer, E.G. Role of intestinal microbiota in transplantation outcomes. *Best Pract. Res. Clin. Haematol.* **2015**, *28*, 155–161. [CrossRef]
10. Annavajhala, M.K.; Gomez-Simmonds, A.; Macesic, N.; Sullivan, S.B.; Kress, A.; Khan, S.D.; Giddins, M.J.; Stump, S.; Kim, G.I.; Narain, R.; et al. Colonizing multidrug-resistant bacteria and the longitudinal evolution of the intestinal microbiome after liver transplantation. *Nat. Commun.* **2019**, *10*, 1–12. [CrossRef]
11. Eisenga, M.F.; Gomes-Neto, A.W.; Van Londen, M.; Ziengs, A.L.; Douwes, R.M.; Stam, S.P.; Osté, M.C.J.;

Knobbe, T.J.; Hessels, N.R.; Buunk, A.M.; et al. Rationale and design of TransplantLines: A prospective cohort study and biobank of solid organ transplant recipients. *BMJ Open* **2018**, *8*, 1–13. [CrossRef] [PubMed]

12. Gavin, J.R.; Alberti, K.G.M.M.; Davidson, M.B.; DeFronzo, R.A.; Drash, A.; Gabbe, S.G.; Genuth, S.; Harris, M.I.; Kahn, R.; Keen, H.; et al. Report of the expert committee on the diagnosis and classification of diabetes mellitus. *Diabetes Care* **2002**, *25*, 5–20.

13. De Goffau, M.C.; Luopajärvi, K.; Knip, M.; Ilonen, J.; Ruohtula, T.; Härkönen, T.; Orivuori, L.; Hakala, S.; Welling, G.W.; Harmsen, H.J.; et al. Fecal microbiota composition differs between children with β-cell autoimmunity and those without. *Diabetes* **2013**, *62*, 1238–1244. [CrossRef]

14. Heida, F.H.; Van Zoonen, A.G.J.F.; Hulscher, J.B.F.; Te Kiefte, B.J.C.; Wessels, R.; Kooi, E.M.W.; Bos, A.F.; Harmsen, H.J.M.; De Goffau, M.C. A necrotizing enterocolitis-associated gut microbiota is present in the meconium: Results of a prospective study. *Clin. Infect. Dis.* **2016**, *62*, 863–870. [CrossRef]

15. Caporaso, J.G.; Kuczynski, J.; Stombaugh, J.; Bittinger, K.; Bushman, F.D.; Costello, E.K.; Fierer, N.; Pena, A.G.; Goodrich, J.K.; Gordon, J.I.; et al. QIIME allows analysis of high-throughput community sequencing data. *Nat. Methods* **2011**, *7*, 1–12. [CrossRef] [PubMed]

16. Masella, A.P.; Bartram, A.K.; Truszkowski, J.M.; Brown, D.G.; Neufeld, J.D. PANDAseq: Paired-end assembler for illumina sequences. *BMC Bioinformatics* **2012**, *13*, 31. [CrossRef] [PubMed]

17. Ludwig, W.; Strunk, O.; Westram, R.; Richter, L.; Meier, H.; Yadhukumar, A.; Buchner, A.; Lai, T.; Steppi, S.; Jacob, G.; et al. ARB: A software environment for sequence data. *Nucleic Acids Res.* **2004**, *32*, 1363–1371. [CrossRef] [PubMed]

18. Oksanen, J.; Blanchet, F.G.; Kindt, R.; Legendre, P.; Minchin, P.R.; O'hara, R.B.; Simpson, G.L.; Solymos, P.; Stevens, M.H.H.; Wagner, H. Package 'vegan'. Community Ecology Package. **2018**. Available online: https://cran.ism.ac.jp/web/packages/vegan/vegan.pdf (accessed on 1 February 2020).

19. Morgan, X.C.; Tickle, T.L.; Sokol, H.; Gevers, D.; Devaney, K.L.; Ward, D.V.; Reyes, J.A.; Shah, S.A.; LeLeiko, N.; Snapper, S.B.; et al. Dysfunction of the intestinal microbiome in inflammatory bowel disease and treatment. *Genome Biol.* **2012**, *13*, R79. [CrossRef]

20. Zhernakova, A.; Kurilshikov, A.; Bonder, M.J.; Tigchelaar, E.F.; Schirmer, M.; Vatanen, T.; Mujagic, Z.; Vila, A.V.; Falony, G.; Vieira-Silva, S.; et al. Population-based metagenomics analysis reveals markers for gut microbiome composition and diversity. *Science* **2016**, *352*, 565–569. [CrossRef]

21. Consortium, T.H.M.P. Structure, Function and Diversity of the Healthy Human Microbiome. *Nature* **2013**, *486*, 1049–1058.

22. Shin, N.R.; Whon, T.W.; Bae, J.W. Proteobacteria: Microbial signature of dysbiosis in gut microbiota. *Trends Biotechnol.* **2015**, *33*, 496–503. [CrossRef] [PubMed]

23. Canani, R.B.; Costanzo, M.; Di Leone, L.; Pedata, M.; Meli, R.; Calignano, A. Potential beneficial effects of butyrate in intestinal and extraintestinal diseases. *World J. Gastroenterol.* **2011**, *17*, 1519–1528. [CrossRef]

24. Flint, H.J.; Duncan, S.H.; Scott, K.P.; Louis, P. Links between diet, gut microbiota composition and gut metabolism. *Proc. Nutr. Soc.* **2014**, *760*, 13–22. [CrossRef] [PubMed]

25. Furusawa, Y.; Obata, Y.; Fukuda, S.; Endo, T.A.; Nakato, G.; Takahashi, D.; Nakanishi, Y.; Uetake, C.; Kato, K.; Kato, T.; et al. Commensal microbe-derived butyrate induces the differentiation of colonic regulatory T cells. *Nature* **2013**, *504*, 446–450. [CrossRef]

26. Sampaio-Maia, B.; Simões-Silva, L.; Pestana, M.; Araujo, R.; Soares-Silva, I.J. The Role of the Gut Microbiome on Chronic Kidney Disease. *Adv. Appl. Microbiol.* **2016**, *96*, 65–94. [PubMed]

27. Mathewson, N.D.; Jenq, R.; Mathew, A.V.; Koenigsknecht, M.; Hanash, A.; Toubai, T.; Oravecz-Wilson, K.; Wu, S.R.; Sun, Y.; Rossi, C.; et al. Gut microbiome-derived metabolites modulate intestinal epithelial cell damage and mitigate graft-versus-host disease. *Nat. Immunol.* **2016**, *17*, 505–513. [CrossRef]

28. Litvak, Y.; Byndloss, M.X.; Tsolis, R.M.; Bäumler, A.J. Dysbiotic Proteobacteria expansion: A microbial signature of epithelial dysfunction. *Curr. Opin. Microbiol.* **2017**, *39*, 1–6. [CrossRef]

29. Tang, Y.; Forsyth, C.B.; Keshavarzian, A. New molecular insights into inflammatory bowel disease-induced diarrhea. *Expert Rev. Gastroenterol. Hepatol.* **2011**, *5*, 615–625. [CrossRef]

30. Imhann, F.; Bonder, M.J.; Vila, A.V.; Fu, J.; Mujagic, Z.; Vork, L.; Tigchelaar, E.F.; Jankipersadsing, S.A.; Cenit, M.C.; Harmsen, H.J.M.; et al. Proton pump inhibitors affect the gut microbiome. *Gut* **2016**, *65*, 740–748. [CrossRef]

31. Spasić, A.; Catić-Đorđević, A.; Veličković-Radovanović, R.; Stefanović, N.; Džodić, P.; Cvetković, T. Adverse effects of mycophenolic acid in renal transplant recipients: Gender differences. *Int. J. Clin. Pharm.* **2019**, *41*,

776–784. [CrossRef] [PubMed]

32. Chu, N.M.; Gross, A.L.; Shaffer, A.A.; Haugen, C.E.; Norman, S.P.; Xue, Q.L.; Sharrett, A.R.; Carlson, M.C.; Bandeen-Roche, K.; Segev, D.L.; et al. Frailty and changes in cognitive function after kidney transplantation. *J. Am. Soc. Nephrol.* **2019**, *30*, 336–345. [CrossRef] [PubMed]

33. Pruett, T. Spectrum of Cancer Risk Among US Solid Organ Transplant Recipients. *Yearb. Surg.* **2012**, *2012*, 105–106. [CrossRef]

34. Appleton, J. The gut-brain axis: Influence of microbiota on mood and mental health. *Integr. Med.* **2018**, *17*, 28–32.

35. Salem, I.; Ramser, A.; Isham, N.; Ghannoum, M.A. The gut microbiome as a major regulator of the gut-skin axis. *Front. Microbiol.* **2018**, *9*, 1–14. [CrossRef]

36. Eisenga, M.F.; Kieneker, L.M.; Soedamah-Muthu, S.S.; Van Den Berg, E.; Deetman, P.E.; Navis, G.J.; Gans, R.O.B.; Gaillard, C.A.J.M.; Bakker, S.J.L.; Joosten, M.M. Urinary potassium excretion, renal ammoniagenesis, and risk of graft failure and mortality in renal transplant recipients1-3. *Am. J. Clin. Nutr.* **2016**, *104*, 1703–1711. [CrossRef]

37. Kalantar-Zadeh, K.; Fouque, D. Nutritional management of chronic kidney disease. *N. Engl. J. Med.* **2017**, *377*, 1765–1776. [CrossRef]

38. Novotný, M.; Klimova, B.; Valis, M. Microbiome and cognitive impairment: Can any diets influence learning processes in a positive way? *Front. Aging Neurosci.* **2019**, *11*, 1–7. [CrossRef]

39. de la Cuesta-Zuluaga, J.; Kelley, S.T.; Chen, Y.; Escobar, J.S.; Mueller, N.T.; Ley, R.E.; McDonald, D.; Huang, S.; Swafford, A.D.; Knight, R.; et al. Age- and Sex-Dependent Patterns of Gut Microbial Diversity in Human Adults. *mSystems* **2019**, *4*, 1–12. [CrossRef]

40. Lozupone, C.A.; Stombaugh, J.I.; Gordon, J.I.; Jansson, J.K.; Knight, R. Diversity, stability and resilience of the human gut microbiota. *Nature* **2012**, *489*, 220–230. [CrossRef]

16

Ischemia and Reperfusion Injury in Kidney Transplantation: Relevant Mechanisms in Injury and Repair

Gertrude J. Nieuwenhuijs-Moeke [1,*], Søren E. Pischke [2], Stefan P. Berger [3], Jan Stephan F. Sanders [3], Robert A. Pol [4], Michel M. R. F. Struys [1,5], Rutger J. Ploeg [4,6] and Henri G. D. Leuvenink [4]

[1] Department of Anesthesiology, University of Groningen, University Medical Centre Groningen, Hanzeplein 1, 9713 GZ Groningen, The Netherlands; m.m.r.f.struys@umcg.nl

[2] Clinic for Emergencies and Critical Care, Department of Anesthesiology, Department of Immunology, Oslo University Hospital, 4950 Nydalen, 0424 Oslo, Norway; s.e.pischke@medisin.uio.no

[3] Department of Nephrology, University of Groningen, University Medical Centre Groningen, Hanzeplein 1, 9713 GZ Groningen, The Netherlands; s.p.berger@umcg.nl (S.P.B.); j.sanders@umcg.nl (J.S.F.S.)

[4] Department of Surgery, University of Groningen, University Medical Centre Groningen, Hanzeplein 1, 9713 GZ Groningen, The Netherlands; r.pol@umcg.nl (R.A.P.); rutger.ploeg@nds.ox.ac.uk (R.J.P.); h.g.d.leuvenink@umcg.nl (H.G.D.L.)

[5] Department of Basic and Applied Medical Sciences, Ghent University, Corneel Heymanslaan 10, 9000 Ghent, Belgium

[6] Nuffield Department of Surgical Sciences, University of Oxford, Headington, Oxford OX3 9DU, UK

* Correspondence: g.j.nieuwenhuijs-moeke@umcg.nl

Abstract: Ischemia and reperfusion injury (IRI) is a complex pathophysiological phenomenon, inevitable in kidney transplantation and one of the most important mechanisms for non- or delayed function immediately after transplantation. Long term, it is associated with acute rejection and chronic graft dysfunction due to interstitial fibrosis and tubular atrophy. Recently, more insight has been gained in the underlying molecular pathways and signalling cascades involved, which opens the door to new therapeutic opportunities aiming to reduce IRI and improve graft survival. This review systemically discusses the specific molecular pathways involved in the pathophysiology of IRI and highlights new therapeutic strategies targeting these pathways.

Keywords: ischemia reperfusion injury; kidney transplantation; delayed graft function; innate immune system; adaptive immune system; apoptosis; necrosis; hypoxic inducible factor; endothelial dysfunction

1. Introduction

To date, 10% of the worldwide population suffers from chronic kidney disease (CKD). The prevalence of the disease will most likely grow over the next decade due to the increase in the elderly population and the growing incidence of diabetes and hypertension. In 2015, CKD was ranked 12th in the global list of causes of death [1]. The population of patients needing renal replacement therapy (RRT) worldwide was estimated to be approximately 4.902 million (95% CI 4.438–5.431 million) in a conservative model and 9.701 million (95% CI 8.544–11.021 million) in a high estimate model, illustrating the magnitude of the disease burden of end stage renal disease (ESRD) [2].

For patients with ESRD, transplantation is still the optimal treatment. Long-term survival with kidney transplantation is dramatically better than dialysis and transplantation provides a sustainably higher quality of life. Unfortunately, there is a worldwide shortage of suitable donor organs for (kidney) transplantation. The number of renal transplantations performed worldwide in 2018 was 75.664 [3]. Due to the persistent shortage of donor kidneys, many transplant centres have established large living donor programmes and transplant teams are also now accepting increasing numbers of older and higher risk organs, retrieved from deceased donors. The use of these extended criteria donors (ECD) has affected outcomes after transplantation due to an often-suboptimal quality of the donor organ [4,5]. As we will face more complex donors in the future with a reduced viability such as unstable donation after brain death (DBD) donors, donation after circulatory death (DCD) donors, and ECD, the challenge in transplantation is to be able to use these donor sources, however, without compromising successful immediate function and long-term graft survival after transplantation. It is therefore imperative that the condition of every graft-to-be is optimised prior to or at the time of transplantation and that additional injury is minimized in order to achieve the best possible post-transplant function and avoid primary non function (PNF), delayed graft function (DGF), and rejection with chronic graft failure.

Ischemia and reperfusion injury (IRI) is inevitable in (kidney) transplantation and one of the most important mechanisms for non- or delayed function immediately after transplantation [6–8]. It is accompanied by a proinflammatory response and is associated with acute rejection due to an increased immunogenicity favouring T-cell mediated rejection as well as anti-body mediated rejection (ABMR) [9,10]. In addition, it may result in progressive interstitial fibrosis and is associated with chronic graft dysfunction due to interstitial fibrosis and tubular atrophy (IFTA) [11]. In the past decade more insight has been gained in the complex molecular pathophysiology of IRI. This may open a door to new therapeutic targets aiming to reduce IRI. The aim of this review is to systematically highlight these molecular mechanisms and to discuss potential therapeutic strategies specifically targeting these molecular pathways.

2. Ischemia and Reperfusion Injury

IRI consists of a complex pathophysiology involving activation of cell death programs, endothelial dysfunction, transcriptional reprogramming and activation of the innate and adaptive immune system [8]. Numerous pathways and signalling cascades are implicated (Figure 1) and it is while worthy to dissect the distinct effects of ischemia and reperfusion (I/R).

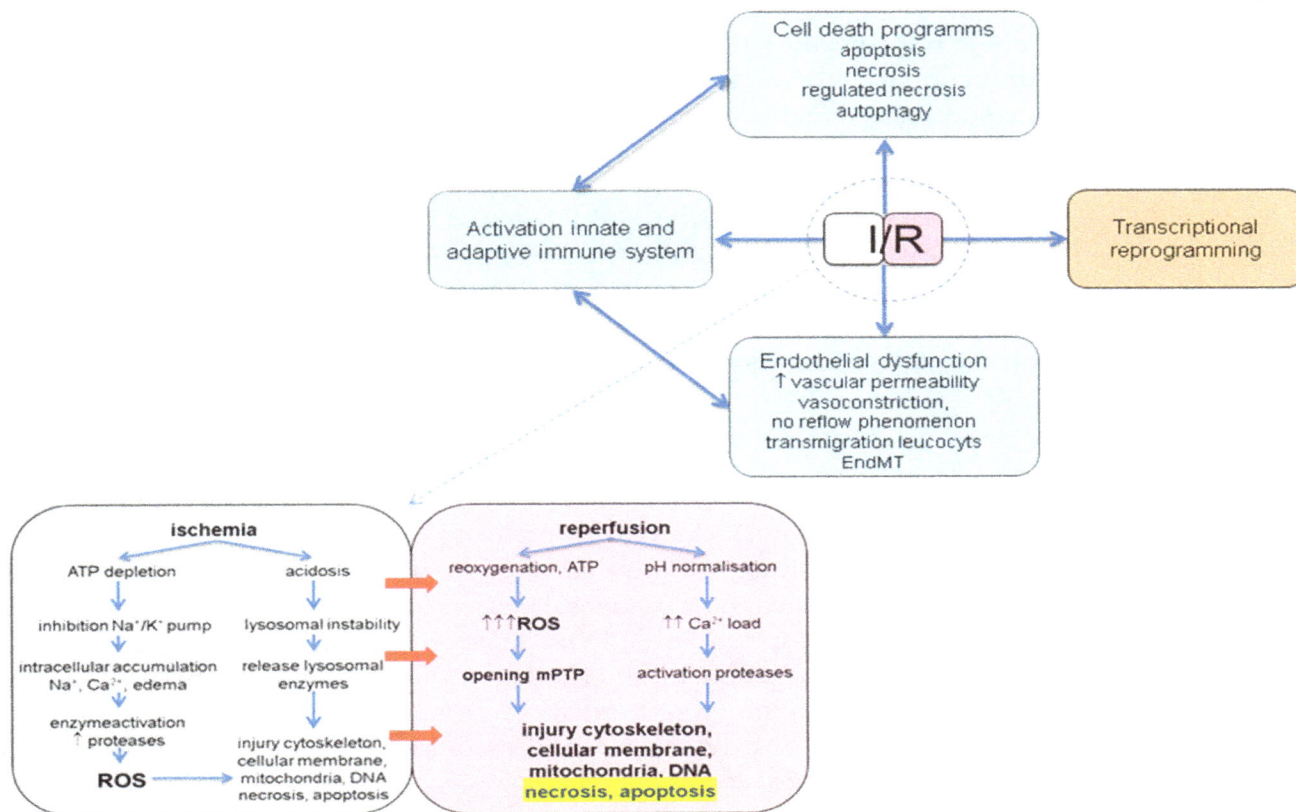

Figure 1. Schematic overview of the pathophysiological consequences of ischemia and reperfusion. I/R: ischemia/reperfusion; ATP: adenosine triphosphate; EndMT: endothelial to mesenchymal transition; ROS: reactive oxygen species; mPTP: mitochondrial permeability transition pore.

2.1. Ischemia

Due to a decrease in oxygen supply, cells will switch from an aerobic to an anaerobic metabolism, which results in a decrease in adenosine triphosphate (ATP) production and intracellular acidosis due to the formation of lactate. This causes destabilisation of lysosomal membranes with leakage of lysosomal enzymes, breakdown of the cytoskeleton and inhibition of membrane-bound Na^+/K^+ ATPase activity [12–14]. This last process gives rise to an intracellular accumulation of Na^+ ions and water with as a consequence cellular oedema. Due to declined Ca^{2+} excretion, there is an intracellular Ca^{2+} accumulation, which causes activation of Ca^{2+} dependant proteases like calpains. Due to the acidosis, these calpains stay inactive during the ischemic period but may damage the cell after normalisation of the pH during reperfusion. The remaining ATP is broken down to hypoxanthine, which will accumulate in the cell, since further metabolism into xanthine requires oxygen [15]. In the mitochondria, the Ca^{2+} overload is responsible for generation of reactive oxygen species (ROS) [8]. This will lead to opening of the mitochondrial permeability transition pores (mPTP) after reperfusion. During the ischemic period, only small amounts of ROS are produced compared to the entire I/R due to the reduction of cytochromes, nitric oxide synthases, xanthine oxidase and reduced nicotinamide adenine dinucleotide phosphate (NADPH) oxidase activation [16–19].

2.2. Reperfusion

During reperfusion, oxygen levels increase, and the pH normalises which is harmful for the previously ischemic cells. The intracellular Ca^{2+} level further increases, which activates the calpains causing injury to the cell structure and cell death [8]. Restoration of normoxemia leads to the production of large amounts of ROS, together with a reduction in the antioxidant capacity [20]. This burst of

ROS production was thought to be due to a generalised dysregulation of the electron transport chain with electrons leaking out at non-specific sites [21]. Recently, however, Chouchani et al. [22] showed that this superoxide production is generated by reverse action of complex I of the electron transport chain driven by a pool of succinate, a metabolite of the citric acid cycle, accumulated during ischemia. This massive amount of mitochondrially produced ROS is responsible for the activation of various injurious pathways through carbonylation of proteins or lipid peroxidation. This may contribute to injury of the cell membranes, the cytoskeleton and DNA and may lead to a disruption of ATP generation and induction of mPTP [20]. Additionally, the combination of ROS, dysfunctioning of the mitochondrial machinery and increase in mitochondrial Ca^{2+} load causes opening of the mPTP and release of substances like cytochrome C, succinate and mitochondrial DNA (mtDNA), which are able to induce cell death through apoptosis and necrosis and may act as danger/damage associated molecular patterns (DAMPs) entailing activation of the innate and subsequently the adaptive immune system [23–26].

Recent insights in the pathophysiological mitochondrial mechanisms and general understanding of the pivotal role of the mitochondria in IRI has led to various strategies targeting mitochondria with the aim to reduce IRI including limiting oxidative stress and mitochondrial ROS generation [20]. Both lipophilic cations and mitochondrial targeted proteins have been developed to deliver antioxidants to the mitochondria [27]. Triphenylphosphonium (TTP), a lipophilic cation, is rapidly taken up by mitochondria where it releases covalently bonded bioactive compounds. MitoQ, with its bioactive compound ubiqinone, is the most investigated of these molecules. In the mitochondria ubiqinone is reduced to ubiquinol, a powerful ROS scavenger. Administration of MitoQ in renal I/R models resulted in reduced markers of oxidative stress, reduced renal injury and improved function [28–30]. Regarding the mitochondrial targeted proteins, the Szeto-Schiller (SS) proteins are the best known. Exact mechanism of action is poorly understood but a possible explanation of action is through interaction with cardiolipin, an important component of the inner mitochondrial membrane. SS peptides have shown to reduce renal IRI in rodents [31], and its lead compound SS-31 (Elamipretide, Stealth BioTherapeutics-Alexion Pharmaceuticals) is currently being investigated in humans for its efficacy in reducing IRI post-angioplasty for renal artery stenosis. A pilot study administration of SS-31 before and during percutaneous transluminal renal angioplasty and stenting has shown to attenuate post-procedural hypoxia, increased renal blood flow and improved kidney function [32].

Another strategy to reduce ROS generation is reduction of succinate formation by inhibition of succinate dehydrogenase, preventing the accumulation of succinate, a driving force of reverse action of complex I. This has been shown to be effective in various in vivo models of IRI including the heart but has yet been unexplored in renal IRI [22,33].

3. Pathophysiological Consequences of IRI

3.1. Cell Death: Necrosis, Apoptosis, Regulated Necrosis and Autophagy

3.1.1. Necrosis

I/R leads to the activation of cell death programs. Of these programs, necrosis is the most uncontrolled form. It is due to swelling of the cell and subsequent rupture of the cellular membrane [34]. This will lead to an uncontrolled release of cellular fragments into the extracellular space. These fragments act as DAMPs and are able to activate the innate and adaptive immune system, entailing infiltration of inflammatory cells into the tissue and release of different cytokines.

3.1.2. Apoptosis

In contrast to the uncontrolled process of necrosis, apoptosis is a highly regulated and controlled process in which activation of the caspase signalling cascade results in a self-limiting programmed cell death. These caspases, a family of proteases, are essential in this process. There are two types of caspases: initiator caspases (2,8,9,10) and effector caspases (3,6,7) [35,36]. The initiator caspases are activated by binding to a specific activator protein complex (death-inducing signalling complex (DISC), apoptosome) [37]. The formed complexes then activate the effector caspases through proteolytic cleavage upon which these proteolytically degenerate various intracellular proteins. Apoptosis gives rise to apoptotic bodies, containing these intracellular protein fragments, via the process of membrane blebbing. The apoptotic bodies will undergo phagocytosis before they can spill their content into the extracellular space and therefore will generate a less immune stimulating impulse compared to necrosis. Apoptosis can be initiated through the intrinsic pathway (mitochondrial dependent pathway) in which the initiating signal comes from within the cell (e.g., damaged DNA, hypoxia, metabolic stress) or the extrinsic pathway (cell death receptor pathway) due to signals from out of the cell (tumor necrosis factor-α (TNF-α), first apoptosis signal (Fas)-ligand, FasL) (Figure 2) [37].

A protein family playing an important role in the regulation of apoptosis is the B-cell lymphoma 2 (BcL-2) family [38]. Members of this family can act as protectors (BcL-2, BcL-xL) inhibiting apoptosis, sensors (BH3 only proteins, Bad, Bim, Bid) inhibiting the protectors, or effectors (Bax, Bad) initiating apoptosis by enhancing the permeability of the mitochondrial membrane [39]. In case of intrinsic signalling, intracellular signals of cell stress will lead to an increase in the BH3 only proteins resulting in inhibition of the protectors and activation of the effectors. These effectors increase the permeability of the mitochondrial membrane resulting in leakage of pro-apoptotic proteins upon which a caspase activator complex, the apoptosome, is formed in the intracellular space [40–43]. The apoptosome cleaves procaspase-9 to its active form of caspase-9, which in turn is able to activate the effector caspase-3. In case of the extrinsic signalling, binding of TNF-α (TNF path) or the FasL, expressed on cytotoxic T lymphocytes, (Fas path) to receptors of the TNF receptor (TNFR) family will lead to the formation of a complex called the death-inducing signalling complex (DISC) [44–46]. The DISC, amongst others, consisting of a death effector domain and three procaspase-8 or -10 molecules, cleaves and activates the procaspases [47]. Activation of the initiator caspase-8 by both paths directly activates other members of the caspase signalling cascade such as the effector caspase-3 but also can lead to an increase in BH3-only proteins (Bim, Bid) and trigger the intrinsic pathway (Figure 2) [48].

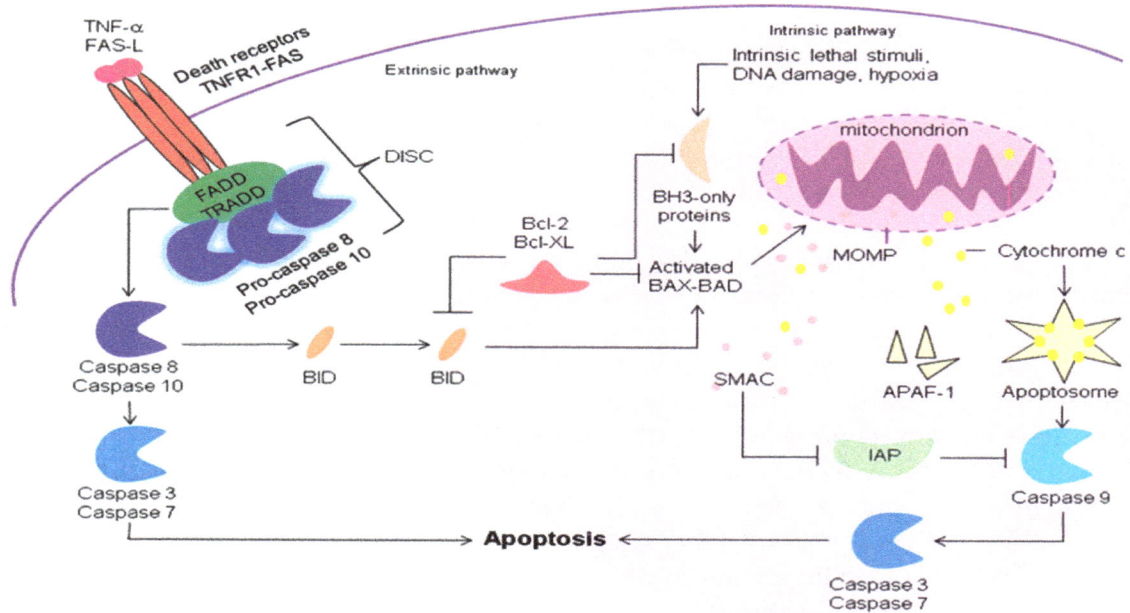

Figure 2. Extrinsic and intrinsic apoptotic pathway. The intrinsic pathway is mediated by intracellular signals of cell stress leading to an increase in the BH3 only proteins (members of the B-cell lymphoma 2 (Bcl-2) family) resulting in an inhibition of the protectors and activation of the effectors. The effectors Bax and Bad increase the permeability of the mitochondrial membrane (MOMP: mitochondrial outer membrane permeabilisation) resulting in leakage of apoptotic proteins. One of these proteins, known as second mitochondria-derived activator of caspases (SMAC), binds to proteins that inhibit apoptosis (IAPs, by suppression of the caspase proteins) causing an inactivation of these IAPs. Another protein released from the mitochondria is cytochrome c, which binds to Apoptotic protease activating factor-1 (Apaf-1) and ATP. This complex binds to procaspase-9 creating a complex, the apoptosome. The apoptosome cleaves procaspase-9 to its active form of caspase-9, which in turn is able to activate the effector caspase-3. The extrinsic pathway is mediated through receptors of the tumor necrosis factor (TNF) receptor (TNFR) family either via the TNF path or the Fas (first apoptosis signal) path. In the TNF path binding of TNF-α to a trimeric complex of TNFR1 molecules induces activation of the intracellular death domain and the formation of the receptor-bound complex 1 made up of TNF receptor-associated death domain (TRADD), receptor-interacting protein kinase 1 (RIPK1), two ubiquitin ligases (TNFR-associated factor (TRAF)-2 and cellular inhibitors of apoptosis (cIAP)1/2) and the linear ubiquitin assembly complex (LUBAC). This complex 1 can lead to a pro-survival pathway or to apoptosis. In case of apoptosis the TRADD dependant complex IIa (consisting of TRADD, Fas-associated death domain protein (FADD) and caspase-8) or the RIPK-1 dependant complex IIb also known as the ripoptosome (consisting FADD, RIPK1, RIPK3 and caspase-8) is formed. In the Fas path, presence of the Fas ligand (FasL, expressed on cytotoxic T lymphocytes) causes three Fas receptors (CD95) to trimirize. This clustering and binding to the FasL initiates binding of FADD. Three procaspase-8 or -10 molecules can then interact with the complex by their own death effector domains. The complex formed is the death-inducing signalling complex (DISC) which cleaves and activates procaspase-8 and 10. Activation of the initiator caspase-8 by both paths directly activates other members of the caspase signalling cascade such as the effector caspase-3 but also can lead to an increase in BH3-only proteins (Bim, Bid) and trigger the intrinsic pathway).

3.1.3. Regulated Necrosis

Recently, new pathways of a more regulated form of necrosis have been described. These processes show features of apoptosis as well as necrosis. One of the best-known pathways of regulated necrosis is via TNFR-1 and is called necroptosis [46]. In the absence of active caspase-8, phosphorylation of receptor-interacting protein kinase 1 (RIPK1) and RIPK3 in complex IIb leads to formation of a complex called the necrosome. The necrosome recruits Mixed Kinase Domain-Like protein (MLKL), which is then phosphorylated by RIPK3 [46]. MLKL activates the necrosis phenotype by entering the bilipid membranes of organelles and the cellular membrane. This causes formation of pores in these membranes and leads to release of cellular contents, functioning as DAMPs, into the extracellular space [49]. As in necrosis the DAMPs are able to activate both the innate and adaptive immune system promoting proinflammatory responses that activate rejection pathways [50,51]. A recent study in a kidney transplant mouse model showed that RIPK3-deficient kidneys had better function and longer rejection-free survival [52]. Therefore RIPK3-inhibiting drugs might be of interest in the reduction of IRI in organ transplantation. Next to TNFR-1, other death receptors and toll like receptors (TLR) have also shown to be able to induce necroptosis [46]. Other forms of regulated necrosis include mitochondrial permeability transition (MPT)-associated death (involving opening of mPTP leading to necrosis instead of apoptosis), ferroptosis (involving iron and gluthation metabolism), parthanatos (also known as PARP-1 (Poly(ADP-ribose) polymerase-1) dependent cell death, involving the accumulation of PAR (poly(ADP-ribose)) and the nuclear translocation of apoptosis-inducing factor (AIF) from mitochondria) and pyroptosis (involving caspase-1 and -11 in mice and caspase-4 and -5 in humans) [53]. The role of pyroptosis in IRI in the kidney, however, is unclear.

3.1.4. Autophagy

Cells can preserve their metabolic function and escape cellular death. This is due to autophagy of damaged cell parts. There are several pathways of autophagy, namely, macro-autophagy, micro-autophagy and chaperone-mediated autophagy—the last two are beyond the scope of this review. Macro-autophagy (hereafter called autophagy) involves formation of autophagosomes containing damaged cell parts or unused proteins. These double membrane autophagosomes travel through the cytoplasm to fuse with lysosomes (autolysosome) leading to degradation of the damaged cell parts. This process is continuously active at low basal levels, preserving cellular homeostasis, but stimulated upon stress through various signals like nutrient deprivation, ROS formation, hypoxia, free amino acids, etc. [54–56]. Cellular building blocks obtained from recycling of damaged cell parts by autophagy may serve as anti-stress responses and energy source promoting cell survival.

The first step in autophagy, the initiation, is regulated by two kinases: mammalian target of rapamycin complex 1 (mTOR, mTORC1) and adenosine monophosphate-activated protein kinase (AMPK) [54,57,58]. Together, they regulate the activity of the Unc-51 like autophagy activating kinase 1/2 (ULK1/2) complex [59,60]. Activation of mTOR leads to the phosphorylation of this complex and inhibition of autophagy (for instance, through the phosphatidylinositol 3-kinase (PI3K)/Protein kinase B (AKT) or the mitogen-activated protein kinase (MAPK)/extracellular signal–regulated kinase (Erk) 1/2 signalling pathway). On the other hand, activation of AMPK, upon intracellular AMP increase, activates autophagy [61]. This occurs by inhibition of the mTORC1 through dissociation of mTORC1 from ULK1/2 (indirect) or in a direct way by phosphorylation of ULK1/2 forming the ULK1/2-complex [62,63]. Next to the ULK1/2 complex, inducible beclin-1 complex (or class III PI3K complex) is involved in initiation of autophagy. This complex is activated by the ULK-1/2 complex and inhibited by Bcl-2 and Bcl-XL. The ULK1/2 and class III PI3K complexes join to form the phagopore and eventually the autophagosme which will fuse with a lysosome [64–69]. The content of this formed autolysosome is degenerated, and the components are released to be reused to synthesise new proteins or to function as an energy source for the cell (Figure 3) [70].

In renal IRI, autophagy is considered a doubled-edged sword. Upon I/R, it is mostly upregulated, but both protective and harmful effects are observed, proposing a dual role for autophagy in renal IRI [71,72]. Decuypere et al. [71] hypothesize that autophagy can switch roles depending on the severity of the ischemic injury. The exact mechanism behind this switch is unclear but may depend on the survival vs death properties of beclin1 and its interaction with the Bcl-2 family proteins [71,73]. Autophagy can be considered a protective mechanism in (oxidative) stress injured cells through restoring cellular homeostasis. Kidneys from older donors are at increased risk of DGF.

The age-dependent decline in autophagy activity and age-dependant autophagic dysfunction may be one of the underlying mechanisms of this phenomenon [74]. Extensive oxidative stress (amount or duration), however, may have detrimental effects which eventually could trigger the switch to aggravation of the injury through autophagy dependant cell death. Excessive or prolonged ROS exposure may lead to the oxidative modification of macromolecules making them only partially degradable by the autolysosome [75]. Furthermore, an energy dependent process of autophagy could deprive the cell of necessary energy. In this light, excessive autophagy seen after prolonged cold ischemia time in particular in DCD donors seems to be one of the underlying mechanisms behind augmentation of reperfusion injury seen in these circumstances, thereby increasing the risk of DGF [71,76]. Based on this dual role of autophagy in renal IRI and transplantation the goal would be to restrict autophagy levels within a protective window. Upon severe ischemia (prolonged cold ischemia time (CIT)) autophagy inhibitors most likely outweigh the activators [71]. Continuing efforts have to be made to elucidate the mechanism of autophagic transition from protective to harmful function.

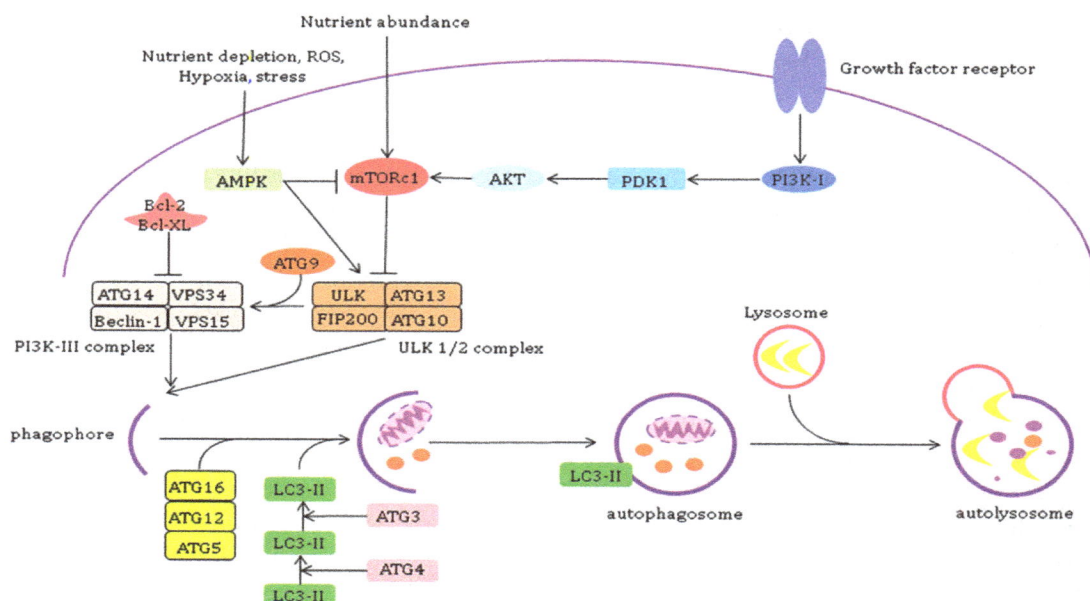

Figure 3. Pathways of macro-autophagy. Initiation of autophagy is regulated by mTORC1 (mammalian target of rapamycin complex 1) and AMPK (AMP-activated kinase). Together, they regulate the activity of the ULK1/2 complex consisting of ULK1/2 (Unc-51 like autophagy activating kinase), FIP200 (FAK family kinase interacting protein of 200 kDa) and the autophagy related proteins (ATG) ATG13 and ATG10. Activation of mTOR leads to the phosphorylation of this complex and inhibition of autophagy (for instance, through the phosphatidylinositol 3-kinase (PI3K)/ Protein kinase B (AKT) or the mitogen-activated protein kinase (MAPK)/ extracellular signal–regulated kinase (Erk) 1/2 signalling pathway) whereas activation of AMPK activates autophagy. AMPK, activated upon intracellular AMP increase, is able to activate autophagy by inhibition of the mTORC1 through dissociation of mTORC1 from ULK1/2 allowing ULK1/2 to be activated. AMPK, is also able to initiate autophagy in a direct way by phosphorylation of ULK1/2 forming the ULK1/2-complex. Another complex involved in the initiation is the autophagy inducible beclin-1 complex (or class III PI3K complex) which consists of Vps34 (phosphatidylinositol 3-kinase), beclin-1 (a BH3 only domain protein member of the Bcl-2 family), vps15 and ATG14. This complex is activated by the ULK-1 complex and inhibited by Bcl-2 and Bcl-XL. The ULK1/2 and class III PI3K complexes join to form the phagopore and eventually the autophagosme. This process is mediated by the ATG5-ATG12-ATG16 complex and the formation of phosphatidylethanolamine-conjugated Light Chain (LC) 3 (LC3-II) facilitating elongation of the bilipid membrane to form a closed autophagosme. The autophagosome fuses with a lysosome and the content of the autolysosome is degenerated and the components are released to be reused to synthesise new proteins or to function as an energy source for the cell. PDK-1: pyruvate dehydrogenase kinase-1.

The different cell death programs described above are induced in response to common stimuli. Several proteins in the autophagy and apoptosis pathway are shared resulting in an intimate crosstalk between apoptosis and autophagy. Regulation of these proteins determines cellular fate to cell survival or cell death. Caspase-mediated degradation of several autophagy regulation proteins limits autophagosome formation and therefore autophagy [77–79]. Apoptosis inhibitors Bcl-2 and Bcl-XL also inhibit autophagy by binding to Beclin-1 limiting its availability to form the classIII PI3K complex [80,81]. Inhibition of cisplatin induced autophagy enhanced caspase-3 activation and apoptosis in renal proximal tubular cells [82,83]. On the other hand, overexpression of ATG5 and beclin-1 prevented cisplatinum induced caspase activation and apoptosis [84]. Additionally, there is evidence that autophagy induction regulates necroptosis. Inhibition of autophagy has shown to prevent necroptosis and vice versa inhibition of necroptosis is able to supress autophagy [85,86].

3.1.5. Targeting Cell Death Programs

Targeting pathways of cell death programs to reduce IRI seems very attractive, since it directly preserves cellular function. Secondly, dead cells releasing DAMPs elicit a strong immune response not only in the organ exposed to I/R but also in other organs of the individual, so called remote organ injury. Therefore, interfering with this process might be immunosuppressive and organ protective. The relative contribution of each of the cell death programs to IRI and outcome in transplantation, however, has to be elucidated.

Nydam et al. [87] showed in a syngeneic mouse transplant model that administration of the pan-caspase inhibitor Q-VD-OPh during graft retrieval and cold preservation resulted in decreased caspase-3 expression and activity, reduced apoptosis in renal tubular cells and improved renal function post-transplantation. The pro-apoptotic gene p53 is activated upon hypoxia, oxidative stress and DNA damage and is able to induce cell cycle arrest, which enables DNA-repair proteins to repair the sustained injury. However, in case of severe DNA damage it induces apoptosis by initiating the intracellular pathway.

Inhibition of P53 in proximal tubular cells has been shown to decrease apoptotic cell death and provide protection against IRI [88,89]. QPI-1002 is a synthetic small interfering ribonucleic acid (siRNA) designed to reversibly and temporarily inhibit p53. In pre-clinical models it has been shown that QPI undergoes rapid glomerular filtration and uptake by proximal tubular epithelial cells [89]. Administration of QPI-1002 has shown to be safe in humans. Two phase I dose escalating safety and pharmacokinetics studies in patients undergoing major cardiovascular surgery (NCT00554359, NCT00683553) has been executed without dose-limiting toxicities or safety issues. A phase I/II study has been executed to evaluate QPI-1002 for the prevention of DGF in recipients of kidneys from deceased donors (NCT00802347) in which treatment with QPI-1002 resulted in lower incidence and severity of DGF [90]. Recently, a phase 3 randomized, double-blind, placebo-controlled study in recipients ($n = 594$) of (older) DBD donor kidneys (>45 years) has been completed (NCT02610296, ReGIFT-study). Results have not been reported yet.

Various pharmacological substances like necrostatins (RIPK1 inhibitors, necroptosis), ferrostatins (ferroptosis), sanglifehrin A (MPT-associated death) and olaparib (parthanatos) and many others have been developed to target specific key molecules of the different programs of regulated necrosis and are currently tested in various animal and disease models (Figure 4) [91,92]. The question remains how safe it will be to inhibit non-apoptocic cell death pathways in patients, since these pathways also function as a backup system when apoptosis fails or is inhibited for instance, by caspase inhibitor expressing viruses. Of these molecules, RIPK1 inhibitors have now entered clinical trials and their safety is being tested in healthy volunteers [93,94].

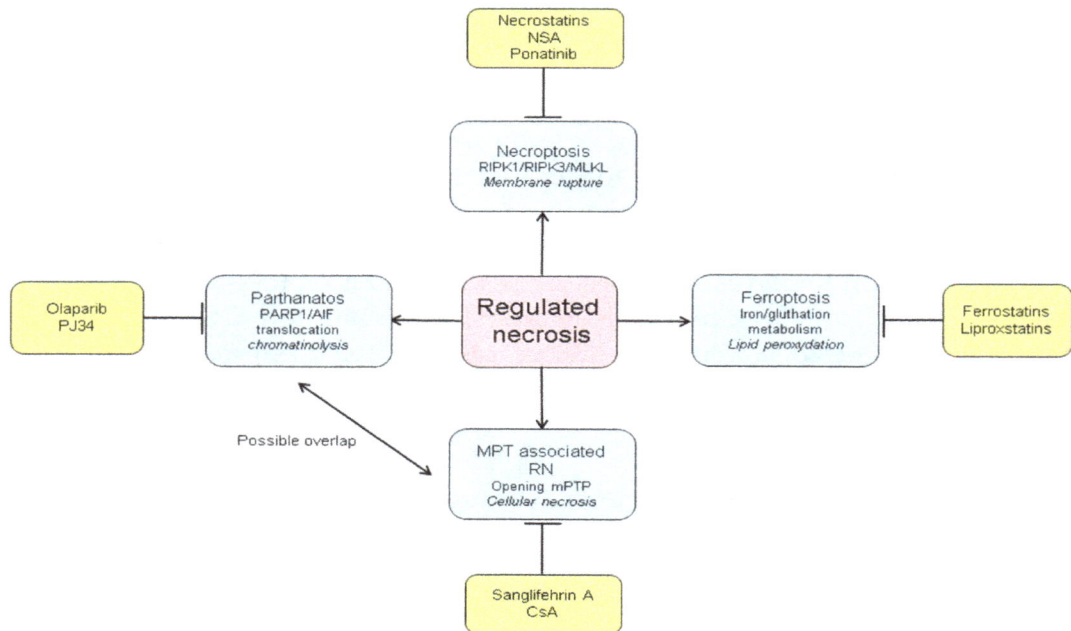

Figure 4. Programs of regulated necrosis and their inhibitors. RIPK1: receptor-interacting protein kinase 1; RIPK3: receptor-interacting protein kinase 3; MLKL: Mixed Kinase Domain-Like protein; MPT: mitochondrial permeability transition; mPTP: mitochondrial permeability transition pore; RN: regulated necrosis; CsA: cyclosporin A; PARP1: poly (ADP-ribose) polymerase-1; AIF: apoptosis-inducing factor.

3.2. Endothelial Dysfunction

At a vascular level, I/R leads to swelling of the endothelial cells (ECs), loss of the glycocalyx and degradation of the cytoskeleton. As a consequence, intercellular contact of endothelial cells is lost, increasing vascular permeability and fluid loss to the interstitial space [95]. Furthermore, the endothelium will produce vasoactive substances like platelet-derived growth factor (PDGF) and Endothelin-1 (ET-1), causing vasoconstriction [96]. This vasoconstriction can be enhanced by a reduced nitric oxide (NO) production during reperfusion due to decreased endothelial nitric oxide synthase (eNOS) expression and increased sensitivity of the arterioles for vasoactive substances like angiotensin II, thromboxane A2 and prostaglandin H2 [97–99]. Eventually this can lead to the so called no reflow phenomenon characterized by the absence of adequate perfusion on microcirculatory level despite reperfusion.

The regenerative capacity of ECs in peritubular capillaries is limited and injury to the microcirculation may lead to permanent peritubular capillary rarefaction [100,101]. Chronic hypoxia in these regions may induce transcription of fibrogenic genes like transforming growth factor-β (TGF-β) and connective tissue growth factor (CTGF) together with an accumulation of α-smooth muscle actin (α-SMA) [101]. In the end, this may lead to development of IFTA, a process which has mainly been attributed to resident fibroblasts. More recently, however, the role of endothelial-to-mesenchymal transition (EndMT) in this process has been described [102,103]. During EndMT, ECs lose their endothelial phenotype (such as expression of specific endothelial markers like Von Willebrand factor (VWF)) and acquire the phenotype of multipotent mesenchymal cells (MSC). These cells show an increased expression of α-SMA, neuronal (N)-cadherin, vimentin and fibroblast-specific protein-1 and exhibit enhanced migratory potential and increased extracellular matrix production [104–106]. In a porcine I/R model Curci et al. [102] showed that 20%–30% of the total α-SMA+ cells emerging after IRI were also CD31+ suggesting a different origin compared to resident activated fibroblasts. Man et al. [107] showed that in kidney transplant recipients experiencing IFTA and allograft dysfunction, progression of EndMT plays an important role. EndMT is controlled by complex signalling pathways and networks. In their porcine I/R model, Curci et al. [102] showed a critical role of complement in this process. Kidneys of pigs treated with recombinant C1 inhibitor (C1-INH) showed preserved EC density, significant reduction of α-SMA expression and limited collagen deposition 24 h after I/R compared to untreated pigs. The ECs in the treated pigs showed preserved physiological conformation and position tight to the basal layer of the vessels. The number of transitioning ECs was significantly lower in the treated animals. In an additional in vitro experiment activating ECs with the anaphylatoxin C3a, they showed that C3a induced down regulation of the expression of VWF whilst upregulating α-SMA, by activating the Akt pathway. Activation of the ECs with C5a showed a similar response [102]. Targeting signalling pathways in EndMT in kidney transplantation could be of interest to reduce IFTA and enhance long-term graft survival. More insight however has to be gained to the exact role of EndMT in renal transplantation and what suitable targets to aim for. Furthermore, since EndMT gives rise to multipotent MSC this placidity could be of interest to push these MSCs in the direction of regeneration rather than fibrosis.

An important feature of IRI is the chemotaxis of leukocytes, endothelial adhesion and transmigration of these cells into the interstitial compartment [108]. This process is initiated by increased expression of P-selectin on the endothelial cells and interaction of P-selectin with P-selectin glycoprotein 1 (PSGL-) expressed on the leukocytes. This interaction results in rolling of the leukocytes on the endothelium. Subsequently, firm adherence of the leucocytes to the endothelium is achieved by the interaction of the β2-integrins lymphocyte function-associated antigen 1(LFA-1) and macrophage-1 antigen (MAC-1 or complement receptor 3, CR3) on the leukocyte and the intracellular adhesion molecule 1 (ICAM-1) on the endothelial cells. Platelet endothelial cell adhesion molecule 1 (PECAM-1) thereafter facilitates transmigration into the interstitial space. Once activated, these leukocytes will release several toxic substances like ROS, proteases, elastases and different cytokines in the interstitial compartment which will result in further injury like increased vascular permeability, oedema, thrombosis and parenchymal cell death (Figure 5) [109].

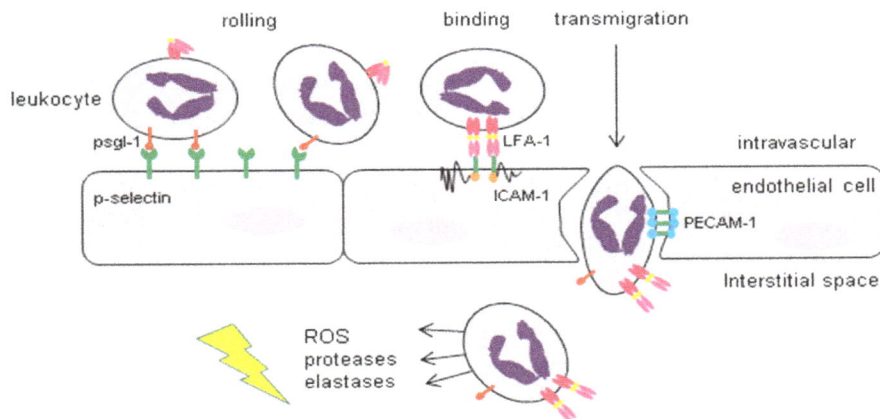

Figure 5. Interaction of leukocytes and endothelial cells in the process of transmigration of leukocytes. The increased expression of P-selectin on the endothelial cells upon I/R facilitates interaction with P-selectin glycoprotein 1 (PSGL-) expressed on the leukocytes. This results in rolling of the leukocytes on the endothelium. Subsequently, firm adherence of the leucocytes to the endothelium is achieved by interaction of lymphocyte function-associated antigen 1(LFA-1) and macrophage-1 antigen (MAC-1 or complement receptor 3, CR3) on the leukocyte and the intracellular adhesion molecule 1 (ICAM-1) on the endothelial cells. Finally, platelet endothelial cell adhesion molecule 1 (PECAM-1) facilitates transmigration of the leukocytes into the interstitial space. Once activated, these leukocytes will release several toxic substances like ROS, proteases, elastases and different cytokines in the interstitial compartment resulting in further injury like increased vascular permeability, oedema, thrombosis and parenchymal cell death.

3.3. Innate and Adaptive Immune Response

IRI is accompanied by sterile inflammation in which the innate as well as the adaptive immune system are involved.

3.3.1. Innate Immune Response

The innate, or non-specific, immune system is evolutionary the oldest part of the immune system. It acts on infection or injury with a fast, short-lasting and non-specific response in which different cells and systems are involved.

Toll-Like Receptor Signalling

In the innate immune response, the toll-like receptors (TLRs) play an important role [110]. TLRs are transmembrane proteins and members of the interleukin-1 receptor (IL-IR) superfamily. They function as pattern recognition receptors (PRR) and are present on the cellular membrane and in the cytosol of cells like leukocytes, endothelial cells and tubular cells [111]. The human TLR family contains 10 members, TLR1–TLR10 [112]—of which, TLR2 and TLR4 have shown to be upregulated in tubular epithelial cells upon ischemia [113–117]. Both are attributed an equal importance in initiating apoptosis in a genetic knock-out renal I/R mouse model [115]. TLR activation leads to the downstream recruitment of various adapter molecules (TNF receptor-associated factor 6 (TRAF6), Myeloid differentiation primary-response protein 88 (MyD88), toll-interleukin 1 receptor (TIR) domain containing adaptor protein (TIRAP), TIR-domain-containing adapter-inducing interferon-β (TRIF), TRIF-related adaptor molecule (TRAM)) activating different kinases (IL-1 receptor-associated kinase (IRAK)-1 (IRAK-1), IRAK-4, inhibitor of nuclear factor-κB kinase (IKK), TANK-binding Kinase-1 (TBK1)), leading to activation of transcription factors (nuclear factor kappa-light-chain-enhancer of activated B cells (NF-κB), IFN-regulatory factor 3 (IRF3) resulting in transcription of proinflammatory genes and the subsequent inflammatory response [8,112].

TLR2 and TLR4 have polyvalent ligand binding activity and can be activated by exogeneous (e.g., lipopolysaccharide, LPS) and endogenous ligands comprising DAMPs released upon I/R. These DAMPs vary depending on type of injury and tissue involved. High-mobility group box-1 (HMGB-1), an intracellular protein involved in the organisation of DNA and the regulation of gene transcription, is one of the DAMPs linked to the pathogenesis of IRI [118–120]. From the nucleus, HMGB-1 can be released into the cytosol or extracellular space by passive leakage from injured cells or through active secretion by immune cells [121,122].

In IRI in the kidney, TLR4 plays an important role. Bergler et al. [123] showed that TLR4 is highly upregulated after renal IRI, and that high TLR4 expression is strongly correlated with graft dysfunction in an allogenic renal transplant model in rats. Furthermore, TLR4-deficient mice are protected against renal IRI and kidneys from donors with a TLR4-loss of function allele show less pro inflammatory cytokines in the kidney after transplantation and a higher percentage of immediate graft function [118,124]. Activation of TLR4 in renal IRI has various consequences on the graft. First of all it promotes the release of different proinflammatory mediators like IL-6, IL-1β and TNF-α, accompanied by an increased expression of macrophage inflammatory protein-2 (MIP-2) and monocyte chemo attractant protein-1 (MCP-1) involved in the recruitment of neutrophils and macrophages [124]. Second, TLR-4 activation leads to increased expression of adhesion molecules ICAM-1, vascular cell adhesion molecule 1 (VCAM-1) and E-selectin facilitating leukocyte migration and infiltration into the interstitial space. TLR-4 signalling seems mandatory for this increased expression. Chen et al. [125]

showed that increased expression of adhesion molecules after renal IRI was absent in TLR4 knockout mice in vivo and the addition of HMGB-1 to isolated endothelial cells increased adhesion molecule expression on cells from wild-type but not from TLR4 knockout mice. Thirdly, activation of TLR4 on circulating immune cells of the innate immune system leads to activation of these cells. Neutrophils and macrophages are involved in an early stage after reperfusion. Neutrophils are regarded as the primary mediators of injury and their activation leads to ROS release, secretion of different proteases and renal tissue injury [126]. Upon activation, macrophages release proteolytic enzymes and proinflammatory cytokines like TNF-α, IL-1β and interferon-γ (IFN-γ) [127]. In TLR-4 knockout mice subjected to IRI, neutrophil and macrophage infiltration was reduced [124]. Finally, the TLR4-facilitated immune response is linked to renal fibrosis. The upregulation of TLR4 upon I/R induces a strong inflammatory response accompanied by tubular necrosis, loss of brush border, formation of casts and tubular dilatation [124]. Such a robust inflammation is known to potentiate interstitial fibrosis [128].

Proposed endogenous ligands for TLR-4 in renal IRI include HMGB-1, extracellular matrix (ECM) components like biglycan, heparin sulphate and soluble hyaluronan, and heat shock proteins (Hsps) [129–134]. Upon ligand binding, activation of TLR4 leads to downstream signalling via the MyD88-dependent and MyD88 independent pathway (Figure 6). The MyD88-dependent pathway in which MyD88 and TIRAP or MyD88 adapter-like (Mal) recruits and activates members of the IRAK family is considered to be the dominant pathway [124,135]. Wang et al. [136] demonstrated that MyD88- and TRIF-deficient mice showed a significant reduction in interstitial fibrosis reflected by α-SMA and collagen I and II accumulation Furthermore, Administration of the MyD88 specific inhibitor TJ-M2010-2, a small molecular compound, inhibiting the homodimerisation of MyD88, in a renal I/R model in mice has shown to prolong the survival rate, preserve renal function and attenuate the inflammatory responses and apoptosis in the kidney. In the long term, inhibition of the TLR/MyD88 signalling pathway with TJ-M2010-2 attenuated renal fibrosis via inhibition of TGF-β-induced epithelial to mesenchymal transition [137]. Liu et al. [138] showed that pre-treatment with the synthetic TLR4 inhibitor eritoran (Eisai co., Ltd, Tokyo, Japan) in an renal I/R rat model resulted in reduced expression of TNF-α, IL-1β and MCP-1, attenuated monocyte infiltration in the kidney and improved renal outcome Altogether in view of the pivotal role of TLR4 in renal IRI, inhibition of TLR4 or upstream or downstream mediators could be an interesting target in reducing IRI and optimising graft survival.

Next to TLR4, TLR 2 is markedly upregulated upon ischemic injury in the kidney and its upregulation is associated with the initiation of an inflammatory response [139]. Kidneys of TLR2-/- mice subjected to I/R showed less tubular damage compared to TLR2+/+ mice. Reduced levels of MIP-2, MCP-1, and IL-6 and reduced levels of infiltrating leucocytes were seen [140]. The role of TLR2 in the development or progression of renal fibrosis, however, is less clear. Leemans et al. [139] showed that in a mouse model of obstructive nephropathy TLR2 does not play a significant role in renal progressive injury and fibrosis. In addition to this de Groot et al. [141] showed in human allograft biopsies that TLR2 expression 6, 12 and 24 months after transplantation is associated with superior graft outcome in the long run Currently, the humanized immune globuline (Ig) G4 (IgG4) monoclonal antibody against TLR2 OPN-305 (Tomaralimab, Opsona Therapeutics Ltd, Dublin, Ireland) has entered phase 2 trials (NCT01794663) with the aim to reduce delayed graft function in recipients of post-mortal donor kidneys. In the first part (A) of this study a single dose of 0.5 mg/kg administered 1h before reperfusion was associated with full inhibition of TLR2 and an 80% reduction of IL-6 [142]. Subsequently, this dose has been used in part B of the study, which has been completed but results have not been reported yet.

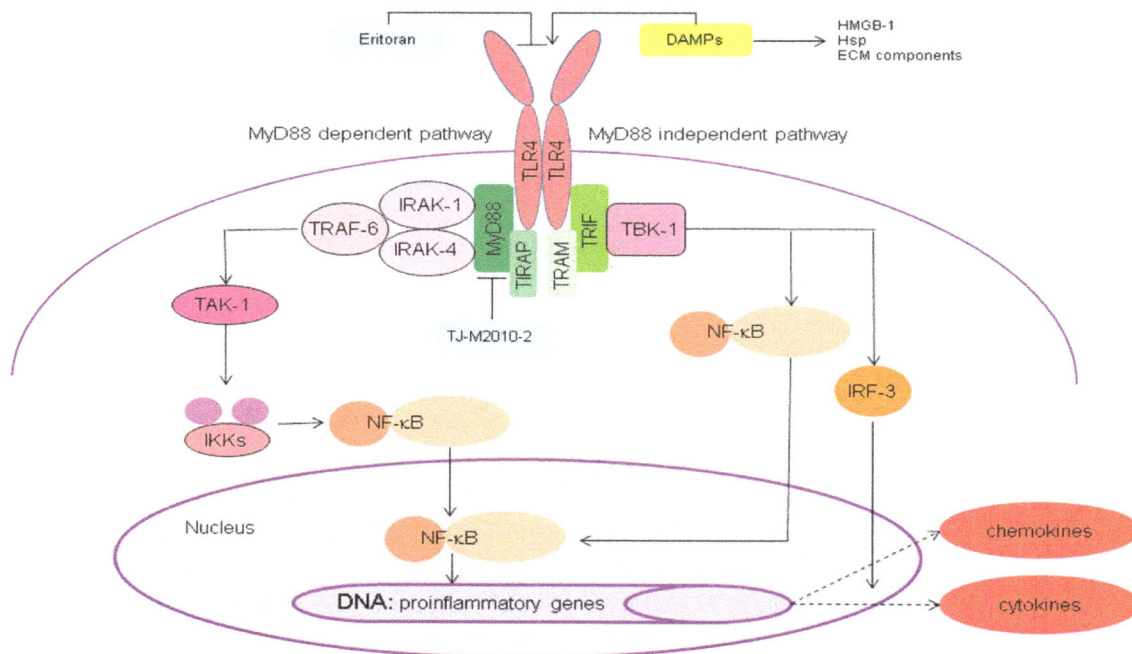

Figure 6. Toll-like receptor 4 signalling. Activation of toll-like receptor 4 (TLR4) by danger associated molecular patterns (DAMPs), like high mobility group box-1 (HMGB-1), heat shock proteins (hsp) and extracellular matrix (ECM) components, leads to downstream signalling via the MyD88 (Myeloid differentiation primary-response protein 88) dependent and MyD88 independent pathway. The MyD88-dependent pathway in which MyD88 and TIRAP (toll-interleukin 1 receptor (TIR) domain containing adaptor protein) or MyD88 adapter-like (Mal) recruits and activates members of the IL-1 receptor-associated kinase (IRAK) family is considered to be the dominant pathway. IRAK activation leads to recruitment of TRAF6 (TNF receptor-associated factor 6) and subsequently activation of transforming growth factor beta-activated kinase 1 (TAK1). Activation of TAK1 then leads to the activation of inhibitor of nuclear factor-κB kinase (IKK), which results in the release of nuclear factor kappa-light-chain-enhancer of activated B cells (NF-κB) from its inhibitor, promoting translocation to the nucleus. The MyD88 independent pathway is mediated by the adapter molecules TIR-domain-containing adapter-inducing interferon-β (TRIF)/TRIF-related adaptor molecule (TRAM) and downstream signalling leads to activation of 2 inhibitor of nuclear factor-κB kinase (IKK) homologs IKKε and TANK-binding Kinase-1 (TBK1), which possibly form a complex together and activate transcription factors NF-κB and IFN-regulatory factor 3 (IRF3). From here, proinflammatory gene transcription is initiated. TLR4 signalling is inhibited by Eritoran and TJ-M2010-2.

Complement System

The complement system is the second crucial player in the innate immune response in IRI. The system consists of soluble proteins, regulatory proteins and membrane-bound receptors and comprises three pathways. DAMPs released upon I/R are able to activate all three pathways via binding to C1q (classical pathway), C3 (alternative pathway) or PRRs of the lectin pathway (LP).

Recently, the LP has been pointed out as the primary route of renal complement activation after I/R [143]. Activation of the LP can take place through various PRRs like collectins (manose binding lectin (MBL) and collectin-11) [144] and ficolins (ficolin 1-3) [145]. Upon binding of the collectin–mannan-binding lectin serine protease (MASP) complex to carbohydrate-bearing ligands (for instance, mannose or fructose expressed on stressed cells) the MASPs are activated to cleave complement component (C) 4 (C4) and C2. LP activation is critically dependant on the action of MASP-2 [146,147]. In an isograft transplantation model in wild-type and MASP-2-deficient mice, Asgari et al. [147] showed that renal function was preserved with MASP-2 deficiency After complex-ligand interaction,

LP proceeds with cleavage of C4 and C2, mediated by MASP-2, leading to the synthesis of the classical pathway C3 convertase. Recently, a C4 independent bypass in the LP pathway was also demonstrated [122]. This could explain why C4-deficient mice are not protected against renal I/R and cellular mediated rejection [148,149]. One of the PRRs assigned an important role in the LP is collectin-11 (CL-11), a soluble C-type lectin containing a carbohydrate recognition domain and MASP binding domain [150]. In renal tissue, tubular cells are the main source of CL-11 and expression increases after IRI [151]. CL-11 has been appointed an important role in complement activation in the kidney. It has been shown that CL-11 engages L-fucose at sites of ischemic stress and inflammation initiating the LP [147]. In a renal I/R model, CL-11-deficient mice showed no post-ischemic and complement mediated injury supporting the importance of CL-11 in triggering renal complement activation.

All activating routes converge and lead to the formation of the C3 convertase (C4b2b, C3bBbP). C3 convertase cleaves and activates additional C3, creating C3a and C3b. C3b together with C4b2b forms the C5 convertase, which will cleave C5 into C5a and C5b. C5b together with C6–9 will then form the Membrane Attack Complex (MAC, C5b-9). The formed complement effectors will lead to opsonisation (C3b), chemotaxis of neutrophils and macrophages (C3a, C5a) [143]. The formed MAC inserted into the cellular membrane is associated with a proinflammatory response via noncanonical NF-KB signalling (Figure 7) [152,153].

Next to inducing inflammation and cell death, the complement system is able to modulate antigen presentation and T cell priming via C3a and C5a and is therefore playing a role in donor antigen sensitisation and rejection [154]. Antigen-presenting cells (APC) express C3 and C5 along with complement receptors C3aR and C5aR1. Upon complement activation in the extracellular space, C3a and C5a increase the presentation of alloantigens and expression of co-stimulatory molecules on the APC enhancing APC priming of T cells [143]. Furthermore, C3a and C5a promote T-cell differentiation of CD4+ and CD8+ T-cells. CD8+ cells mediate vascular and cellular T-cell mediated rejection. Upon activation, CD4+ T-cells can stimulate further CD8+ T-cell differentiation, they can proliferate and differentiate to memory and effector CD4+ cells which can activate macrophages, recruit leukocytes and stimulate inflammation and finally CD4+ cells stimulate B-cell differentiation and in the end antibody production [143]. The B-cells response can also be enhanced in a direct manner via C3b and C3d on the APC and the complement receptor 2 (CR2) on the B-cell. Activation of the B-cell by binding to the donor alloantigen induces class switching of the donor specific antibody from IgM to IgG. Subsequently, ABMR occurs when IgG donor specific antibodies (DSA) recognizes antigens in the kidney graft and engage with C1q, C1r and C1s to activate the classical pathway [143]. Under normal physiological circumstances, formation of the complement effectors is controlled by proteins (soluble or surface bound) that mediate break down of the C3 and C5 convertases. After I/R this balance shifts to uncontrolled complement activation predisposing the graft to complement mediated injury and rejection [155].

Many interventions on the level of C3, C5, and regulatory proteins in I/R injury and especially kidney transplantation have been evaluated in pre- and clinical studies [156]. Eculizumab (Soliris®, Alexion Pharmaceuticals, New Haven, CT, USA) is to date the best studied complement inhibitor in kidney transplantation. Therapeutic inhibition of C5 with the use of eculizumab, an anti-human C5 micro antibody, showed potential in the prevention and/or treatment in AMBR [157–159] and has been investigated as such in several phase 2/3 clinical trials (NCT01567085, NCT01106027, NCT01399593). All studies report a safety profile of the drug that is consistent with that reported for eculizumab's approved indications like atypical haemolytic uremic syndrome. Results of these trials suggest a potential role of eculizumab in the prevention and treatment of ABMR in patients with DSA [160,161]. Next to ABMR, eculizumab has been investigated for the prevention of DGF (NCT01919346, NCT02145182). Again, the safety profile was good but pre-treatment with eculizumab had no effect on the incidence of DGF. Groups in these studies, however, were rather small [162]. Another anti-C5 antibody Tesidolumab (LFG-316, MorphoSys, Novartis) has currently entered phase 1 studies (NCT02878616).

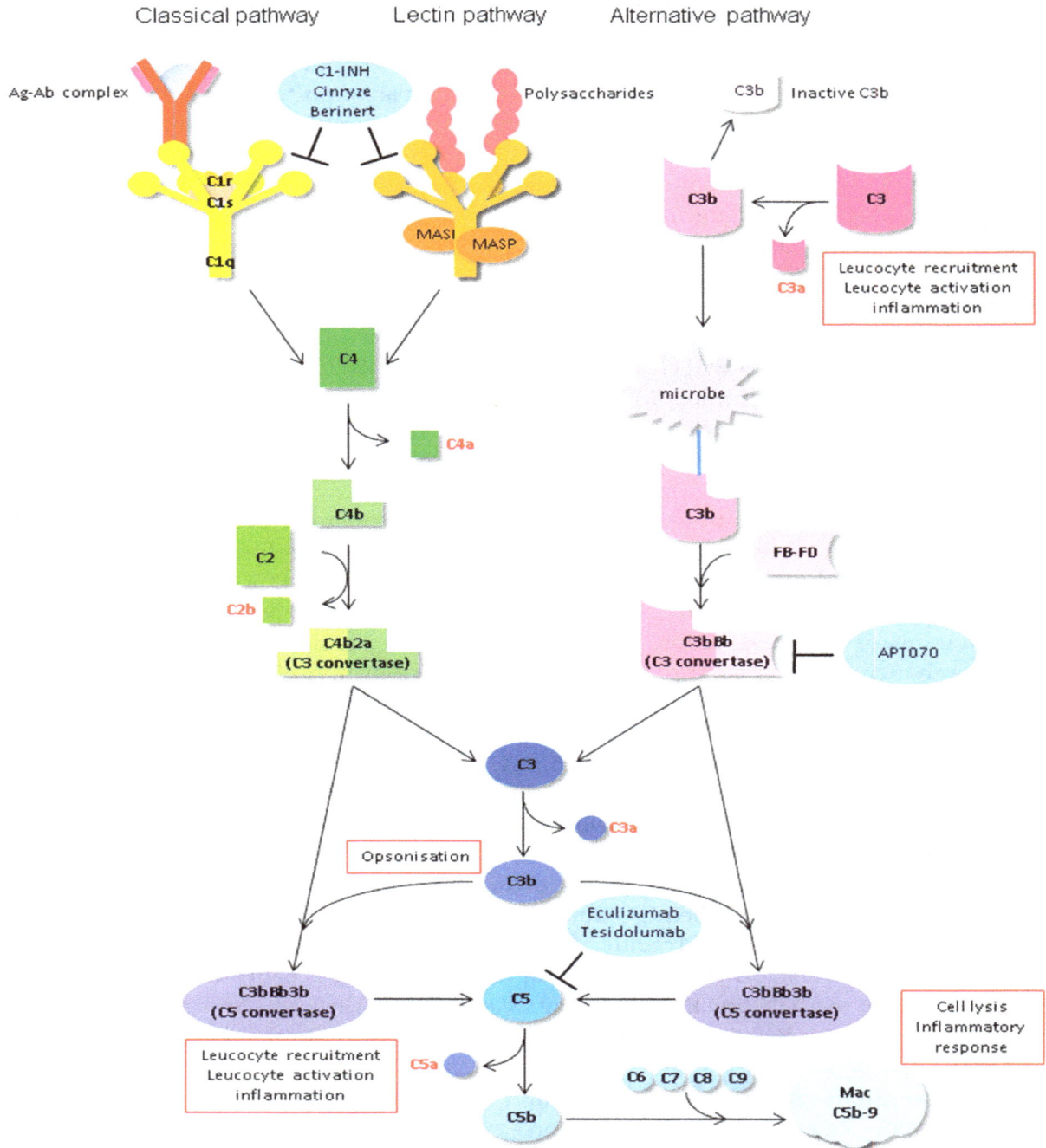

Figure 7. Routes of the complement system with its inhibitors currently studied in kidney transplantation. Damps released upon I/R are able to activate all three pathways via binding to C1q (classical pathway), C3 (alternative pathway) or pattern recognition receptors (PRRs) of the lectin path. All activating routes converge and lead to the formation of the complement component (C) 3 (C3) convertase (C4b2b, C3bBbP). C3 convertase cleaves and activates additional C3, creating C3a and C3b. C3b together with C4b2b forms the C5 convertase, which will cleave C5 into C5a and C5b. C5b together with C6–9 will then form the Membrane Attack Complex (MAC, C5b-9). The formed complement effectors will lead to opsonisation (C3b), chemotaxis of neutrophils and macrophages (C3a, C5a). The formed MAC inserted into the cellular membrane is associated with a proinflammatory response via noncanonical NF-KB signalling. C1-inhibitors (C1-INH), Cinryze®and Berinert®target complement initiation and APT070 complement amplification. Eculizumab and Tesidolumab inhibit complement activation at the level of C5.

In addition to targeting terminal complement pathways, therapeutics targeting complement initiation (C1) and amplification (C3, convertases) have been developed. C1 esterase inhibitors (C1-INH) should not be considered complement-specific inhibitors, since these broad protease inhibitors and their functions extend beyond the classical pathway and even beyond the complement system [163]. The C1INH Cinryze®(Shire US Inc., Lexington, MA, USA) is recently being evaluated for treatment of ABMR (NCT02547220). The study was terminated May 2019 following a pre-scheduled interim analysis, it was determined that the study met the pre-specified criteria for futility. Cinryze®is still listed to be tested as a pre-treatment to reduce IRI and DGF (NCT02435732). Another C1INH, Berinert®(CSL Behring, King of Prussia, PA, USA), has been evaluated in a phase 1/2, double-blind, placebo-controlled study assessing its safety and efficacy for prevention of delayed graft function in recipients of deceased donor kidneys [164]. Although the primary outcome measure (DGF) was not met, treatment with Berinert®was associated with significantly fewer dialysis sessions 2 to 4 weeks post-transplantation. In addition, a better renal function was seen at 1 year compared with the placebo treated group. No significant adverse events were noted in this study [164]. Finally, Mirococept (APT070) a membrane-localising C3 convertase inhibitor is currently being evaluated in a double-blind randomised controlled investigation its efficacy for preventing IRI deceased donor kidneys (EMPIRIKAL-trial, ISRCTN49958194) [165].

Translation to the Adaptive Immune System

The link between the innate and adaptive immune response is made by dendritic cells (DCs, Figure 8). DCs are APCs and play an essential role in the pathogenesis of IRI. Immature DCs can be activated by DAMPs via TLRs and the complement system. After maturation, they are able to activate the adaptive immune system in a direct manner by antigen presentation to B- and T-cells or indirectly via cytokine signalling [8,166]. This process can already start in the donor in which in case of a DBD donor, DCs are activated by oxidative stress or C5a and present donor antigens to T-cells of the recipient [167]. Furthermore, it is thought that DCs (subtype CDC11c+ and F4/80+) play an important role in the early pathophysiology of IRI by secretion of TNF-α, Chemokine (C-C motif) ligand 5 (CCL5), IL-6 and MCP-1within the first 24h after IRI [168]. Further, at a later stage, DCs contribute to allograft dysfunction. Batal et al. [169] looked at kidney transplant biopsies performed > 15 days after transplantation and found that a high DC density was independently associated with poor graft survival. Additionally, they found that high DC density was correlated with an increased T-cell proliferation and poor patient outcome in patients with high total inflammation scores of biopsies, including inflammation in areas of tubular atrophy. In these patients, DC density could predict allograft loss. When looking at the origin of the DCs they showed that initially donor DC predominated but found that in late biopsies the majority of DCs were of recipient origin. These data suggest a potential rationale to target DCs influx in the kidney to improve long-term allograft survival.

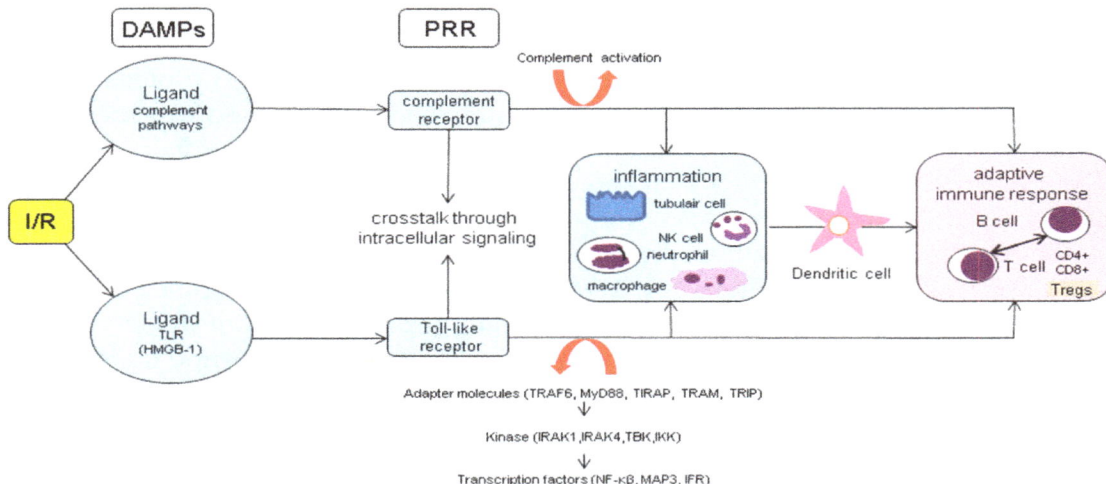

Figure 8. Interaction of the innate and adaptive immune system in the pathophysiology of ischemia and reperfusion injury. DAMPs released upon I/R are able to activate the innate immune system by binding to PRRs like complement receptors and TLRs. Activation of these receptors will lead to production of pro-inflammatory cytokines and chemokines and chemotaxis, opsonisation and activation of leucocytes like macrophages, neutrophils and natural killer (NK) cells. Additionally, immature dendritic cells can be activated, which, after maturation, are able to activate the adaptive immune system in a direct manner by antigen presentation to B- and T-cells or indirectly via cytokine signalling. Treg: regulatory T-cell.

3.3.2. Adaptive Immune Response

In contrast to the non-specific nature of the innate immune response, the role of the adaptive immune system is to recognize alloantigens and to react with an alloantigen-specific response, simultaneously generating immunological memory. Involved cells are B- and T-cells.

T-Cells

Activation of T-cells occurs through binding of the T-cell receptor (TCR) on the surface of the T-cell, to the major histocompatibility complex (MHC, in case of humans the human leucocyte antigen (HLA) system) on the APC. This can be in a direct way when the TCR binds to unprocessed allogenic MHC on the APC of the donor or in an indirect manner when MHC proteins of the donor have been taken up by APC of the recipient, processed and presented by the MHC of the recipient [170]. In case of IRI, CD4+ T helper (Th) cells as well as CD8+ cytotoxic T-cells are found in the kidney and are important mediators of IRI [171–174]. T-cell-deficient mice showed attenuated renal IRI and adoptive T-cell transfer experiments in athymic mice resulted in acute kidney injury (AKI) [175–177].

The TCR on CD4+ T-cells can only bind to MHC class 2 molecules (HLA DP, DQ, DR). Upon activation, these CD4+ T-cells become cytokine producing effector cells harming the graft through cytokine mediated inflammation [170]. The effector CD4+ Th cells can differentiate into three major subtypes Type 1 (Th1), Type 2 (Th2) and Th17 cells depending on the cytokines they produce and the transcription factors they express. This differentiation process, referred to as polarisation, starts with induction in lymphoid tissue. Cytokines produced by APCs (DCs and macrophages), NK cells, basophils and mast cells act on T-cells stimulated by the antigen and co-stimulators. This induces transcription of cytokine genes characteristic for the particular subset. Upon continued activation, genetic modifications occur, keeping the characteristic cytokine genes in a transcriptionally active state (commitment). The cytokines produced by the subset promote development of this subset and inhibit differentiation toward other subsets (amplification) [170]. The main effector cytokine of Th1 cells is IFN-γ and the key Th1 transcription factors are signal transducer and activator of transcription (STAT) 4 (STAT-4) and the T-box transcription factor T-bet. Main effector cells are macrophages, B-cells,

CD8+ T-cells and CD4+ T-cells (amplification). IFN-γ secreted by Th1 cells will activate macrophages leading to secretion of inflammatory cytokines (TNF, IL-1 and IL-2), an increased production of toxic substances like ROS, NO and lysosomal enzymes and finally stimulation of expression of costimulatory molecules enhancing the efficiency of the macrophage as APC [170]. The main effector cytokines of Th2 are IL-4, IL-5 and IL-13 and key transcription factors are GATA binding protein 3 (GATA-3) and STAT-6. IL-4 act on B-cells to stimulate production of IgE antibodies which can lead to mast cell degranulation upon binding of IgE with mast cells. IL-5 activates eosinophils, inducing defence against helminthic infections. IL-4 and IL-13 are involved in alternative macrophage activation promoting development of M2 macrophages which have anti-inflammatory effects and may promote tissue repair and fibrosis [170]. Signature cytokines of Th17 are IL-17 and IL-22. Differentiation into this subtype is mediated by IL-6 and TGF-β leading to activation of transcription factors STAT-3 and retinoic acid-related orphan receptor γt (RORγt) respectively. IL-17 act on leukocytes and tissue cells and stimulates production of several chemokines and cytokines (TNF-α, IL-1β, IL-6) that recruit neutrophils and to a lesser extend monocytes to generate an inflammatory response. IL-22 produced in epithelial cells is primarily involved in maintaining the barrier function of epithelia [170]. Th17 T-cell most likely play a significant role in IRI-induced inflammation. STAT-3 KO mice are protected from renal IRI via downregulation of Th17 activity [178]. The differentiated T-cells can convert from one subtype to another by changes in activation circumstances [179]. It is suggested that Th1/Th2 ratio plays an important role in the pathogenesis of IRI [180,181]. Yokota et al. [181] demonstrated that STAT-6-deficient mice with a defective Th2 phenotype have enhanced renal I/R injury whereas STAT-4-deficient mice have mild improved function In addition, Loverre et al. [182] showed that kidney transplant recipients experiencing DGF predominantly expressed Th1 phenotype within the graft In literature both Th1 and Th17 cells are associated with T-cell mediated rejection [183–188].

The TCR on CD8+ T-cells can only bind to MHC class 1 molecules (HLA A, B, C) presented on APCs. Upon activation in lymphoid tissue, they differentiate into cytotoxic T-cells (CTLs) or memory cells. This differentiation is facilitated by CD4+ Th1 cells by secreting cytokines that act directly on the CD8+ cells [170]. The main cytokines involved are IL-2 (proliferation, differentiation CTL/memory cell), IL-12/IFN (differentiation CTL), IL-15 (memory cell survival), IL-21 (memory cell induction). The CTLs are able to kill cells which present the allogenic class 1 MHC of the donor in the graft. This through binding on the target cell and release of granule content into the immune synapse. These granules contain perforin and granzymes. Perforin induces the uptake of granzymes into the target cell. These granzymes are capable of activating caspases and inducing apoptosis. The killing of the target cell can also be Fas/Fas-L mediated in which the CTL expose the Fas ligand on the membrane which will bind to the Fas receptor on the target cell inducing apoptosis. Only CTLs that are activated in the direct way (by donor MHC on donor APC) are able to kill graft cells [170]. Like CD4+ Th cells, CTL secrete inflammatory cytokines, (predominantly IFN-γ) that attribute to inflammation and injury of the graft. The role of CD8+ cells in early phase of renal IRI is unclear, in a mouse model CD4+ deficient mouse was protected from IRI but CD8+ deficient mouse was not [176].

Ko et al. [189] showed that already 6 h after renal IRI, transcriptional activity occurs in T-cells and that these gene expression changes persist up to 4 weeks after the event. Genes involved in immune cell trafficking and cellular movement were most upregulated in the early phase (6 h, 3 days). On day 10 this was shifted to genes related to cellular development products involved in immune responses and on day 28 to genes involved in cellular and humoral immune response involved in antigen presentation. In addition, they found that the CC motif chemokine receptor 5 (CCR5) was one of the most upregulated genes at all time points, which was confirmed at a protein level. Subsequently, the addition of CCR5 antibody attenuated IRI and led to decreased T-cell activation [189].

B-Cells

Next to alloreactive CD4+ and CD8+ T-cells, antibodies (immune globulins, Ig) against the graft contribute to rejection. Most of these Igs are produced by Th dependant alloreactive B-cells. The naive

B-cell recognizes allogenic MHC-molecules, processes these MHC-molecules and presents them to Th cells that were activated previously by the same alloantigen presented by APCs. The produced Igs (IgM/IgG) are then able to induce complement activation, and activation of neutrophils, NK cells and macrophages. The T-cells are responsible for T-cell mediated rejection and B-cells together with complement activation for ABMR [170].

Regulatory T-Cells

The T-cells which most likely play a protective role in renal IRI are regulatory T-cells (Tregs), a subset of CD4+ T-cells whose function is to supress the innate as well as the adaptive immune response and maintain self-tolerance. Tregs can be discriminated from other T-cells by expression of FoxP3 amongst other proteins like CD25. FoxP3 is probably the most important transcription factor for Treg differentiation. The mechanism of action of Tregs is production of immune suppressive cytokines IL-10 and TGF-β, reduction of APC is to stimulate T-cells (possibly by binding to B7 proteins on the APC) and finally consumption of IL-2, an important growth factor for other T-cells [170]. TGF-β inhibits various immune cells amongst which: proliferation and effector functions of T-cells, macrophages, neutrophils and endothelial cells. It regulates differentiation of FoxP3+ Tregs and promotes polarisation towards Th17 cells. Furthermore, TGF-β promotes tissue repair by the ability to stimulate collagen synthesis and matrix modifying enzyme by macrophages and fibroblasts. IL-10 inhibits the production of IL-12 by activated macrophages and DCs, therefore inhibiting these cells and their IFN-γ production. It also inhibits T-cell activation by inhibiting the expression of co-stimulators and MHC-II molecules on DCs and macrophages [170].

Tregs play a potentially promising role in the reduction of IRI and graft tolerance [190–193]. Currently, several clinical trials are running evaluating the safety and effecaicy of FoxP3 cellular therapy in kidney transplantation (NCT02091232, NCT03284242, NCT01446484) [194,195]. However, all that glitters is not gold, since recent studies have shown that human FoxP3+ T-cells show great variations in gene expression phenotype and function [196–199]. Furthermore, recently a subset of FoxP3+ Tregs mimicking Th cells was discovered that secreted pro-inflammatory cytokines [200]. Also, the effect of different immune suppressive agents on the Treg phenotype needs to be elucidated, since these drugs might influence Treg phenotype [200,201]. Altogether, more insight in function and biology is needed before this therapy finds its way to clinical settings.

3.4. Transcriptional Reprogramming

Finally, cells can protect themselves from hypoxia and ischemia and maintain homeostasis via an evolutionary conserved mechanism with the use of oxygen sensors and activation of specific transcription factors. These so called hypoxic inducible factors (HIFs) regulate various genes involved in the metabolic cell cycle, angiogenesis, erythropoiesis, energy conservation and cell survival and are therefore able to induce a protective cell response to hypoxia [202].

HIFs are heterodimeric transcription factors consisting of an α and β subunit. There are two types of α subunits, HIF-1α and HIF-2α, which have common, but also subunit-specific target genes. In the kidney, HIF-1α is predominantly localized in tubular and glomerular cells, whereas HIF-2α can be found in glomerular cells, peritubular endothelial cells and fibroblasts [203–205]. In aerobic circumstances, HIFs are inactive. Oxygen-sensing prolylhydroxylase (PHD) hydroxylates the amino acid proline on the HIF-1α/HIF-2α subunit. This induces a conformational change enabling von Hippel–Lindau tumour suppressor protein (pVHL) to bind with the α-subunit, leading to degradation of the HIF-α subunit. Ischemia/hypoxia will lead to inhibition of the oxygen-dependent PHD, which enables nuclear translocation of the α subunit, binding of the α and β subunit and formation of HIF. In the nucleus HIF binds with the hypoxia response promotor element (HRE) leading to the transcription of various genes like glycolysis enzymes Glut-1 and aldolase (enabling ATP production under hypoxic circumstances), NF-κB, TLRs, adenosine receptors, vascular endothelial growth factor (VGEF), CD73 and erythropoietin. Activation of HIF can also occur in normoxemic circumstances, for instance, by ROS, LPS, various cytokines and TCR-CD28 stimulation. Transcriptional reprogramming is a consequence of I/R that should be considered a protective mechanism (Figure 9) [206].

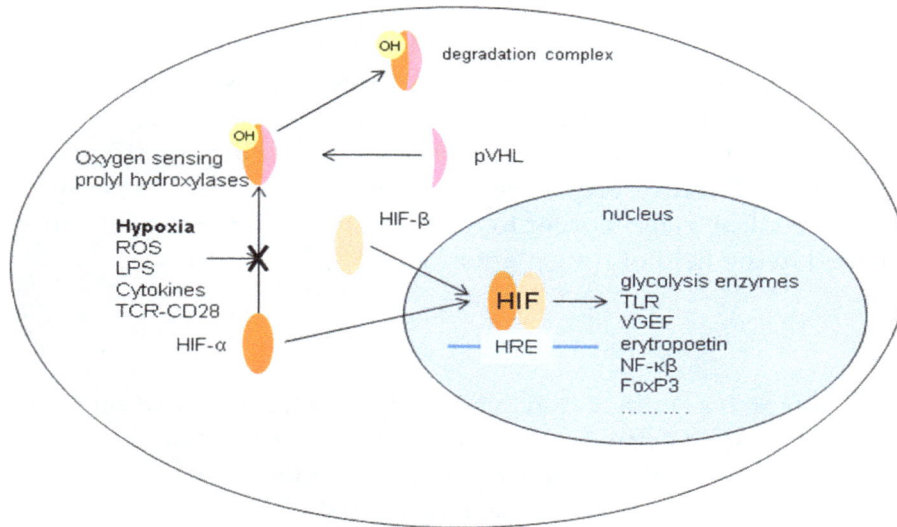

Figure 9. Intracellular stabilisation and activation of hypoxic inducible factor. Under normoxemic conditions, proline on the hypoxic inducible factor (HIF) α (HIFα) subunit is rapidly hydroxylated by oxygen-sensing prolyl hydroxylase (PHD). This induces a conformational change enabling von Hippel–Lindau tumour suppressor protein (pVHL) to bind with the α-subunit, leading to degradation of the HIF-α subunit. Ischemia (or other signals like lipopolysaccharide (LPS), various cytokines, etc.) will lead to inhibition of the oxygen-dependent PHD, enabling nuclear translocation of the α subunit, binding of the α and β subunit and formation of HIF. In the nucleus, HIF binds with the hypoxia response promotor element (HRE) leading to the transcription of various genes. VGEF: vascular endothelial growth factor.

Conde et al. [207] showed in various models and human post-transplantation biopsies that HIF-1α is induced in a biphasic manner namely during the hypoxic as well as the reperfusion phase. They pointed out the PI3K/Akt mTOR pathway to be responsible for this HIF-1α accumulation during the normoxemic reperfusion phase. In their study, this second increase (e.g., during reperfusion) seemed crucial for tubular cell survival and recovery. During the hypoxic phase, an increase in HIF-1 resulted predominantly in the upregulation of PHD3 and VGEF mRNA, which remained elevated during oxygenation. EPO mRNA was upregulated upon reperfusion. EPO and VGEF have been suggested to be involved in proximal tubular regeneration [208–210]. Their human post-transplantation biopsies revealed HIF-1α expression in proximal tubular cells without ischemic damage or features of regeneration suggesting a protective role for HIF-1α during I/R [207]. Oda et al. [211] had similar findings in patients receiving a DBD/DCD donor kidney. Their analysis of 46 post-transplant biopsies, gained 1h after reperfusion, showed that expression levels of PI3K, Akt, mTOR and HIF-1α were significantly higher in patients without DGF compared to patients experiencing DGF (76% of the patients). The expression levels of HIF-1α and donor type (DCD) were independently associated with DGF HIF-2α expression in renal endothelial cells is suggested in several studies to be protective against renal IRI via protection and preservation of the vasculature endothelium by upregulation of angiogenic factors like VGEF and their receptors Tie2 and VGEFreceptor-2 (FLK-1) [212–215]. Increased production of HIF in myeloid and lymphoid cells influences the innate and adaptive immune response. T-cell activation and proliferation is reduced under hypoxic conditions [216]. A study of Zhang et al. [217] revealed a hypoxia/HIF-2α/adenosine2A receptor axis to be responsible in reduction of NK T-cells activation and renal IRI upon I/R. HIF-1α induces a shift from Th1 to Th2 cells (decrease

Th1/Th2 ratio) accompanied by a decrease in excretion of inflammatory cytokines. Furthermore, HIF-1α promotes transcription of FoxP3 and therefore generation activation of Tregs.

Various PHD inhibitors have been developed and tested in animal I/R models. In a rat model, Wang et al. [218] showed that use of the PHD-1 inhibitor acetate prior to the ischemic event was able to stabilize HIF in a dose-dependent manner and was associated with improved renal outcome. In addition, in an allogenic renal transplant model in rats, the use of the PHD inhibitor FD-4497 pre-donation was associated with increased HIF expression and improved graft outcome and reduced mortality of recipients [219]. Hence, activation and/or upregulation of HIF could be an interesting approach to reduce renal IRI and improve renal transplant outcome. Several PHD inhibitors are currently being tested in clinical trials in order to treat anaemia in patients with chronic kidney disease but have not been tested in the field of transplantation yet.

4. Summary

The past decade's research in kidney transplant recipients has focussed on post-transplant patient management, with a predominant emphasis on immunosuppression. However, the biggest 'hit' to the donor organ is encountered during the process of donation and reperfusion at time of transplantation, i.e., ischemia and reperfusion injury. An important initiating step in IRI is the uncontrolled ROS formation during reperfusion and dysfunction of the mitochondrial machinery leading to the opening of mPTP and the release of DAMPs in the intra- and extracellular space. From here, several injury cascades are activated, including activation of cell death programs like apoptosis and (regulated) necrosis, endothelial dysfunction implicating increased vasoconstriction upon reperfusion, loss of specific phenotype of endothelial cells and transmigration of leucocytes into the interstitial space. Activation of the innate and subsequently the adaptive immune system will take place through binding of DAMPs to the toll-like receptors and activation of the complement system, leading to further injury of the graft, increased immunogenicity favouring T-cell and antibody mediated rejection and the initiation of fibrosis associated with chronic graft dysfunction. Currently, several novel agents targeting various pathways are tested and, although most are still in the preclinical phase, some have already entered clinical trials. Intervention early in this cascade of events (e.g., on a mitochondrial level), seems very attractive, since mitochondrial dysfunction plays a pivotal role in the initiation of IRI. Due to the complexity of the pathophysiological mechanisms, however, it may be predicted that a multiple treatment strategy using a combination of agents given at various time points during the donation, preservation and transplantation process will most likely be the best strategy to reduce IRI.

Author Contributions: G.J.N.-M.: participated in conceptualisation, investigation, visualisation, and writing—original draft preparation. S.E.P.: participated in conceptualisation, investigation, and writing—original draft preparation. S.P.B.: writing—original draft preparation. J.S.F.S.: writing—original draft preparation. R.A.P.: writing—original draft preparation. M.M.R.F.S.: writing—original draft preparation. R.J.P.: participated in conceptualisation, investigation, and writing—original draft preparation. H.G.D.L.: participated in conceptualisation, investigation, and writing—original draft preparation. All authors have read and agreed to the published version of the manuscript.

References

1. World Health Organisation. *Disease Burden and Mortality Estimates*; WTO: Geneva, Switzerland, 2015. Available online: https://www.who.int/healthinfo/global_burden_disease/estimates/en/index1.html (accessed on 15 January 2020).
2. Liyanage, T.; Ninomiya, T.; Jha, V.; Neal, B.; Patrice, H.M.; Okpechi, I.; Zhao, M.H.; Lv, J.; Garg, A.X.; Knight, J.; et al. Worldwide access to treatment for end-stage kidney disease: A systematic review. *Lancet* **2015**, *385*, 1975–1982. [CrossRef]

3. Global Observatory on Donation and Transplantation. 2019. Available online: http://www.transplant-observatory.org (accessed on 15 January 2020).

4. Cooper, J.T.; Chin, L.T.; Krieger, N.R.; Fernandez, L.A.; Foley, D.P.; Becker, Y.T.; Odorico, J.S.; Knechtle, S.J.; Kalayoglu, M.; Sollinger, H.W.; et al. Donation after cardiac death: The university of Wisconsin experience with renal transplantation. *Am. J. Transplant.* **2004**, *4*, 1490–1494. [CrossRef] [PubMed]

5. Koffman, G.; Gambaro, G. Renal transplantation from non-heart-beating donors: A review of the European experience. *J. Nephrol.* **2003**, *16*, 334–341. [PubMed]

6. Ponticelli, C. Ischemia-reperfusion injury: A major protagonist in kidney transplantation. *Nephrol. Dial. Transplant.* **2014**, *29*, 1134–1140. [CrossRef] [PubMed]

7. Cooper, J.E.; Wiseman, A.C. Acute kidney injury in kidney transplantation. *Curr. Opin. Nephrol. Hypertens.* **2013**, *22*, 698–703. [CrossRef]

8. Salvadori, M.; Rosso, G.; Bertoni, E. Update on ischemia-reperfusion injury in kidney transplantation: Pathogenesis and treatment. *World J. Transplant.* **2015**, *5*, 52–67. [CrossRef]

9. Erpicum, P.; Detry, O.; Weekers, L.; Bonvoisin, C.; Lechanteur, C.; Briquet, A. Mesenchymal stromal cell therapy in conditions of renal ischemia/reperfusion. *Nephrol. Dial. Transplant.* **2014**, *29*, 1487–1493. [CrossRef]

10. Denecke, C.; Tullius, S.G. Innate and adaptive immune responses subsequent to ischemia-reperfusion injury in the kidney. *Prog. Urol.* **2014**, *24*, S13–S19. [CrossRef]

11. Yarlagadda, S.G.; Coca, S.G.; Formica, R.N.; Poggio, E.D.; Parikh, C.R. Association between delayed graft function and allograft and patient survival: A systematic review and meta-analysis. *Nephrol. Dial. Transplant.* **2009**, *24*, 1039–1047. [CrossRef]

12. Sugiyama, S.; Hanaki, Y.; Ogawa, T.; Hieda, N.; Taki, K.; Ozawa, T. The effects of SUN 1165, a novel sodium channel blocker, on ischemia-induced mitochondrial dysfunction and leakage of lysosomal enzymes in canine hearts. *Biochem. Biophys. Res. Commun.* **1988**, *157*, 433–439. [CrossRef]

13. Kako, K.; Kato, M.; Matsuoka, T.; Mustapha, A. Depression of membrane-bound Na+-K+-ATPase activity induced by free radicals and by ischemia of kidney. *Am. J. Physiol.* **1988**, *254*, C330–C337. [CrossRef] [PubMed]

14. Kato, M.; Kako, K.J. Effects of N-(2-mercaptopropionyl) glycine on ischemic-reperfused dog kidney in vivo and membrane preparation in vitro. *Mol. Cell Biochem.* **1987**, *78*, 151–159. [CrossRef]

15. Edelstein, C.L.; Ling, H.; Schrier, R.W. The nature of cell injury. *Kidney Int.* **1997**, *51*, 1341–1351. [CrossRef] [PubMed]

16. Becker, L.B. New concepts in reactive oxygen species and cardiovascular reperfusion physiology. *Cardiovasc. Res.* **2004**, *61*, 461–470. [CrossRef] [PubMed]

17. Alkaitis, M.S.; Crabtree, M.J. Recoupling the cardiac nitric oxide synthases: Tetrahydrobiopterin synthesis and recycling. *Curr. Heart Fail. Rep.* **2012**, *9*, 200–210. [CrossRef] [PubMed]

18. Li, C.; Jackson, R.M. Reactive species mechanisms of cellular hypoxia-reoxygenation injury. *Am. J. Physiol. Cell Physiol.* **2002**, *282*, C227–C241. [CrossRef]

19. Simone, S.; Rascio, F.; Castellano, G.; Divella, C.; Chieti, A.; Ditonno, P.; Battaglia, M.; Crovace, A.; Staffieri, F.; Oortwijn, B.; et al. Complement-dependent NADPH oxidase enzyme activation in renal ischemia/reperfusion injury. *Free Radic. Biol. Med.* **2014**, *74*, 263–273. [CrossRef]

20. Martin, J.L.; Gruszczyk, A.V.; Beach, T.E.; Murphy, M.P.; Saeb-Parsy, K. Mitochondrial mechanisms and therapeutics in ischaemia reperfusion injury. *Pediatr. Nephrol.* **2019**, *34*, 1167–1174. [CrossRef]

21. Chouchani, E.T.; Pell, V.R.; James, A.M.; Work, L.M.; Saeb-Parsy, K.; Frezza, C.; Krieg, T.; Murphy, M.P. A unifying mechanism for mitochondrial superoxide production during ischemia-reperfusion injury. *Cell Metab.* **2016**, *23*, 254–263. [CrossRef]

22. Chouchani, E.T.; Pell, V.R.; Gaude, E.; Aksentijevic, D.; Sundier, S.Y.; Robb, E.L.; Logan, A.; Nadtochiy, S.M.; Ord, E.N.J.; Smith, A.C.; et al. Ischaemic accumulation of succinate controls reperfusion injury through mitochondrial ROS. *Nature* **2014**, *515*, 431–435. [CrossRef]

23. Mills, E.L.; Kelly, B.; O'Neill, L.A. Mitochondria are the powerhouses of immunity. *Nat. Immunol.* **2017**, *18*, 488–498. [CrossRef] [PubMed]

24. Zhang, Q.; Raoof, M.; Chen, Y.; Sumi, Y.; Sursal, T.; Junger, W.; Brohi, K.; Itagaki, K.; Hauser, C.J. Circulating mitochondrial DAMPs cause inflammatory responses to injury. *Nature* **2010**, *464*, 104–107. [CrossRef] [PubMed]

25. Krysko, D.V.; Agostinis, P.; Krysko, O.; Garg, A.D.; Bachert, C.; Lambrecht, B.N.; Vandenabeele, P. Emerging role of damage-associated molecular patterns derived from mitochondria in inflammation. *Trends Immunol.* **2011**, *32*, 157–164. [CrossRef]

26. Kang, J.W.; Kim, S.J.; Cho, H.I.; Lee, S.M. DAMPs activating innate immune responses in sepsis. *Ageing Res. Rev.* **2014**, *24*, 54–65. [CrossRef] [PubMed]

27. Smith, R.A.; Hartley, R.C.; Cocheme, H.M.; Murphy, M.P. Mitochondrial pharmacology. *Trends Pharmacol. Sci.* **2012**, *33*, 341–352. [CrossRef] [PubMed]

28. Dare, A.J.; Logan, A.; Prime, T.A.; Rogatti, S.; Goddard, M.; Bolton, E.M.; Bradley, J.A.; Pettigrew, G.J.; Murphy, M.P.; Saeb-Parsy, K. The mitochondria-targeted antioxidant MitoQ decreases ischemia-reperfusion injury in a murine syngeneic heart transplant model. *J. Heart Lung Transplant.* **2015**, *34*, 1471–1480. [CrossRef]

29. Liu, X.; Murphy, M.P.; Xing, W.; Wu, H.; Zhang, R.; Sun, H. Mitochondria-targeted antioxidant MitoQ reduced renal damage caused by ischemia-reperfusion injury in rodent kidneys: Longitudinal observations of T2-weighted imaging and dynamic contrast-enhanced MRI. *Magn. Reson. Med.* **2018**, *79*, 1559–1567. [CrossRef]

30. Dare, A.J.; Bolton, E.A.; Pettigrew, G.J.; Bradley, J.A.; Saeb-Parsy, K.; Murphy, M.P. Protection against renal ischemia-reperfusion injury in vivo by the mitochondria targeted antioxidant MitoQ. *Redox Biol.* **2015**, *5*, 163–168. [CrossRef]

31. Szeto, H.H.; Liu, S.; Soong, Y.; Alam, N.; Prusky, G.T.; Seshan, S.V. Protection of mitochondria prevents high-fat diet-induced glomerulopathy and proximal tubular injury. *Kidney Int.* **2016**, *90*, 997–1011. [CrossRef]

32. Saad, A.; Herrmann, S.M.S.; Eirin, A.; Ferguson, C.M.; Glockner, J.F.; Bjarnason, H. Phase 2a clinical trial of mitochondrial protection (Elamipretide) during stent revascularization in patients with atherosclerotic renal artery stenosis. *Circ. Cardiovasc. Interv.* **2017**, *10*. [CrossRef]

33. Valls-Lacalle, L.; Barba, I.; Miro-Casas, E.; Alburquerque-Bejar, J.J.; Ruiz-Meana, M.; Fuertes-Agudo, M.; Fuertes-Agudo, M.; Rodríguez-Sinovas, A.; García-Dorado, D. Succinate dehydrogenase inhibition with malonate during reperfusion reduces infarct size by preventing mitochondrial permeability transition. *Cardiovasc. Res.* **2016**, *109*, 374–384. [CrossRef] [PubMed]

34. Hotchkiss, R.S.; Strasser, A.; McDunn, J.E.; Swanson, P.E. Cell death. *N. Eng. J. Med.* **2009**, *361*, 1570–1583. [CrossRef] [PubMed]

35. Cohen, J.J. Programmed cell death in the immune system. *Adv. Immunol.* **1991**, *50*, 55–85. [PubMed]

36. Rai, N.K.; Tripathi, K.; Sharma, D.; Shukla, V.K. Apoptosis: A basic physiologic process in wound healing. *Int. J. Low Extrem. Wounds* **2005**, *4*, 138–144. [CrossRef]

37. Elmore, S. Apoptosis: A review of programmed cell death. *Toxicol. Pathol.* **2007**, *35*, 495–516. [CrossRef] [PubMed]

38. Cory, S.; Adams, J.M. The Bcl2 family: Regulators of the cellular life-or-death switch. *Nat. Rev. Cancer* **2002**, *2*, 647–656. [CrossRef]

39. Reed, J.C.; Zha, H.; Aime-Sempe, C.; Takayama, S.; Wang, H.G. Structure-function analysis of Bcl-2 family proteins. Regulators of programmed cell death. *Adv. Exp. Med. Biol.* **1996**, *406*, 99–112.

40. Saelens, X.; Festjens, N.; Vande Walle, L.; van Gurp, M.; van Loo, G.; Vandenabeele, P. Toxic proteins released from mitochondria in cell death. *Oncogene* **2004**, *23*, 2861–2874. [CrossRef]

41. Chinnaiyan, A.M. The apoptosome: Heart and soul of the cell death machine. *Neoplasia* **1999**, *1*, 5–15. [CrossRef]

42. Hill, M.M.; Adrain, C.; Duriez, P.J.; Creagh, E.M.; Martin, S.J. Analysis of the composition, assembly kinetics and activity of native Apaf-1 apoptosomes. *EMBO. J.* **2004**, *23*, 2134–2145. [CrossRef]

43. Dejean, L.M.; Martinez-Caballero, S.; Kinnally, K.W. Is MAC the knife that cuts cytochrome c from mitochondria during apoptosis? *Cell Death Differ.* **2006**, *13*, 1387–1395. [CrossRef]

44. Locksley, R.M.; Killeen, N.; Lenardo, M.J. The TNF and TNF receptor superfamilies: Integrating mammalian biology. *Cell* **2001**, *104*, 487–501. [CrossRef]

45. Ashkenazi, A.; Dixit, V.M. Death receptors: Signaling and modulation. *Science* **1998**, *281*, 1305–1308. [CrossRef] [PubMed]

46. Pasparakis, M.; Vandenabeele, P. Necroptosis and its role in inflammation. *Nature* **2015**, *517*, 311–320. [CrossRef] [PubMed]

47. Kischkel, F.C.; Hellbardt, S.; Behrmann, I.; Germer, M.; Pawlita, M.; Krammer, P.H.; Peter, M.E. Cytotoxicity dependent APO-1 (Fas/CD95)-associated proteins form a death-inducing signaling complex (DISC) with the receptor. *EMBO J.* **1995**, *14*, 5579–5588. [CrossRef] [PubMed]

48. Igney, F.H.; Krammer, P.H. Death and anti-death: Tumour resistance to apoptosis. *Nat. Rev. Cancer* **2002**, *2*, 277–288. [CrossRef] [PubMed]

49. Murphy, J.M.; Czabotar, P.E.; Hildebrand, J.M.; Lucet, I.S.; Zhang, J.G.; Alvarez-Diaz, S.; Lewis, R.; Lalaoui, N.; Metcalf, D.; Webb, A.I. The pseudokinase MLKL mediates necroptosis via a molecular switch mechanism. *Immunity* **2013**, *39*, 443–453. [CrossRef] [PubMed]

50. Linkermann, A.; Hackl, M.J.; Kunzendorf, U.; Walczak, H.; Krautwald, S.; Jevnikar, A.M. Necroptosis in immunity and ischemia-reperfusion injury. *Am. J. Transplant.* **2013**, *13*, 2797–2804. [CrossRef]

51. Mannon, R.B. Necroptosis in solid organ transplantation: A missing link to immune activation? *Am. J. Transplant.* **2013**, *13*, 2785–2786. [CrossRef]

52. Lau, A.; Wang, S.; Jiang, J.; Haig, A.; Pavlosky, A.; Linkermann, A.; Zhang, Z.X.; Jevnikar, A.M. RIPK3-mediated necroptosis promotes donor kidney inflammatory injury and reduces allograft survival. *Am. J. Transplant.* **2013**, *13*, 2805–2818. [CrossRef]

53. Kers, J.; Leemans, J.C.; Linkermann, A. An Overview of Pathways of Regulated Necrosis in Acute Kidney Injury. *Semin. Nephrol.* **2016**, *36*, 139–152. [CrossRef] [PubMed]

54. Kroemer, G.; Marino, G.; Levine, B. Autophagy and the integrated stress response. *Mol. Cell* **2010**, *40*, 280–293. [CrossRef] [PubMed]

55. Kundu, M.; Thompson, C.B. Autophagy: Basic principles and relevance to disease. *Annu. Rev. Pathol.* **2008**, *3*, 427–455. [CrossRef] [PubMed]

56. Rubinsztein, D.C.; Codogno, P.; Levine, B. Autophagy modulation as a potential therapeutic target for diverse diseases. *Nat. Rev. Drug Discov.* **2012**, *11*, 709–730. [CrossRef]

57. Mizushima, N.; Komatsu, M. Autophagy: Renovation of cells and tissues. *Cell* **2011**, *147*, 728–741. [CrossRef]

58. Russell, R.C.; Yuan, H.X.; Guan, K.L. Autophagy regulation by nutrient signaling. *Cell Res.* **2014**, *24*, 42–45. [CrossRef]

59. Lamb, C.A.; Yoshimori, T.; Tooze, S.A. The autophagosome: Origins unknown, biogenesis complex. *Nat. Rev. Mol. Cell Biol.* **2013**, *14*, 759–774. [CrossRef] [PubMed]

60. Mizushima, N. The role of the Atg1/ULK1 complex in autophagy regulation. *Curr. Opin. Cell Biol.* **2010**, *22*, 132–139. [CrossRef] [PubMed]

61. Chan, E.Y.; Longatti, A.; McKnight, N.C.; Tooze, S.A. Kinase-inactivated ULK proteins inhibit autophagy via their conserved C-terminal domains using an Atg13-independent mechanism. *Mol. Cell Biol.* **2009**, *29*, 157–171. [CrossRef]

62. Kim, J.; Kundu, M.; Viollet, B.; Guan, K.L. AMPK and mTOR regulate autophagy through direct phosphorylation of Ulk1. *Nat. Cell Biol.* **2011**, *13*, 132–141. [CrossRef] [PubMed]

63. Dunlop, E.A.; Tee, A.R. mTOR and autophagy: A dynamic relationship governed by nutrients and energy. *Semin. Cell Dev. Biol.* **2014**, *36*, 121–129. [CrossRef] [PubMed]

64. Yang, Z.; Klionsky, D.J. Mammalian autophagy: Core molecular machinery and signaling regulation. *Curr. Opin. Cell Biol.* **2010**, *22*, 124–131. [CrossRef] [PubMed]

65. Feng, Y.; He, D.; Yao, Z.; Klionsky, D.J. The machinery of macroautophagy. *Cell Res.* **2014**, *24*, 24–41. [CrossRef] [PubMed]

66. Rubinsztein, D.C.; Shpilka, T.; Elazar, Z. Mechanisms of autophagosome biogenesis. *Curr. Biol.* **2012**, *22*, R29–R34. [CrossRef] [PubMed]

67. Dooley, H.C.; Razi, M.; Polson, H.E.; Girardin, S.E.; Wilson, M.I.; Tooze, S.A. WIPI2 links LC3 conjugation with PI3P, autophagosome formation, and pathogen clearance by recruiting Atg12-5-16L1. *Mol. Cell* **2014**, *55*, 238–252. [CrossRef] [PubMed]

68. Dooley, H.C.; Wilson, M.I.; Tooze, S.A. WIPI2B links PtdIns3P to LC3 lipidation through binding ATG16L1. *Autophagy* **2015**, *11*, 190–191.

69. Vergne, I.; Deretic, V. The role of PI3P phosphatases in the regulation of autophagy. *FEBS Lett.* **2010**, *584*, 1313–1318. [CrossRef]

70. Kaushal, G.P.; Shah, S.V. Autophagy in acute kidney injury. *Kidney Int.* **2016**, *89*, 779–791. [CrossRef]

71. Decuypere, J.P.; Ceulemans, L.J.; Agostinis, P.; Monbaliu, D.; Naesens, M.; Pirenne, J.; Jochmans, I. Autophagy and the kidney: Implications for ischemia-reperfusion injury and therapy. *Am. J. Kidney Dis.* **2015**, *66*, 699–709. [CrossRef]

72. Ma, S.; Wang, Y.; Chen, Y.; Cao, F. The role of the autophagy in myocardial ischemia/reperfusion injury. *Biochim. Biophys. Acta (BBA)-Mol. Basis Dis.* **2012**, *1852*, 271–276. [CrossRef]

73. Sciarretta, S.; Hariharan, N.; Monden, Y.; Zablocki, D.; Sadoshima, J. Is Autophagy in Response to Ischemia and Reperfusion Protective or Detrimental for the Heart? *Pediatr. Cardiol.* **2011**, *32*, 275–281. [CrossRef]

74. Slegtenhorst, B.R.; Dor, F.M.J.F.; Elkhal, A.; Rodriguez, H.; Yang, X.; Edtinger, K.; Quante, M.; Chong, A.S.; Tullius, S.G. Mechanisms and consequences of injury and repair in older organ transplants. *Transplantation* **2014**, *97*, 1091–1099. [CrossRef] [PubMed]

75. Kiffin, R.; Bandyopadhyay, U.; Cuervo, A.M. Oxidative stress and autophagy. *Antioxid. Redox Signal.* **2006**, *8*, 152–162. [CrossRef] [PubMed]

76. Decuypere, J.P.; Pirenne, J.; Jochmans, I. Autophagy in renal ischemia-reperfusion injury: Friend or foe? *Am. J. Transplant.* **2014**, *14*, 1464–1465. [CrossRef] [PubMed]

77. Pyo, J.O.; Jang, M.H.; Kwon, Y.K.; Lee, H.J.; Jun, J.I.; Woo, H.N.; Cho, D.H.; Choi, B.; Lee, H.; Kim, J.H.; et al. Essential roles of Atg5 and FADD in autophagic cell death: Dissection of autophagic cell death into vacuole formation and cell death. *J. Biol. Chem.* **2005**, *280*, 20722–20729. [CrossRef]

78. Bell, B.D.; Leverrier, S.; Weist, B.M.; Newton, R.H.; Arechiga, A.F.; Luhrs, K.A.; Morrissette, N.S.; Walsh, C.M. FADD and caspase-8 control the outcome of autophagic signaling in proliferating T cells. *Proc. Natl. Acad. Sci. USA* **2008**, *105*, 16677–16682. [CrossRef]

79. Laussmann, M.A.; Passante, E.; Düssmann, H.; Rauen, J.A.; Würstle, M.L.; Delgado, M.E.; Devocelle, M.; Prehn, J.H.M.; Rehm, M.; et al. Proteasome inhibition can induce an autophagy-dependent apical activation of caspase-8. *Cell Death Differ.* **2011**, *18*, 1584–1597. [CrossRef]

80. Pattingre, S.; Tassa, A.; Qu, X.; Garuti, R.; Liang, X.H.; Mizushima, N.; Packer, M.; Schneider, M.D.; Levine, B. Bcl-2 antiapoptotic proteins inhibit Beclin 1-dependent autophagy. *Cell* **2005**, *122*, 927–939. [CrossRef]

81. Erlich, S.; Mizrachy, L.; Segev, O.; Lindenboim, L.; Zmira, O.; Adi-Harel, S.; Hirsch, J.A.; Stein, R.; Kramarski, R.P. Differential interactions between Beclin 1 and Bcl-2 family members. *Autophagy* **2007**, *3*, 561–568. [CrossRef]

82. Yang, C.; Kaushal, V.; Shah, S.V.; Kaushal, G.P. Autophagy is associated with apoptosis in cisplatin injury to renal tubular epithelial cells. *Am. J. Physiol. Renal. Physiol.* **2008**, *294*, F777–F787. [CrossRef]

83. Kaushal, G.P.; Kaushal, V.; Herzog, C.; Yang, C.A. Autophagy delays apoptosis in renal tubular epithelial cells in cisplatin cytotoxicity. *Autophagy* **2008**, *4*, 710–720. [CrossRef] [PubMed]

84. Herzog, C.; Yang, C.; Holmes, A.; Kaushal, G.P. z-VAD-fmk prevents cisplatininduced cleavage of autophagy proteins but impairs autophagic flux and worsens renal function. *Am. J. Physiol. Renal. Physiol.* **2012**, *303*, F1239–F1250. [CrossRef] [PubMed]

85. Khan, M.J.; Alam, M.R.; Waldeck-Weiermair, M.; Karsten, F.; Groschner, L.; Riederer, M.; Hallstrom, S.; Rockenfeller, P.; Konya, V.; Heinemann, A.; et al. Inhibition of autophagy rescues palmitic acid-induced necroptosis of endothelial cells. *J. Biol. Chem.* **2012**, *287*, 21110–21120. [CrossRef] [PubMed]

86. Wang, Y.Q.; Wang, L.; Zhang, M.Y.; Wang, T.; Bao, H.J.; Liu, W.L.; Dai, D.K.; Zhang, L.; Chang, P.; Dong, W.W.; et al. Necrostatin-1 suppresses autophagy and apoptosis in mice traumatic brain injury model. *Neurochem. Res.* **2012**, *37*, 1849–1858. [CrossRef] [PubMed]

87. Nydam, T.L.; Plenter, R.; Jain, S.; Lucia, S.; Jani, A. Caspase Inhibition During Cold Storage Improves Graft Function and Histology in a Murine Kidney Transplant Model. *Transplantation* **2018**, *102*, 1487–1495. [CrossRef] [PubMed]

88. Kelly, K.J.; Plotkin, Z.; Vulgamott, S.L.; Dagher, P.C. P53 mediates the apoptotic response to GTP depletion depletion after renal ischemia-reperfusion: Protective role of a p53 inhibitor. *J. Am. Soc. Nephrol.* **2003**, *14*, 128–138. [CrossRef]

89. Molitoris, B.A.; Dagher, P.C.; Sandoval, R.M.; Campos, S.B.; Ashush, H.; Fridman, E.; Brafman, A.; Faerman, A.; Atkinson, S.J.; Thompson, J.D.; et al. siRNA targeted to p53 attenuates ischemic and cisplatin-induced acute kidney injury. *J. Am. Soc. Nephrol.* **2009**, *20*, 1754–1764. [CrossRef]

90. Tchervenkov, J.; Squiers, E.; Stratta, R.; Odenheimer, D.; Rothenstein, D. QPI-1002 DGF Study Group QPI-1002, a siRNA Targeting p53: Improvement in Outcomes Following Acute Kidney Injury (AKI): Cardiac Surgery to AKI Donors. Available online: https://atcmeetingabstracts.com/abstract/qpi-1002-a-sirna-targeting-p53-improvement-in-outcomes-following-acute-kidney-injury-aki-cardiac-surgery-to-aki-donors/ (accessed on 15 January 2020).

91. Garg, J.P.; Vucic, D. Targeting Cell Death Pathways for Therapeutic Intervention in Kidney Diseases. *Semin. Nephrol.* **2016**, *36*, 153–161. [CrossRef]

92. Linkermann, A. Nonapoptotic cell death in acute kidney injury and transplantation. *Kidney Int.* **2016**, *89*, 46–57. [CrossRef]

93. Grievink, H.W.; Heuberger, J.A.A.C.; Huang, F.; Chaudhary, R.; Birkhoff, W.A.J.; Tonn, G.R.; Mosesova, S.; Erickson, R.; Moerland, M.; Haddick, P.C.G.; et al. DNL104, a Centrally Penetrant RIPK1 Inhibitor, Inhibits RIP1 Kinase Phosphorylation in a Randomized Phase I Ascending Dose Study in Healthy Volunteers. *Clin. Pharmacol. Ther.* **2019**, *22*. [CrossRef]

94. Weisel, K.; Scott, N.E.; Tompson, D.J.; Votta, B.J.; Madhavan, S.; Povey, K.; Wolstenholme, A.; Simeoni, M.; Rudo, T.; Peterson, L.R.; et al. Randomized clinical study of safety, pharmacokinetics, and pharmacodynamics of RIPK1 inhibitor GSK2982772 in healthy volunteers. *Pharmacol. Res. Perspect.* **2017**, *5*. [CrossRef] [PubMed]

95. Basile, D.P.; Friedrich, J.L.; Spahic, J.; Knipe, N.; Mang, H.; Leonard, E.C.; Changizi-Ashtiyani, S.; Bacallao, R.L.; Molitoris, B.A.; Sutton, T.A. Impaired endothelial proliferation and mesenchymal transition contribute to vascular rarefaction following acute kidney injury. *Am. J. Physiol. Renal. Physiol.* **2011**, *300*, 721–733. [CrossRef] [PubMed]

96. Faller, D.V. Endothelial cell responses to hypoxic stress. *Clin. Exp. Pharmacol. Physiol.* **1999**, *26*, 74–84. [CrossRef] [PubMed]

97. Kwon, O.; Hong, S.M.; Ramesh, G. Diminished NO generation by injured endothelium and loss of macula densa nNOS may contribute to sustained acute kidney injury after ischemia-reperfusion. *Am. J. Physiol. Renal. Physiol.* **2009**, *296*, 25–33. [CrossRef] [PubMed]

98. Bonventre, J.V.; Yang, L. Cellular pathophysiology of ischemic acute kidney injury. *J. Clin. Investig.* **2011**, *121*, 4210–4221. [CrossRef] [PubMed]

99. Legrand, M.; Mik, E.G.; Johannes, T.; Payen, D.; Ince, C. Renal hypoxia and dysoxia after reperfusion of the ischemic kidney. *Mol. Med.* **2008**, *14*, 502–516. [CrossRef] [PubMed]

100. Kwon, O.; Hong, S.M.; Sutton, T.A.; Temm, C.J. Preservation of peritubular capillary endothelial integrity and increasing pericytes may be critical to recovery from postischemic acute kidney injury. *Am. J. Physiol. Renal. Physiol.* **2008**, *295*, F351–F359. [CrossRef]

101. Basile, D.P.; Donohoe, D.; Roethe, K.; Osborn, J.L. Renal ischemic injury results in permanent damage to peritubular capillaries and influences long-term function. *Am. J. Physiol. Renal. Physiol.* **2001**, *281*, F887–F899. [CrossRef]

102. Curci, C.; Castellano, G.; Stasi, A.; Divella, C.; Loverre, A.; Gigante, M.; Simone, S.; Cariello, M.; Montinaro, V.; Lucarelli, G.; et al. Endothelial-to-mesenchymal transition and renal fibrosis in ischaemia/reperfusion injury are mediated by complement anaphylatoxins and Akt pathway. *Nephrol. Dial. Transplant.* **2014**, *29*, 799–808. [CrossRef]

103. Wang, Z.; Han, Z.; Tao, J.; Wang, J.; Liu, X.; Zhou, W.; Xu, Z.; Zhao, C.; Wang, Z.; Tan, R.; et al. Role of endothelial-to-mesenchymal transition induced by TGF-β1 in transplant kidney interstitial fibrosis. *J. Cell Mol. Med.* **2017**, *21*, 2359–2369. [CrossRef]

104. Frid, M.G.; Kale, V.A.; Stenmark, K.R. Mature vascular endothelium can give rise to smooth muscle cells via endothelial mesenchymal transdifferentiation: In vitro analysis. *Circ. Res.* **2002**, *90*, 1189–1196. [CrossRef] [PubMed]

105. Moonen, J.R.A.; Krenning, G.; Brinker, M.G.L.; Koerts, J.A.; Van Luyn, M.J.A.; Harmsen, M.C. Endothelial progenitor cells give rise to pro-angiogenic smooth muscle-like progeny. *Cardiovasc. Res.* **2010**, *86*, 506–515. [CrossRef] [PubMed]

106. Potenta, S.; Zeisberg, E.; Kalluri, R. The role of endothelial-to-mesenchymal transition in cancer progression. *Br. J. Cancer* **2008**, *99*, 1375–1379. [CrossRef] [PubMed]

107. Man, S.; Sanchez Duffhues, G.; Ten Dijke, P.; Baker, D. The therapeutic potential of targeting the endothelial-to-mesenchymal transition. *Angiogenesis* **2019**, *22*, 3–13. [CrossRef] [PubMed]

108. Eltzschig, H.K.; Collard, C.D. Vascular ischemia and reperfusion injury. *Br. Med. Bull.* **2004**, *70*, 71–86. [CrossRef] [PubMed]

109. Carden, D.L.; Granger, D.N. Pathophysiology of ischemia reperfusion injury. *J. Pathol.* **2000**, *190*, 255–266. [CrossRef]

110. O'Neill, L.A.; Bowie, A.G. The family of five: TIR-domain-containing adaptors in Toll-like receptor signalling. *Nat. Rev. Immunol.* **2007**, *7*, 353–364. [CrossRef]

111. Delneste, Y.; Beauvillain, C.; Jeannin, P. Innate immunity: Structure and function of TLRs. *Med. Sci.* **2007**, *23*, 67–73.

112. Kawasaki, T.; Kawai, T. Toll-Like receptor signaling pathways. *Front. Immunol.* **2014**, *5*, 461. [CrossRef]

113. Assadiasl, S.; Mousavi, M.J.; Amirzargar, A. Toll-Like Receptor 4 in Renal Transplant. *Exp. Clin. Transplant.* **2018**, *16*, 245–252.

114. Zhao, H.; Watts, H.R.; Chong, M.; Huang, H.; Tralau-Stewart, C.; Maxwell, P.H.; Maze, M.; George, A.J.; Ma, D. Xenon treatment protects against cold ischemia associated delayed graft function and prolongs graft survival in rats. *Am. J. Transplant.* **2013**, *13*, 2006–2018. [CrossRef] [PubMed]

115. Rusai, K.; Sollinger, D.; Baumann, M.; Wagner, B.; Strobl, M.; Schmaderer, C.; Roos, M.; Kirschning, C.; Heemann, U.; Lutz, J. Toll-like receptors 2 and 4 in renal ischemia/reperfusion injury. *Pediatr. Nephrol.* **2010**, *25*, 853–860. [CrossRef] [PubMed]

116. Wolfs, T.G.A.M.; Buurman, W.A.; van Schadewijk, A.; de Vries, B.; Daemen, M.A.R.C.; Hiemstra, P.S.; van't Veer, C. In vivo expression of Toll-like receptor 2 and 4 by renal epithelial cells: IFN-gamma and TNF-alpha mediated up-regulation during inflammation. *J. Immunol.* **2002**, *168*, 1286–1293. [CrossRef] [PubMed]

117. Zahedi, K.; Barone, S.; Wang, Y.; Murray-Stewart, T.; Roy-Chaudhury, P.; Smith, R.D.; Casero, R.A., Jr.; Soleimani, M. Proximal tubule epithelial cell specific ablation of the spermidine/spermine N1-acetyltransferase gene reduces the severity of renal ischemia/reperfusion injury. *PLoS ONE* **2014**, *9*, e110161. [CrossRef] [PubMed]

118. Kruger, B.; Krick, S.; Dhillon, N.; Lerner, S.M.; Ames, S.; Bromberg, J.S.; Lin, M.; Walsh, L.; Vella, J.; Fischereder, M.; et al. Donor Toll-like receptor 4 contributes to ischemia and reperfusion injury following human kidney transplantation. *Proc. Natl. Acad. Sci. USA* **2009**, *106*, 3390–3395. [CrossRef] [PubMed]

119. Zhao, H.; Ning, J.; Savage, S.; Kang, H.; Lu, K.; Zheng, X.; George, A.J.; Ma, D. A novel strategy for preserving renal grafts in an ex vivo setting: Potential for enhancing the marginal donor pool. *FASEB J.* **2013**, *27*, 4822–4833. [CrossRef]

120. Chen, C.B.; Liu, L.S.; Zhou, J.; Wang, X.P.; Han, M.; Jiao, X.Y.; He, X.S.; Yuan, X.P. Up-Regulation of HMGB1 Exacerbates Renal Ischemia-Reperfusion Injury by Stimulating Inflammatory and Immune Responses through the TLR4 Signaling Pathway in Mice. *Cell Physiol. Biochem.* **2017**, *41*, 2447–2460. [CrossRef]

121. Harris, H.E.; Andersson, U.; Pisetsky, D.S. HMGB1: A multifunctional alarmin driving autoimmune and inflammatory disease. *Nat. Rev. Rheumatol.* **2012**, *8*, 195–202. [CrossRef]

122. Lotze, M.T.; Tracey, K.J. High-mobility group box 1 protein (HMGB1): Nuclear weapon in the immune arsenal. *Nat. Rev. Rheumatol.* **2005**, *5*, 331–342. [CrossRef]

123. Bergler, T.; Hoffmann, U.; Bergler, E.; Jung, B.; Banas, M.C.; Reinhold, S.W.; Krämer, B.K.; Banas, B. Toll-like receptor 4 in experimental kidney transplantation: Early mediator of endogenous danger signals. *Nephron. Exp. Nephrol.* **2012**, *121*, e59–e70. [CrossRef]

124. Wu, H.; Chen, G.; Wyburn, K.R.; Yin, J.; Bertolino, P.; Eris, J.M.; Alexander, S.I.; Alexander, S.I.; Sharland, A.F.; Chadban, S.J. TLR4 activation mediates kidney ischemia/reperfusion injury. *J. Clin. Invest.* **2007**, *117*, 2847–2859. [CrossRef] [PubMed]

125. Chen, J.; John, R.; Richardson, J.A.; Shelton, J.M.; Zhou, X.J.; Wang, Y.; Wu, Q.Q.; Hartono, J.R.; Winterberg, P.D.; Lu, C.Y. Toll-like receptor 4 regulates early endothelial activation during ischemic acute kidney injury. *Kidney Int.* **2011**, *79*, 288–299. [CrossRef] [PubMed]

126. Jang, H.R.; Rabb, H. The innate immune response in ischemic acute kidney injury. *Clin. Immunol.* **2009**, *130*, 41–50. [CrossRef]

127. Jo, S.K.; Sung, S.A.; Cho, W.Y.; Go, K.J.; Kim, H.K. Macrophages contribute to the initiation of ischemic acute renal failure in rats. *Nephrol. Dial. Transplant.* **2006**, *21*, 1231–1239. [CrossRef] [PubMed]

128. Liu, Y. Cellular and molecular mechanisms of renal fibrosis. *Nat. Rev. Nephrol.* **2011**, *7*, 684–696. [CrossRef] [PubMed]

129. Ali, S.; Malik, G.; Burns, A.; Robertson, H.; Kirby, J.A. Renal transplantation: Examination of the regulation of chemokine binding during acute rejection. *Transplantation* **2005**, *79*, 672–679. [CrossRef]

130. Snoeijs, M.G.; Vink, H.; Voesten, N.; Christiaans, M.H.; Daemen, J.W.; Peppelenbosch, A.G.; Tordoir, J.H.; Peutz-Kootstra, C.J.; Buurman, W.A.; Schurink, G.W.; et al. Acute ischemic injury to the renal microvasculature in human kidney transplantation. *Am. J. Physiol. Renal. Physiol.* **2010**, *299*, F1134–F1140. [CrossRef]

131. Tuuminen, R.; Nykanen, A.I.; Saharinen, P.; Gautam, P.; Keranen, M.A.; Arnaudova, R.; Rouvinen, E.; Helin, H.; Tammi, R.; Rilla, K.; et al. Donor simvastatin treatment prevents ischemia-reperfusion and acute kidney injury by preserving microvascular barrier function. *Am. J. Transplant.* **2013**, *13*, 2019–2034. [CrossRef]

132. Zhang, W.; Gao, L.; Qi, S.; Liu, D.; Xu, D.; Peng, J.; Daloze, P.; Chen, H.; Buelow, R. Blocking of CD44-hyaluronic acid interaction prolongs rat allograft survival. *Transplantation* **2000**, *69*, 665–667. [CrossRef]

133. Ben Mkaddem, S.; Pedruzzi, E.; Werts, C.; Coant, N.; Bens, M.; Cluzeaud, F.; Goujon, J.M.; Ogier-Denis, E.; Vandewalle, A. Heat shock protein gp96 and NAD(P)H oxidase 4 play key roles in Toll-like receptor 4-activated apoptosis during renal ischemia/reperfusion injury. *Cell Death Differ.* **2010**, *17*, 1474–1485. [CrossRef]

134. Kim, B.S.; Lim, S.W.; Li, C.; Kim, J.S.; Sun, B.K.; Ahn, K.O.; Han, S.W.; Kim, J.; Yang, C.W. Ischemia-reperfusion injury activates innate immunity in rat kidneys. *Transplantation* **2005**, *79*, 1370–1377. [CrossRef] [PubMed]

135. Zhao, H.; Perez, J.S.; Lu, K.; George, A.J.; Ma, D. Role of Toll-like receptor-4 in renal graft ischemia-reperfusion injury. *Am. J. Physiol. Renal. Physiol.* **2014**, *306*, F801–F811. [CrossRef] [PubMed]

136. Wang, S.; Schmaderer, C.; Kiss, E.; Schmidt, C.; Bonrouhi, M.; Porubsky, S.; Gretz, N.; Schaefer, L.; Kirschning, C.J.; Popovic, Z.V.; et al. Recipient Toll-like receptors contribute to chronic graft dysfunction by both MyD88- and TRIF-dependent signaling. *Dis. Model. Mech.* **2010**, *3*, 92–103. [CrossRef] [PubMed]

137. Zhang, L.M.; Liu, J.H.; Xue, C.B.; Li, M.Q.; Xing, S.; Zhang, X.; He, W.T.; Jiang, F.C.; Lu, X.; Zhou, P. Pharmacological inhibition of MyD88 homodimerization counteracts renal ischemia reperfusion-induced progressive renal injury in vivo and in vitro. *Sci. Rep.* **2016**, *6*, 26954. [CrossRef] [PubMed]

138. Liu, J.H.; He, L.; Zou, Z.M.; Ding, Z.C.; Zhang, X.; Wang, H.; Zhou, P.; Xie, L.; Xing, S.; Yi, C.Z. A Novel Inhibitor of Homodimerization Targeting MyD88 Ameliorates Renal Interstitial Fibrosis by Counteracting TGF-β1-Induced EMT in Vivo and in Vitro. *Kidney Blood Press Res.* **2018**, *43*, 1677–1687. [CrossRef]

139. Leemans, J.C.; Butter, L.M.; Pulskens, W.P.; Teske, G.J.D.; Claessen, N.; van der Poll, T.; Florquin, S. The role of Toll-like receptor 2 in inflammation and fibrosis during progressive renal injury. *PLoS ONE* **2009**, *4*, e5704. [CrossRef]

140. Leemans, J.C.; Stokman, G.; Claessen, N.; Rouschop, K.M.; Teske, G.J.D.; Kirschning, C.J.; Akira, S.; van der Poll, T.; Weening, J.J.; Florquin, S. Renal-associated TLR2 mediates ischemia/reperfusion injury in the kidney. *J. Clin. Investig.* **2005**, *115*, 2894–2903. [CrossRef]

141. de Groot, K.; Kuklik, K.; Bröcker, V.; Schwarz, A.; Gwinner, W.; Kreipe, H.; Haller, H.; Fliser, D.; Mengel, M. Toll-like receptor 2 and renal allograft function. *Am. J. Nephrol.* **2008**, *28*, 583–588. [CrossRef]

142. Reilly, M.; Miller, R.M.; Thomson, M.H.; Patris, V.; Ryle, P.; McLoughlin, L.; Mutch, P.; Gilboy, P.; Miller, C.; Broekema, M.; et al. Randomized, double-blind, placebo-controlled, dose-escalating phase I, healthy subjects study of intravenous OPN-305, a humanized Anti-TLR2 antibody. *Clin. Pharmacol. Ther.* **2013**, *94*, 593–600. [CrossRef]

143. Nauser, C.L.; Farrar, C.A.; Sacks, S.H. Complement Recognition Pathways in Renal Transplantation. *J. Am. Soc. Nephrol.* **2017**, *28*, 2571–2578. [CrossRef]

144. Selman, L.; Hansen, S. Structure and function of collectin liver 1 (CL-L1) and collectin 11 (CL-11, CL-K1). *Immunobiology* **2012**, *217*, 851–863. [CrossRef] [PubMed]

145. Garred, P.; Genster, N.; Pilely, K.; Bayarri-Olmos, R.; Rosbjerg, A.; Ma, Y.; Skjoedt, M.O. A journey through the lectin pathway of complement- MBL and beyond. *Immunol. Rev.* **2016**, *274*, 74–97. [CrossRef] [PubMed]

146. Wallis, R. Interactions between mannosebinding lectin and MASPs during complement activation by the lectin pathway. *Immunobiology* **2007**, *212*, 289–299. [CrossRef] [PubMed]

147. Asgari, E.; Farrar, C.A.; Lynch, N.; Ali, Y.M.; Roscher, S.; Stover, C.; Zhou, W.; Schwaeble, W.J.; Sacks, S.H. Mannan-binding lectin-associated serine protease 2 is critical for the development of renal ischemia reperfusion injury and mediates tissue injury in the absence of complement C4. *FASEB J.* **2014**, *28*, 3996–4003. [CrossRef]

148. Zhou, W.; Farrar, C.A.; Abe, K.; Pratt, J.R.; Marsh, J.E.; Wang, Y.; Stahl, G.L.; Sacks, S.H. Predominant role for C5b-9 in renal ischemia/reperfusion injury. *J. Clin. Investig.* **2000**, *105*, 1363–1371. [CrossRef]

149. Lin, T.; Zhou, W.; Farrar, C.A.; Hargreaves, R.E.; Sheerin, N.S.; Sacks, S.H. Deficiency of C4 from donor or recipient mouse fails to prevent renal allograft rejection. *Am. J. Pathol.* **2006**, *168*, 1241–1248. [CrossRef]

150. Ma, Y.J.; Skjoedt, M.O.; Garred, P. Collectin-11/ MASP complex formation triggers activation of the lectin complement pathway–the fifth lectin pathway initiation complex. *J. Innate Immun.* **2013**, *5*, 242–250. [CrossRef]

151. Farrar, C.A.; Tran, D.; Li, K.; Wu, W.; Peng, Q.; Schwaeble, W.; Zhou, W.; Sacks, S.H. Collectin-11 detects stress-induced L-fucose pattern to trigger renal epithelial injury. *J. Clin. Investig.* **2016**, *126*, 1911–1925. [CrossRef]

152. Jane-Wit, D.; Manes, T.D.; Yi, T.; Qin, L.; Clark, P.; Kirkiles-Smith, N.C.; Abrahimi, P.; Devalliere, J.; Moeckel, G.; Kulkarni, S.; et al. Alloantibody and complement promote T cell-mediated cardiac allograft vasculopathy through noncanonical nuclear factor-κB signaling in endothelial cells. *Circulation* **2013**, *128*, 2504–2516. [CrossRef]

153. Jane-wit, D.; Surovtseva, Y.V.; Qin, L.; Li, G.; Liu, R.; Clark, P.; Manes, T.D.; Wang, C.; Kashgarian, M.; Kirkiles-Smith, N.C.; et al. Complement membrane attack complexes activate noncanonical NF-κB by forming an Akt+ NIK+ signalosome on Rab5+ endosomes. *Proc. Natl. Acad. Sci. USA* **2015**, *112*, 9686–9691. [CrossRef]

154. Farrar, C.A.; Kupiec-Weglinski, J.W.; Sacks, S.H. The innate immune system and transplantation. *Cold Spring Harb. Perspect. Med.* **2013**, *3*, a015479. [CrossRef] [PubMed]

155. Yamanaka, K.; Kakuta, Y.; Miyagawa, S.; Nakazawa, S.; Kato, T.; Abe, T.; Imamura, R.; Okumi, M.; Maeda, A.; Okuyama, H.; et al. Depression of complement regulatory factors in rat and human renal grafts is associated with the progress of acute T-cell mediated rejection. *PLoS ONE* **2016**, *11*, e0148881. [CrossRef] [PubMed]

156. Ricklin, D.; Barratt-Due, A.; Mollnes, T.E. Complement in clinical medicine: Clinical trials, case reports and therapy monitoring. *Mol. Immunol.* **2017**, *89*, 10–21. [CrossRef] [PubMed]

157. Stegall, M.D.; Diwan, T.; Raghavaiah, S.; Cornell, L.D.; Burns, J.; Dean, P.G.; Cosio, F.G.; Gandhi, M.J.; Kremers, W.; Gloor, J.M. Terminal complement inhibition decreases antibodymediated rejection in sensitized renal transplant recipients. *Am. J. Transplant.* **2011**, *11*, 2405–2413. [CrossRef] [PubMed]

158. Locke, J.E.; Magro, C.M.; Singer, A.L.; Segev, D.L.; Haas, M.; Hillel, A.T.; King, K.E.; Kraus, E.; Lees, L.M.; Melancon, J.K.; et al. The use of antibody to complement protein C5 for salvage treatment of severe antibodymediated rejection. *Am. J. Transplant.* **2009**, *9*, 231–235. [CrossRef]

159. Montgomery, R.A.; Orandi, B.J.; Racusen, L.; Jackson, A.M.; Garonzik-Wang, J.M.; Shah, T.; Woodle, E.S.; Sommerer, C.; Fitts, D.; Rockich, K.; et al. Plasma-derived C1 esterase inhibitor for acute antibody-mediated rejection following kidney transplantation: Results of a randomized double-blind placebo-controlled pilot study. *Am. J. Transplant.* **2016**, *16*, 3468–3478. [CrossRef]

160. Glotz, D.; Russ, G.; Rostaing, L.; Legendre, C.; Tufveson, G.; Chadban, S.; Grinyó, J.; Mamode, N.; Rigotti, P.; Couzi, L.; et al. C10-002 Study Group. Safety and efficacy of eculizumab for the prevention of antibody-mediated rejection after deceased-donor kidney transplantation in patients with preformed donor-specific antibodies. *Am. J. Transplant.* **2019**, *19*, 2865–2875. [CrossRef]

161. Marks, W.H.; Mamode, N.; Montgomery, R.A.; Stegall, M.D.; Ratner, L.E.; Cornell, L.D.; Rowshani, A.T.; Colvin, R.B.; Dain, B.; Boice, J.A.; et al. Safety and efficacy of eculizumab in the prevention of antibody-mediated rejection in living-donor kidney transplant recipients requiring desensitization therapy: A randomized trial. *Am. J. Transplant.* **2019**, *19*, 2876–2888. [CrossRef]

162. Schröppel, B.; Akalin, E.; Baweja, M.; Bloom, R.D.; Florman, S.; Goldstein, M.; Haydel, B.; Hricik, D.E.; Kulkarni, S.; Levine, M.; et al. Peritransplant eculizumab does not prevent delayed graft function in deceased donor kidney transplant recipients: Results of two randomized controlled pilot trials. *Am. J. Transplant.* **2019**, *26*. [CrossRef]

163. Davis, A.E.; Mejia, P.; Lu, F. Biological activities of C1 inhibitor. *Mol. Immunol.* **2008**, *45*, 4057–4063. [CrossRef]

164. Jordan, S.C.; Choi, J.; Aubert, O.; Haas, M.; Loupy, A.; Huang, E.; Peng, A.; Kim, I.; Louie, S.; Ammerman, N.; et al. A phase I/II, double-blind, placebo-controlled study assessing safety and efficacy of C1 esterase inhibitor for prevention of delayed graft function in deceased donor kidney transplant recipients. *Am. J. Transplant.* **2018**, *18*, 2955–2964. [CrossRef] [PubMed]

165. Kassimatis, T.; Qasem, A.; Douiri, A.; Ryan, E.G.; Rebollo-Mesa, I.; Nichols, L.L.; Greenlaw, R.; Olsburgh, J.; Smith, R.A.; Sacks, S.H.; et al. A double-blind randomised controlled investigation into the efficacy of Mirococept (APT070) for preventing ischaemia reperfusion injury in the kidney allograft (EMPIRIKAL): Study protocol for a randomised controlled trial. *Trials* **2017**, *18*, 255. [CrossRef] [PubMed]

166. Snelgrove, S.L.; Lo, C.; Hall, P.; Lo, C.Y.; Alikhan, M.A.; Coates, P.T.; Holdsworth, S.R.; Hickey, M.J.; Kitching, A.R. Activated Renal Dendritic Cells Cross Present Intrarenal Antigens After Ischemia-Reperfusion Injury. *Transplantation* **2017**, *101*, 1013–1024. [CrossRef] [PubMed]

167. Damman, J.; Daha, M.R.; van Son, W.J.; Leuvenink, H.G.; Ploeg, R.J.; Seelen, M.A. Crosstalk between complement and Toll-like receptor activation in relation to donor brain death and renal ischemia-reperfusion injury. *Am. J. Transplant.* **2011**, *11*, 660–669. [CrossRef] [PubMed]

168. Dong, X.; Swaminathan, S.; Bachman, L.A.; Croatt, A.J.; Nath, K.A.; Griffin, M.D. Resident dendritic cells are the predominant TNF-secreting cell in early renal ischemia-reperfusion injury. *Kidney Int.* **2007**, *71*, 619–628. [CrossRef] [PubMed]

169. Batal, I.; De Serres, S.A.; Safa, K.; Bijol, V.; Ueno, T.; Onozato, M.L.; Iafrate, A.J.; Herter, J.M.; Lichtman, A.H.; Mayadas, T.N.; et al. Dendritic Cells in Kidney Transplant Biopsy Samples Are Associated with T Cell Infiltration and Poor Allograft Survival. *J. Am. Soc. Nephrol.* **2015**, *26*, 3102–3113. [CrossRef] [PubMed]

170. Abbas, A.K.; Lichtman, A.H.; Pillai, S. *Cellular and Molecular Immunology*, 8th ed.; Elsevier Health Sciences: Amsterdam, The Netherlands, 2014.

171. Ysebaert, D.K.; De Greef, K.E.; De Beuf, A.; Van Rompay, A.R.; Vercauteren, S.; Persy, V.P.; De Broe, M.E. T-cells as mediators in renal ischemia/reperfusion injury. *Kidney Int.* **2004**, *66*, 491–496. [CrossRef]

172. de Perrot, M.; Young, K.; Imai, Y.; Liu, M.; Waddell, T.K.; Fischer, S.; Zhang, L.; Keshavjee, S. Recipient T cells mediate reperfusion injury after lung transplantation in the rat. *J. Immunol.* **2003**, *171*, 4995–5002. [CrossRef]

173. Fiorina, P.; Ansari, M.J.; Jurewicz, M.; Barry, M.; Ricchiuti, V.; Smith, R.N.; Shea, S.; Means, T.K.; Auchincloss, H., Jr.; Luster, A.D.; et al. Role of CXC chemokine receptor 3 pathway in renal ischemic injury. *J. Am. Soc. Nephrol.* **2006**, *17*, 716–723. [CrossRef]

174. Rabb, H. The T cell as a bridge between innate and adaptive immune systems: Implications for the kidney. *Kidney Int.* **2002**, *61*, 1935–1946. [CrossRef]

175. Rabb, H.; Daniels, F.; O'Donnell, M.; Haq, M.; Saba, S.R.; Keane, W.; Tang, W.W. Pathophysiological role of T lymphocytes in renal ischemia-reperfusion injury in mice. *Am. J. Physiol. Renal. Physiol.* **2000**, *279*, F525–F531. [CrossRef] [PubMed]

176. Burne, M.J.; Daniels, F.; El Ghandour, A.; Mauiyyedi, S.; Colvin, R.B.; O'Donnell, M.P.; Rabb, H. Identification of the CD4(+) T cell as a major pathogenic factor in ischemic acute renal failure. *J. Clin. Investig.* **2001**, *108*, 1283–1290. [CrossRef] [PubMed]

177. Day, Y.J.; Huang, L.; Ye, H.; Li, L.; Linden, J.; Okusa, M.D. Renal ischemia-reperfusion injury and adenosine 2A receptor-mediated tissue protection: The role of CD4+ T cells and IFN-gamma. *J. Immunol.* **2006**, *176*, 3108–3114. [CrossRef] [PubMed]

178. Lee, J.W.; Bae, E.; Kwon, S.H.; Yu, M.Y.; Cha, R.H.; Lee, H.; Kim, D.K.; Lee, J.P.; Ye, S.K.; Yoo, J.Y.; et al. Transcriptional modulation of the T helper 17/interleukin 17 axis ameliorates renal ischemia-reperfusion injury. *Nephrol. Dial. Transplant.* **2019**, *34*, 1481–1498. [CrossRef] [PubMed]

179. Murphy, K.M.; Stockinger, B. Effector T cell plasticity: Flexibility in the face of changing circumstances. *Nat. Immunol.* **2010**, *11*, 674–680. [CrossRef] [PubMed]

180. Shen, X.D.; Ke, B.; Zhai, Y.; Gao, F.; Anselmo, D.; Lassman, C.R.; Busuttil, R.W.; Kupiec-Weglinski, J.W. Stat4 and Stat6 signaling in hepatic ischemia/reperfusion injury in mice: HO-1 dependence of Stat4 disruption-mediated cytoprotection. *Hepatology* **2003**, *37*, 296–303. [CrossRef]

181. Yokota, N.; Burne-Taney, M.; Racusen, L.; Rabb, H. Contrasting roles for STAT4 and STAT6 signal transduction pathways in murine renal ischemia-reperfusion injury. *Am. J. Physiol. Renal. Physiol.* **2003**, *285*, F319–F325. [CrossRef]

182. Loverre, A.; Divella, C.; Castellano, G.; Tataranni, T.; Zaza, G.; Rossini, M.; Ditonno, P.; Battaglia, M.; Palazzo, S.; Gigante, M.; et al. T helper 1, 2 and 17 cell subsets in renal transplant patients with delayed graft function. *Transpl. Int.* **2011**, *24*, 233–242. [CrossRef]

183. Afzali, B.; Lombardi, G.; Lechler, R.I.; Lord, G.M. The role of T helper 17 (Th17) and regulatory T cells (Treg) in human organ transplantation and autoimmune disease. *Clin. Exp. Immunol.* **2007**, *148*, 32–46. [CrossRef]

184. Harrington, L.E.; Hatton, R.D.; Mangan, P.R.; Turner, H.; Murphy, T.L.; Murphy, K.M.; Weaver, C.T. Interleukin 17-producing CD4+effector T cells develop via a lineage distinct from the T helper type 1 and 2 lineages. *Nat. Immunol.* **2005**, *6*, 1123–1132. [CrossRef]

185. Loong, C.C.; Hsieh, H.G.; Lui, W.Y.; Chen, A.; Lin, C.Y. Evidence for the early involvement of interleukin 17 in human and experimental renal allograft rejection. *J. Pathol.* **2002**, *197*, 322–332. [CrossRef] [PubMed]

186. Tang, J.L.; Subbotin, V.M.; Antonysamy, M.A.; Troutt, A.B.; Rao, A.S.; Thomson, A.W. Interleukin-17 antagonism inhibits acute but not chronic vascular rejection. *Transplantation* **2001**, *72*, 348–350. [CrossRef] [PubMed]

187. Li, J.; Simeoni, E.; Fleury, S.; Dudler, J.; Fiorini, E.; Kappenberger, L.; von Segesser, L.K.; Vassalli, G. Gene transfer of soluble interleukin-17 receptor prolongs cardiac allograft survival in a rat model. *Eur. J. Cardiothorac. Surg.* **2006**, *29*, 779–783. [CrossRef] [PubMed]

188. Yuan, X.; Paez-Cortez, J.; Schmitt-Knosalla, I.; D'Addio, F.; Mfarrej, B.; Donnarumma, M.; Habicht, A.; Clarkson, M.R.; Iacomini, J.; Glimcher, L.H.; et al. A novel role of CD4 Th17 cells in mediating cardiac allograft rejection and vasculopathy. *J. Exp. Med.* **2008**, *205*, 3133–3144. [CrossRef] [PubMed]

189. Ko, G.J.; Linfert, D.; Jang, H.R.; Higbee, E.; Watkins, T.; Cheadle, C.; Liu, M.; Racusen, L.; Grigoryev, D.N.; Rabb, H. Transcriptional analysis of infiltrating T cells in kidney ischemia-reperfusion injury reveals a pathophysiological role for CCR5. *Am. J. Physiol. Renal. Physiol.* **2012**, *302*, F762–F773. [CrossRef] [PubMed]

190. Waldmann, H.; Graca, L.; Cobbold, S.; Adams, E.; Tone, M.; Tone, Y. Regulatory T cells and organ transplantation. *Semin. Immunol.* **2004**, *16*, 119–126. [CrossRef] [PubMed]

191. Waldmann, H.; Hilbrands, R.; Howie, D.; Cobbold, S. Harnessing FOXP3þ regulatory T cells for transplantation tolerance. *J. Clin. Investig.* **2014**, *124*, 1439–1445. [CrossRef]

192. Wood, K.J.; Sakaguchi, S. Regulatory T cells in transplantation tolerance. *Nat. Rev. Rheumatol.* **2003**, *3*, 199–210. [CrossRef]

193. Ferrer, I.R.; Hester, J.; Bushell, A.; Wood, K.J. Induction of transplantation tolerance through regulatory cells: From mice to men. *Immunol. Rev.* **2014**, *258*, 102–116. [CrossRef]

194. Kinsey, G.; Sharma, R.; Huang, L.; Li, L.; Vergis, A.L.; Ye, H.; Ju, S.T.; Okusa, M.D. Regulatory T Cells Suppress Innate Immunity in Kidney Ischemia-Reperfusion Injury. *J. Am. Soc. Nephrol.* **2009**, *20*, 1744–1753. [CrossRef]

195. Hu, M.; Wang, Y.M.; Wang, Y.; Zhang, G.Y.; Zheng, G.; Yi, S.; O'Connell, P.J.; Harris, D.C.; Alexander, S.I. Regulatory T cells in kidney disease and transplantation. *Kidney Int.* **2016**, *90*, 502–514. [CrossRef] [PubMed]

196. Miyara, M.; Yoshioka, Y.; Kitoh, A.; Shima, T.; Wing, K.; Niwa, A.; Parizot, C.; Taflin, C.; Heike, T.; Valeyre, D.; et al. Functional delineation and differentiation dynamics of human CD4þ T cells expressing the FoxP3 transcription factor. *Immunity* **2009**, *30*, 899–911. [CrossRef] [PubMed]

197. Schmidl, C.; Hansmann, L.; Lassmann, T.; Balwierz, P.J.; Kawaji, H.; Itoh, M.; Kawai, J.; Nagao-Sato, S.; Suzuki, H.; Andreesen, R.; et al. The enhancer and promoter landscape of human regulatory and conventional T cell subpopulations. *Blood* **2014**, *123*, e68–e78. [CrossRef] [PubMed]

198. Braza, F.; Dugast, E.; Panov, I.; Paul, C.; Vogt, K.; Pallier, A.; Chesneau, M.; Baron, D.; Guerif, P.; Lei, H.; et al. Central role of CD45RA- Foxp3hi memory regulatory T cells in clinical kidney transplantation tolerance. *J. Am. Soc. Nephrol.* **2015**, *26*, 1795–1805. [CrossRef]

199. Duhen, T.; Duhen, R.; Lanzavecchia, A.; Sallusto, F.; Campbell, D.J. Functionally distinct subsets of human FOXP3þ Treg cells that phenotypically mirror effector Th cells. *Blood* **2012**, *119*, 4430–4440. [CrossRef]

200. Kawai, M.; Kitade, H.; Mathieu, C.; Waer, M.; Pirenne, J. Inhibitory and stimulatory effects of cyclosporine A on the development of regulatory T cells in vivo. *Transplantation* **2005**, *79*, 1073–1077. [CrossRef]

201. Coenen, J.J.; Koenen, H.J.; van Rijssen, E.; Hilbrands, L.B.; Joosten, I. Rapamycin and not cyclosporin A, preserves the highly suppressive CD27þ subset of human CD4þCD25þ regulatory T cells. *Blood* **2006**, *107*, 1018–1023. [CrossRef]

202. Gunaratnam, L.; Bonventre, J.V. HIF in kidney disease and development. *J. Am. Soc. Nephrol.* **2009**, *20*, 1877–1887. [CrossRef]

203. Rosenberger, C.; Griethe, W.; Gruber, G.; Wiesener, M.; Frei, U.; Bachmann, S.; Eckardt, K.U. Cellular responses to hypoxia after renal segmental infarction. *Kidney Int.* **2003**, *64*, 874–886. [CrossRef]

204. Rosenberger, C.; Mandriota, S.; Jurgensen, J.S.; Wiesener, M.S.; Horstrup, J.H.; Frei, U.; Ratcliffe, P.J.; Maxwell, P.H.; Bachmann, S.; Eckardt, K.U. Expression of hypoxia-inducible factor-1alpha and -2alpha in hypoxic and ischemic rat kidneys. *J. Am. Soc. Nephrol.* **2002**, *13*, 1721–1732. [CrossRef]

205. Wiesener, M.S.; Jurgensen, J.S.; Rosenberger, C.; Scholze, C.K.; Horstrup, J.H.; Warnecke, C.; Mandriota, S.; Bechmann, I.; Frei, U.A.; Pugh, C.W.; et al. Widespread hypoxia-inducible expression of HIF-2alpha in distinct cell populations of different organs. *FASEB J.* **2003**, *17*, 271–273. [CrossRef] [PubMed]

206. Eltzschig, H.K.; Carmeliet, P. Hypoxia and inflammation. *N. Engl. J. Med.* **2011**, *364*, 656–665. [CrossRef] [PubMed]

207. Conde, E.; Alegre, L.; Blanco-Sánchez, I.; Sáenz-Morales, D.; Aguado-Fraile, E.; Ponte, B.; Ramos, E.; Sáiz, A.; Jiménez, C.; Ordoñez, A.; et al. Hypoxia inducible factor 1-alpha (HIF-1 alpha) is induced during reperfusion after renal ischemia and is critical for proximal tubule cell survival. *PLoS ONE* **2012**, *7*, e33258. [CrossRef] [PubMed]

208. Johnson, D.W.; Forman, C.; Vesey, D.A. Novel renoprotective actions of erythropoietin: New uses for an old hormone. *Nephrology* **2006**, *11*, 306–312. [CrossRef] [PubMed]

209. Breen, E.C. VEGF in biological control. *J. Cell Biochem.* **2007**, *102*, 1358–1367. [CrossRef] [PubMed]

210. Arcasoy, M.O. The non-haematopoietic biological effects of erythropoietin. *Br. J. Haematol.* **2008**, *141*, 14–31. [CrossRef] [PubMed]

211. Oda, T.; Ishimura, T.; Yokoyama, N.; Ogawa, S.; Miyake, H.; Fujisaw, M. Hypoxia-Inducible Factor-1α Expression in Kidney Transplant Biopsy Specimens After Reperfusion Is Associated with Early Recovery of Graft Function After Cadaveric Kidney Transplantation. *Transplant. Proc.* **2017**, *49*, 68–72. [CrossRef]

212. Peng, J.; Zhang, L.; Drysdale, L.; Fong, G.H. The transcription factor EPAS-1/hypoxia-inducible factor 2alpha plays an important role in vascular remodeling. *Proc. Natl. Acad. Sci. USA* **2000**, *97*, 8386–8391. [CrossRef]

213. Ralph, G.S.; Parham, S.; Lee, S.R.; Beard, G.L.; Craigon, M.H.; Ward, N.; White, J.R.; Barber, R.D.; Rayner, W.; Kingsman, S.M.; et al. Identification of potential stroke targets by lentiviral vector mediated overexpression of HIF-1 alpha and HIF-2 alpha in a primary neuronal model of hypoxia. *J. Cereb. Blood Flow Metab.* **2004**, *24*, 245–258. [CrossRef]

214. Tian, H.; McKnight, S.L.; Russell, D.W. Endothelial PAS domain protein 1 (EPAS1), a transcription factor selectively expressed in endothelial cells. *Genes Dev.* **1997**, *11*, 72–82. [CrossRef]

215. Elvert, G.; Kappel, A.; Heidenreich, R.; Englmeier, U.; Lanz, S.; Acker, T.; Rauter, M.; Plate, K.; Sieweke, M.; Breier, G.; et al. Cooperative interaction of hypoxia-inducible factor-2alpha (HIF-2alpha) and Ets-1 in the transcriptional activation of vascular endothelial growth factor receptor-2 (Flk-1). *J. Biol. Chem.* **2003**, *278*, 7520–7530. [CrossRef] [PubMed]

216. Zhang, J.; Han, C.; Dai, H.; Hou, J.; Dong, Y.; Cui, X.; Xu, L.; Zhang, M.; Xia, Q. Hypoxia-Inducible Factor-2α Limits Natural Killer T Cell Cytotoxicity in Renal Ischemia/Reperfusion Injury. *J. Am. Soc. Nephrol.* **2016**, *27*, 92–106. [CrossRef] [PubMed]

217. McNamee, E.; Johnson, D.K.; Homann, D.; Clambey, E. Hypoxia and hypoxia-inducible factors as regulators of T cell development, differentiation, and function. *Immunol. Res.* **2013**, *55*, 58–70. [CrossRef] [PubMed]

218. Wang, Z.; Schley, G.; Türkoglu, G.; Burzlaff, N.; Amann, K.U.; Willam, C.; Eckardt, K.U.; Bernhardt, W.M. The protective effect of prolyl-hydroxylase inhibition against renal ischaemia requires application prior to ischaemia but is superior to EPO treatment. *Nephrol. Dial. Transplant.* **2012**, *27*, 929–936. [CrossRef] [PubMed]

219. Bernhardt, W.M.; Gottmann, U.; Doyon, F.; Buchholz, B.; Campean, V.; Schödel, J.; Reisenbuechler, A.; Reisenbuechler, A.; Klaus, S.; Arend, M.; et al. Donor treatment with a PHD-inhibitor activating HIFs prevents graft injury and prolongs survival in an allogenic kidney transplant model. *Proc. Natl. Acad. Sci. USA* **2009**, *106*, 21276–21281. [CrossRef] [PubMed]

Permissions

All chapters in this book were first published by MDPI; hereby published with permission under the Creative Commons Attribution License or equivalent. Every chapter published in this book has been scrutinized by our experts. Their significance has been extensively debated. The topics covered herein carry significant findings which will fuel the growth of the discipline. They may even be implemented as practical applications or may be referred to as a beginning point for another development.

The contributors of this book come from diverse backgrounds, making this book a truly international effort. This book will bring forth new frontiers with its revolutionizing research information and detailed analysis of the nascent developments around the world.

We would like to thank all the contributing authors for lending their expertise to make the book truly unique. They have played a crucial role in the development of this book. Without their invaluable contributions this book wouldn't have been possible. They have made vital efforts to compile up to date information on the varied aspects of this subject to make this book a valuable addition to the collection of many professionals and students.

This book was conceptualized with the vision of imparting up-to-date information and advanced data in this field. To ensure the same, a matchless editorial board was set up. Every individual on the board went through rigorous rounds of assessment to prove their worth. After which they invested a large part of their time researching and compiling the most relevant data for our readers.

The editorial board has been involved in producing this book since its inception. They have spent rigorous hours researching and exploring the diverse topics which have resulted in the successful publishing of this book. They have passed on their knowledge of decades through this book. To expedite this challenging task, the publisher supported the team at every step. A small team of assistant editors was also appointed to further simplify the editing procedure and attain best results for the readers.

Apart from the editorial board, the designing team has also invested a significant amount of their time in understanding the subject and creating the most relevant covers. They scrutinized every image to scout for the most suitable representation of the subject and create an appropriate cover for the book.

The publishing team has been an ardent support to the editorial, designing and production team. Their endless efforts to recruit the best for this project, has resulted in the accomplishment of this book. They are a veteran in the field of academics and their pool of knowledge is as vast as their experience in printing. Their expertise and guidance has proved useful at every step. Their uncompromising quality standards have made this book an exceptional effort. Their encouragement from time to time has been an inspiration for everyone.

The publisher and the editorial board hope that this book will prove to be a valuable piece of knowledge for researchers, students, practitioners and scholars across the globe.

List of Contributors

Fernanda G. Rodrigues
Nutrition Post Graduation Program, Universidade Federal de São Paulo, São Paulo 04023-900, Brazil
Department of Nephrology, University of Groningen, University Medical Center Groningen, 9713 Groningen, The Netherlands

Martin H. de Borst
Department of Nephrology, University of Groningen, University Medical Center Groningen, 9713 Groningen, The Netherlands

Ita P. Heilberg
Nutrition Post Graduation Program, Universidade Federal de São Paulo, São Paulo 04023-900, Brazil
Nephrology Division, Universidade Federal de São Paulo, São Paulo 04023-900, Brazil

Andreas Kronbichler, Christian Koppelstätter, Sara Denicolò, Michael Rudnicki, Hannes Neuwirt, Gert Mayer and Paul Perco
Department of Internal Medicine IV (Nephrology and Hypertension), Medical University Innsbruck, Anichstrasse 35, 6020 Innsbruck, Austria

Maria Effenberger and Herbert Tilg
Department of Internal Medicine I (Gastroenterology, Hepatology, Endocrinology and Metabolism), Medical University Innsbruck, Anichstrasse 35, 6020 Innsbruck, Austria

Jae Il Shin
Department of Pediatrics, Yonsei University College of Medicine, 03722 Seoul, Korea
Department of Pediatric Nephrology, Severance Children's Hospital, Seoul 03722, Korea
Institute of Kidney Disease Research, Yonsei University College of Medicine, Seoul 03722, Korea

Maria José Soler
Department of Nephrology, Hospital Universitari Vall d'Hebron, Nephrology Research Group, Vall d'Hebron Research Institute (VHIR), 08035 Barcelona, Spain

Kate Stevens
Glasgow Renal and Transplant Unit, Queen Elizabeth University Hospital, Glasgow G51 4TF, UK

Annette Bruchfeld
Department of Clinical Sciences Interventions and Technology (CLINTEC), Division of Renal Medicine, Karolinska Institutet, Karolinska University Hospital, 171 77 Stockholm, Sweden

Gerold Thölking
Department of Medicine D, Division of General Internal Medicine, Nephrology and Rheumatology, University Hospital of Münster, 48149 Münster, Germany
Department of Internal Medicine and Nephrology, University Hospital of Münster, Marienhospital Steinfurt, 48565 Steinfurt, Germany

Katharina Schütte-Nütgen, Julia Schmitz, Alexandros Rovas, Maximilian Dahmen, Joachim Bautz, Ulrich Jehn, Hermann Pavenstädt, Barbara Suwelack and Stefan Reuter
Department of Medicine D, Division of General Internal Medicine, Nephrology and Rheumatology, University Hospital of Münster, 48149 Münster, Germany

Barbara Heitplatz and Veerle Van Marck
Gerhard-Domagk-Institute of Pathology, University Hospital of Münster, 48149 Münster, Germany

Janine Mihm and Urban Sester
Department of Nephrology and Hypertension, Internal Medicine IV, Saarland University, Kirrberger Street 100, 66421 Homburg/Saar, Germany

Ilias Zompolas, Nasrin El-Bandar, Thorsten Schlomm and Frank Friedersdorff
Department of Urology, Charité-Universitätsmedizin Berlin, Corporate Member of Freie Universität Berlin, Humbold-Universität zu Berlin, and Berlin Institute of Health, Charitéplatz 1, 10117 Berlin, Germany

Lutz Liefeldt and Klemens Budde
Department of Nephrology, Charité-Universitätsmedizin Berlin, Corporate Member of Freie Universität Berlin, Humbold-Universität zu Berlin, and Berlin Institute of Health, Charitéplatz 1, 10117 Berlin, Germany

Robert Öllinger and Paul Ritschl
Department of Surgery, Campus Charité Mitte/ Campus Virchow-Klinikum CCM/CVK, Charité-Universitätsmedizin Berlin, Corporate Member of Freie Universität Berlin, Humbold-Universität zu Berlin, and Berlin Institute of Health, Charitéplatz 1, 10117 Berlin, Germany

Hyeon Seok Hwang, Jin Sug Kim, Yang Gyun Kim, Ju Young Moon, Kyung Hwan Jeong and Sang Ho Lee
Division of Nephrology, Department of Internal Medicine, College of Medicine, Kyung Hee University, Seoul 130-702, Korea

Kyung-Won Hong
Division of Healthcare Innovation, TheragenEtex Bio Institute Co., Ltd., Suwon 443-721, Korea

Philip Zeuschner, Matthias Saar, Johannes Linxweiler, Stefan Siemer and Michael Stöckle
Department of Urology and Pediatric Urology, Saarland University, Kirrberger Street 100, 66421 Homburg/Saar, Germany

Linda Hennig, Robert Peters, Thorsten Schlomm and Frank Friedersdorff
Department of Urology, Charité-Universitätsmedizin Berlin, Corporate Member of Freie Universität Berlin, Humbold-Universität zu Berlin, and Berlin Institute of Health, Charitéplatz 1, 10117 Berlin, Germany

Ahmed Magheli and Jürgen Kramer
Department of Urology, Klinikum am Urban, 10967 Berlin, Germany

Lutz Liefeldt and Klemens Budde
Department of Nephrology, Charité-Universitätsmedizin Berlin, Corporate Member of Freie Universität Berlin, Humbold-Universität zu Berlin, and Berlin Institute of Health, Charitéplatz 1, 10117 Berlin, Germany

Carolien P.J. Deen
Department of Internal Medicine, University of Groningen, University Medical Center Groningen, 9713 GZ Groningen, The Netherlands
Department of Laboratory Medicine, University of Groningen, University Medical Center Groningen, 9713 GZ Groningen, The Netherlands
Top Institute Food and Nutrition, 6709 PA Wageningen, The Netherlands

Anna van der Veen, Martijn van Faassen, Isidor Minović and Ido P. Kema
Department of Laboratory Medicine, University of Groningen, University Medical Center Groningen, 9713 GZ Groningen, The Netherlands

António W. Gomes-Neto
Department of Internal Medicine, University of Groningen, University Medical Center Groningen, 9713 GZ Groningen, The Netherlands
Transplant Lines Food and Nutrition Biobank and Cohort Study, University of Groningen, University Medical Center Groningen, 9713 GZ Groningen, The Netherlands

Johanna M. Geleijnse and Karin J. Borgonjen-van den Berg
Division of Human Nutrition and Health, Wageningen University, 6708 PB Wageningen, The Netherlands

Stephan J.L. Bakker
Department of Internal Medicine, University of Groningen, University Medical Center Groningen, 9713 GZ Groningen, The Netherlands
Top Institute Food and Nutrition, 6709 PA Wageningen, The Netherlands
TransplantLines Food and Nutrition Biobank and Cohort Study, University of Groningen, University Medical Center Groningen, 9713 GZ Groningen, The Netherlands

Manuela Yepes-Calderón, Camilo G. Sotomayor, Ryanne S. Hijmans, Charlotte A. te Velde-Keyzer, Marco van Londen, Marja van Dijk, Stefan P. Berger, Jan-Stephan Sanders and Jacob Van Den Born
Division of Nephrology, Department of Internal Medicine, University Medical Center Groningen, University of Groningen, 9713 AV Groningen, The Netherlands

Daniel Guldager Kring Rasmussen, Morten Asser Karsdal and Federica Genovese
Nordic Bioscience A/S, 2730 Herlev, Denmark

Arjan Diepstra
Department of Pathology and Medical Biology, University Medical Center Groningen, University of Groningen, 9713 AV Groningen, The Netherlands

Frederike J. Bemelman
Department of Nephrology, Amsterdam University Medical Center, University of Amsterdam, 1105 AZ Amsterdam, The Netherlands

Johan W. de Fijter
Department of Nephrology, Leiden University Medical Center, University of Leiden, 2300 RC Leiden, The Netherlands

Jesper Kers
Amsterdam Institute for Infection and Immunity (AII), Amsterdam UMC, University of Amsterdam, 1098 XH Amsterdam, The Netherlands
Amsterdam Cardiovascular Sciences (ACS), Amsterdam UMC, University of Amsterdam, 1098 XH Amsterdam, The Netherlands
Leiden Transplant Center, Department of Pathology, Leiden University Medical Center, 2300 RC Leiden, The Netherlands
Van 't Hoff Institute for Molecular Sciences (HIMS), University of Amsterdam, 1098 XH Amsterdam, The Netherlands

Charles R.V. Tomson
The Newcastle upon Tyne Hospitals NHS Foundation Trust, Newcastle upon Tyne NE7 7DN, UK

Sandrine Florquin
Amsterdam Institute for Infection and Immunity (AII), Amsterdam UMC, University of Amsterdam, 1098 XH Amsterdam, The Netherlands
Amsterdam Cardiovascular Sciences (ACS), Amsterdam UMC, University of Amsterdam, 1098 XH Amsterdam, The Netherlands
Leiden Transplant Center, Department of Pathology, Leiden University Medical Center, 2300 RC Leiden, The Netherlands

Tomás A. Gacitúa, Camilo G. Sotomayor, Dion Groothof, Michele F. Eisenga, Martin H. de Borst, Rijk O.B. Gans, Stefan P. Berger, Gerjan J. Navis and Stephan J.L. Bakker
Department of Internal Medicine, University Medical Center Groningen, University of Groningen, 9713 GZ Groningen, The Netherlands

Robert A. Pol
Department of Surgery, University Medical Center Groningen, University of Groningen, 9713 GZ Groningen, The Netherlands

Ramón Rodrigo
Molecular and Clinical Pharmacology Program, Institute of Biomedical Sciences, Faculty of Medicine, University of Chile, CP 8380453 Santiago, Chile

Katie Wong, Fergus Caskey and Pippa Bailey
Bristol Medical School: Population Health Sciences, University of Bristol, Bristol BS8 2PS, UK
Southmead Hospital, North Bristol NHS Trust, Bristol BS10 5NB, UK

Amanda Owen-Smith, Stephanie MacNeill and Yoav Ben-Shlomo
Bristol Medical School: Population Health Sciences, University of Bristol, Bristol BS8 2PS, UK

Frank J.M.F. Dor
Imperial College Healthcare NHS Trust, London W12 0HS, UK

Soumeya Bouacida
Bristol Health Partners' Chronic Kidney Disease Health Integration Team, Bristol BS1 2NT, UK

Dela Idowu
Gift of Living Donation (GOLD), London NW10 0NS, UK

Somratai Vadcharavivad
Department of Pharmacy Practice, Faculty of Pharmaceutical Sciences, Chulalongkorn University, Bangkok 10330, Thailand

Sudarat Piyasiridej, Kriang Tungsanga, Somchai Eiam-Ong and Kearkiat Praditpornsilpa
Division of Nephrology, Department of Medicine, Faculty of Medicine, Chulalongkorn University and King Chulalongkorn Memorial Hospital, Bangkok 10330, Thailand

Natavudh Townamchai and Suwasin Udomkarnjananun
Division of Nephrology, Department of Medicine, Faculty of Medicine, Chulalongkorn University and King Chulalongkorn Memorial Hospital, Bangkok 10330, Thailand
Excellence Center for Solid Organ Transplantation, King Chulalongkorn Memorial Hospital, Bangkok 10330, Thailand
Renal Immunology and Renal Transplant Research Unit, Department of Medicine, Chulalongkorn University, Bangkok 10330, Thailand

Krit Pongpirul
Department of Preventive and Social Medicine, Faculty of Medicine, Chulalongkorn University, Bangkok 10330, Thailand
Department of International Health, Johns Hopkins Bloomberg School of Public Health, Johns Hopkins University, Baltimore, MD 21205, USA

Salin Wattanatorn
Division of Nephrology, Department of Medicine, Faculty of Medicine, Chulalongkorn University and King Chulalongkorn Memorial Hospital, Bangkok 10330, Thailand
Excellence Center for Solid Organ Transplantation, King Chulalongkorn Memorial Hospital, Bangkok 10330, Thailand

Boonchoo Sirichindakul
Excellence Center for Solid Organ Transplantation, King Chulalongkorn Memorial Hospital, Bangkok 10330, Thailand
Department of Surgery, Faculty of Medicine, Chulalongkorn University and King Chulalongkorn Memorial Hospital, Bangkok 10330, Thailand

Yingyos Avihingsanon
Division of Nephrology, Department of Medicine, Faculty of Medicine, Chulalongkorn University and King Chulalongkorn Memorial Hospital, Bangkok 10330, Thailand
Renal Immunology and Renal Transplant Research Unit, Department of Medicine, Chulalongkorn University, Bangkok 10330, Thailand

Christoph Weber, Lena Röschke, Boris Betz and Michael Kiehntopf
Department of Clinical Chemistry and Laboratory Diagnostics and Integrated Biobank Jena (IBBJ), Jena University Hospital, 07747 Jena, Germany

Luise Modersohn, Christina Lohr, Tobias Kolditz and Udo Hahn
Jena University Language & Information Engineering (JULIE) Lab, Friedrich Schiller University Jena, 07743 Jena, Germany

Danny Ammon
Data Integration Center, Jena University Hospital, 07743 Jena, Germany

Alwin Tubben, Camilo G. Sotomayor, Adrian Post, Martin H. de Borst, M. Yusof Said, Rianne M. Douwes, Else van den Berg, Stefan P. Berger, Gerjan J. Navis and Stephan J. L. Bakker
Department of Internal Medicine, University Medical Center Groningen, University of Groningen, Hanzeplein 1, 9700 RB Groningen, The Netherlands

Isidor Minovic
Department of Laboratory Medicine, University Medical Center Groningen, University of Groningen, Hanzeplein 1, 9700 RB Groningen, The Netherlands

Timoer Frelink
Metrohm Applikon B.V., 3125 AE Schiedam, The Netherlands

Johannes von Einsiedel, Christian Wilms, Elena Vorona, Arne Bokemeyer, Hartmut H. Schmidt, Iyad Kabar and Anna Hüsing-Kabar
Department of Medicine B, Gastroenterology and Hepatology, University Hospital Münster, 48149 Münster, Germany

Gerold Thölking
Department of Internal Medicine and Nephrology, University Hospital of Münster Marienhospital Steinfurt, 48565 Steinfurt, Germany

J. Casper Swarte
Department of Internal Medicine, Division of Nephrology, University Medical Center Groningen, University of Groningen, 9700RB Groningen, The Netherlands

Rianne M. Douwes, Michele F. Eisenga, Marco van Londen and António W. Gomes-Neto
Department of Internal Medicine, Division of Nephrology, University Medical Center Groningen, University of Groningen, 9700RB Groningen, The Netherlands

Shixian Hu and Arnau Vich Vila
Department of Gastroenterology and Hepatology, University Medical Center Groningen, University of Groningen, 9700RB Groningen, The Netherlands
Department of Genetics, University Medical Center Groningen, University of Groningen, 9700RB Groningen, The Netherlands

Rinse K. Weersma
Department of Gastroenterology and Hepatology, University Medical Center Groningen, University of Groningen, 9700RB Groningen, The Netherlands

Hermie J.M. Harmsen
Department of Medical Microbiology, University Medical Center Groningen, University of Groningen, 9700RB Groningen, The Netherlands

Gertrude J. Nieuwenhuijs-Moeke
Department of Anesthesiology, University of Groningen, University Medical Centre Groningen, Hanzeplein 1, 9713 GZ Groningen, The Netherlands

Søren E. Pischke
Clinic for Emergencies and Critical Care, Department of Anesthesiology, Department of Immunology, Oslo University Hospital, 4950 Nydalen, 0424 Oslo, Norway

Stefan P. Berger and Jan Stephan F. Sanders
Department of Nephrology, University of Groningen, University Medical Centre Groningen, Hanzeplein 1, 9713 GZ Groningen, The Netherlands

Robert A. Pol and Henri G. D. Leuvenink
Department of Surgery, University of Groningen, University Medical Centre Groningen, Hanzeplein 1, 9713 GZ Groningen, The Netherlands

Michel M. R. F. Struys
Department of Anesthesiology, University of Groningen, University Medical Centre Groningen, Hanzeplein 1, 9713 GZ Groningen, The Netherlands
Department of Basic and Applied Medical Sciences, Ghent University, Corneel Heymanslaan 10, 9000 Ghent, Belgium

Rutger J. Ploeg
Department of Surgery, University of Groningen, University Medical Centre Groningen, Hanzeplein 1, 9713 GZ Groningen, The Netherlands
Nuffield Department of Surgical Sciences, University of Oxford, Headington, Oxford OX3 9DU, UK

Index

www.ingramcontent.com/pod-product-compliance
Lightning Source LLC
Chambersburg PA
CBHW080522200326
41458CB00012B/4296